Advances in Mucoadhesive Polymers and Formulations for Transmucosal Drug Delivery

Advances in Mucoadhesive Polymers and Formulations for Transmucosal Drug Delivery

Special Issue Editor
Vitaliy V. Khutoryanskiy

MDPI • Basel • Beijing • Wuhan • Barcelona • Belgrade • Manchester • Tokyo • Cluj • Tianjin

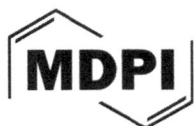

Special Issue Editor
Vitaliy V. Khutoryanskiy
Reading School of Pharmacy,
University of Reading
UK

Editorial Office
MDPI
St. Alban-Anlage 66
4052 Basel, Switzerland

This is a reprint of articles from the Special Issue published online in the open access journal *Polymers* (ISSN 2073-4360) (available at: https://www.mdpi.com/journal/polymers/special_issues/Advances_in_Mucoadhesive_Polymers_and_Formulations_for_Transmucosal_Drug_Delivery).

For citation purposes, cite each article independently as indicated on the article page online and as indicated below:

LastName, A.A.; LastName, B.B.; LastName, C.C. Article Title. *Journal Name* **Year**, *Article Number*, Page Range.

ISBN 978-3-03928-752-9 (Pbk)
ISBN 978-3-03928-753-6 (PDF)

Cover image courtesy of Vitaliy V. Khutoryanskiy.

© 2020 by the authors. Articles in this book are Open Access and distributed under the Creative Commons Attribution (CC BY) license, which allows users to download, copy and build upon published articles, as long as the author and publisher are properly credited, which ensures maximum dissemination and a wider impact of our publications.

The book as a whole is distributed by MDPI under the terms and conditions of the Creative Commons license CC BY-NC-ND.

Contents

About the Special Issue Editor vii

Preface to "Advances in Mucoadhesive Polymers and Formulations for Transmucosal Drug Delivery" ix

Marcelle Silva-Abreu, Lupe Carolina Espinoza, Lyda Halbaut, Marta Espina, María Luisa García and Ana Cristina Calpena
Comparative Study of Ex Vivo Transmucosal Permeation of Pioglitazone Nanoparticles for the Treatment of Alzheimer's Disease
Reprinted from: *Polymers* **2018**, *10*, 316, doi:10.3390/polym10030316 1

Jéssica Bassi da Silva, Sabrina Barbosa de Souza Ferreira, Adriano Valim Reis, Michael Thomas Cook and Marcos Luciano Bruschi
Assessing Mucoadhesion in Polymer Gels: The Effect of Method Type and Instrument Variables
Reprinted from: *Polymers* **2018**, *10*, 254, doi:10.3390/polym10030254 15

Leire Ruiz-Rubio, María Luz Alonso, Leyre Pérez-Álvarez, Rosa Maria Alonso, Jose Luis Vilas and Vitaliy V. Khutoryanskiy
Formulation of Carbopol®/Poly(2-ethyl-2-oxazoline)s Mucoadhesive Tablets for Buccal Delivery of Hydrocortisone
Reprinted from: *Polymers* **2018**, *10*, 175, doi:10.3390/polym10020175 35

Elisabetta Esposito, Maddalena Sguizzato, Christian Bories, Claudio Nastruzzi and Rita Cortesi
Production and Characterization of a Clotrimazole Liposphere Gel for Candidiasis Treatment
Reprinted from: *Polymers* **2018**, *10*, 160, doi:10.3390/polym10020160 49

Sajjad Khan and Joshua Boateng
Effects of Cyclodextrins (β and γ) and L-Arginine on Stability and Functional Properties of Mucoadhesive Buccal Films Loaded with Omeprazole for Pediatric Patients
Reprinted from: *Polymers* **2018**, *10*, 157, doi:10.3390/polym10020157 65

Venera R. Garipova, Chiara G. M. Gennari, Francesca Selmin, Francesco Cilurzo and Rouslan I. Moustafine
Mucoadhesive Interpolyelectrolyte Complexes for the Buccal Delivery of Clobetasol
Reprinted from: *Polymers* **2018**, *10*, 85, doi:10.3390/polym10010085 85

Fabíola Garavello Prezotti, Fernanda Isadora Boni, Natália Noronha Ferreira, Daniella de Souza e Silva, Sérgio Paulo Campana-Filho, Andreia Almeida, Teófilo Vasconcelos, Maria Palmira Daflon Gremião, Beatriz Stringhetti Ferreira Cury and Bruno Sarmento
Gellan Gum/Pectin Beads Are Safe and Efficient for the Targeted Colonic Delivery of Resveratrol
Reprinted from: *Polymers* **2018**, *10*, 50, doi:10.3390/polym10010050 99

Andrea Kovács, Balázs Démuth, Andrea Meskó and Romána Zelkó
Preformulation Studies of Furosemide-Loaded Electrospun Nanofibrous Systems for Buccal Administration
Reprinted from: *Polymers* **2017**, *9*, 643, doi:10.3390/polym9120643 113

Janine Griesser, Gergely Hetényi and Andreas Bernkop-Schnürch
Thiolated Hyaluronic Acid as Versatile Mucoadhesive Polymer: From the Chemistry Behind to Product Developments—What Are the Capabilities?
Reprinted from: *Polymers* **2018**, *10*, 243, doi:10.3390/polym10030243 . . . . **123**

Shaked Eliyahu, Anat Aharon and Havazelet Bianco-Peled
Acrylated Chitosan Nanoparticles with Enhanced Mucoadhesion
Reprinted from: *Polymers* **2018**, *10*, 106, doi:10.3390/polym10020106 . . . . **139**

Twana Mohammed M. Ways, Wing Man Lau and Vitaliy V. Khutoryanskiy
Chitosan and Its Derivatives for Application in Mucoadhesive Drug Delivery Systems
Reprinted from: *Polymers* **2018**, *10*, 267, doi:10.3390/polym10030267 . . . . **157**

About the Special Issue Editor

Vitaliy V. Khutoryanskiy has been Professor of Formulation Science since 2014, having previously been Associate Professor in Pharmaceutical Materials (2010–2014) and Lecturer in Pharmaceutics (2005–2010) at University of Reading School of Pharmacy. Prior to University of Reading, he worked as a Research Associate in the School of Pharmacy and Pharmaceutical Sciences, University of Manchester (2004–2005), and as Research Fellow in the Department of Pharmaceutical Sciences, University of Strathclyde (2002–2005). Prof Khutoryanskiy has researched broadly in the area of new biomaterials for pharmaceutical and biomedical applications, with a particular emphasis on drug delivery, mucoadhesive materials, hydrogels, and stimuli-responsive polymers. He was the recipient of the 2012 McBain Medal from the Society of Chemical Industry and Royal Society of Chemistry for his imaginative use of colloid, polymer and interface science in the development of novel biomedical materials. He has published 151 original research articles and 22 reviews. He also edited 3 books and filed 2 patent applications. He serves as a member of EPSRC peer-review college and sits on editorial boards for several journals (e.g., European Polymer Journal, Pharmaceutics, Polymers, Journal of Pharmaceutical Sciences, Gels, etc.).

Preface to "Advances in Mucoadhesive Polymers and Formulations for Transmucosal Drug Delivery"

Mucoadhesion, defined as the ability of materials to stick to mucosal tissues in the human body, has attracted substantial interest of researchers over the past few decades. The applicability of mucoadhesion in the drug delivery has been first demonstrated in 1947 but received wide recognition only in the early 1980th. Currently there are several routes of administration established for transmucosal drug delivery, where mucoadhesive materials increasingly find some applications. These include ocular, nasal, oromucosal, gastrointestinal, esophageal, vaginal, rectal and intravesical drug delivery. Each route will have some specific physiological features that will determine the possibility of drug administration and the design of suitable dosage forms. Mucoadhesive dosage forms have been formulated as tablets, lozenges, wafers, pessaries, films, gels, liquid and semi-solid systems as well as suspensions of various nano- and microparticles.

Hydrophilic polymers have been shown to exhibit mucoadhesive properties due to specific interactions with mucins as well as because of their ability to form viscous solutions and penetration into mucus gel. There is currently a continuously increased interest in the design of novel mucoadhesive materials and dosage forms. These dosage forms could be formulated using conventional hydrophilic polymers, their combinations and complexes. Additionally there is currently a strong interest of researchers in chemical modification of existing polymers to enhance their mucoadhesive properties.

This book represents a collection of reviews and original research papers, focusing on mucoadhesive polymers and formulations for transmucosal drug delivery. It includes some contributions reporting the design of nanoparticles, gels, tablets, films, beads, and nanofibrous systems. Additionally some of the contributions describe methodologies for chemical modification of chitosan and hyaluronic acid to enhance their mucoadhesive properties.

Vitaliy V. Khutoryanskiy
Special Issue Editor

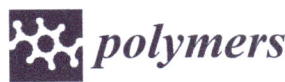

Article

Comparative Study of Ex Vivo Transmucosal Permeation of Pioglitazone Nanoparticles for the Treatment of Alzheimer's Disease

Marcelle Silva-Abreu [1,2], Lupe Carolina Espinoza [1,3], Lyda Halbaut [1], Marta Espina [1,2], María Luisa García [1,2] and Ana Cristina Calpena [1,2,*]

1. Department of Pharmacy, Pharmaceutical Technology and Physical Chemistry, Faculty of Pharmacy and Food Sciences, University of Barcelona, 08028 Barcelona, Spain; marcellesabreu@gmail.com (M.S.-A.); lcespinoza@utpl.edu.ec (L.C.E.); halbaut@ub.edu (L.H.); m.espina@ub.edu (M.E.); rdcm@ub.edu (M.L.G.)
2. Institute of Nanoscience and Nanotechnology (IN2UB), University of Barcelona, 08028 Barcelona, Spain
3. Departamento de Química y Ciencias Exactas, Universidad Técnica Particular de Loja, Loja 1101608, Ecuador
* Correspondence: anacalpena@ub.edu; Tel.: +34-93-402-4560

Received: 27 February 2018; Accepted: 13 March 2018; Published: 14 March 2018

Abstract: Pioglitazone has been reported in the literature to have a substantial role in the improvement of overall cognition in a mouse model. With this in mind, the aim of this study was to determine the most efficacious route for the administration of Pioglitazone nanoparticles (PGZ-NPs) in order to promote drug delivery to the brain for the treatment of Alzheimer's disease. PGZ-loaded NPs were developed by the solvent displacement method. Parameters such as mean size, polydispersity index, zeta potential, encapsulation efficacy, rheological behavior, and short-term stability were evaluated. Ex vivo permeation studies were then carried out using buccal, sublingual, nasal, and intestinal mucosa. PGZ-NPs with a size around of 160 nm showed high permeability in all mucosae. However, the permeation and prediction parameters revealed that lag-time and vehicle/tissue partition coefficient of nasal mucosa were significantly lower than other studied mucosae, while the diffusion coefficient and theoretical steady-state plasma concentration of the drug were higher, providing biopharmaceutical results that reveal more favorable PGZ permeation through the nasal mucosa. The results suggest that nasal mucosa represents an attractive and non-invasive pathway for PGZ-NPs administration to the brain since the drug permeation was demonstrated to be more favorable in this tissue.

Keywords: nanoparticles; pioglitazone; PLGA-PEG; transmucosal permeations; Alzheimer's disease

1. Introduction

Alzheimer's disease (AD) is a progressive neurodegenerative disease that is considered the most common cause of dementia [1,2]. AD is characterized by a gradual decline in cognition and neuropsychiatric disorders that affect the ability to perform activities of daily living [3,4]. Chronic neuroinflammation has been described as a pathological feature which may contribute to amyloid plaque progression and neurodegeneration [5,6].

PPAR-γ is a nuclear receptor whose activation regulates genes involved in glucose homeostasis, lipid metabolism, and inflammation [7–9]. Recent studies have shown that PPAR-γ ligands inhibit proinflammatory gene expression, regulate amyloidogenic pathways, and exhibit neuroprotective effects [10–12]. Pioglitazone (PGZ) is a PPAR-γ activator that increases tissue sensitivity to insulin and is widely used to treat type 2 diabetes mellitus (T2DM) [13]. Other pharmacological effects reported for PGZ include selective suppression of the T-helper 17 (Th17) cells differentiation and improvements in overall cognition using a mouse model, suggesting that PGZ is a viable treatment option not only for T2DM but also for autoimmune diseases, inflammatory conditions, and neurodegenerative diseases such as multiple sclerosis, rosacea, and AD [14–17].

PGZ is classified as a biopharmaceutical classification system (BCS) Class II drug with low solubility and high permeability which limits its absorption rate [18]. PGZ is available in conventional tablets for oral administration [19]. However, oral delivery of this dosage form has notable disadvantages such as prolonged disintegration time, first-pass metabolism, poor solubility, and low intestinal bioavailability, consequently demonstrating the need to develop new drug delivery systems and their administration by alternative routes [20].

Drugs administered via mucosal surfaces (buccal, sublingual, nasal, and intestinal tissues) provide local and/or systemic pharmacological action [21,22]. Novel mucosal delivery systems have been developed to optimize the efficacy and safety of drugs administered by these routes. Nanostructured systems are considered the most promising strategies [23,24]. Polymeric and solid lipid nanoparticles, nanostructured lipid carriers, and nanoemulsions are examples of nanotechnologies that offer numerous benefits including improved solubility for hydrophobic drugs, controlled drug release, and enhanced stability and bioavailability [25,26]. Polymeric nanoparticles (PNPs) are extensively employed due to their favorable properties, not the least of which include their ease of manufacture, low toxicity, biocompatibility, protection of drug, and biodegradation [27,28]. PNPs are defined as particles with a size ranging from 10 nm to 1000 nm that are composed of either natural polymers (gelatin, albumin, chitosan) or synthetic polymers such as polylactides (PLA), poly(lactic-co-glycolic) acid (PLGA), and polyglycolides (PGA) [28,29]. The incorporation of mucoadhesive polymers that adhere to a mucosal surface prolongs the residence time at the administration site of these drug delivery systems, increasing the local or systemic bioavailability [30]. Polyethylene glycol (PEG) is a hydrophilic polymer that is non-toxic and used in many pharmaceutical formulations. Surface coating with PEG is reported to prevent non-specific interactions of serum proteins with NPs [31]. PLGA-PEG copolymer nanoparticles are composed of a hydrophilic surface of PEG around a hydrophobic core of PLGA [32]. This structure allows the encapsulation of hydrophobic drugs into the core region and prolongs the circulation time while the PEG hydrophilic shield around the particle core augments mucus-penetrating properties [33,34].

The purpose of this study was to determine the best mucosal route for the administration of NPs of PGZ on the basis of their biopharmaceutical parameters in order to provide drug delivery to the brain for optimal treatment of AD. Additionally, rheological behavior and short-term stability were analyzed.

2. Materials and Methods

2.1. Materials

PGZ was purchased from Capot Chemical (Hangzhou, China), and Diblock copolymer PLGA-PEG (Resomer® Select 5050 DLG mPEG 5000–5 wt % PEG) was purchased from Evonik Corporation (Birmingham, AL, USA). Tween (Tw) 80 and acetone were obtained from Sigma-Aldrich (Madrid, Spain) and Fisher Scientific (Pittsburgh, PA, USA), respectively. The dialysis membrane MWCO 12,000–14,000 Da was obtained from Medicell International Ltd. (London, UK) and the Transcutol was obtained from Gattefossé (Barcelona, Spain). Water filtered through a Millipore MilliQ system was used for all the experiments and reagents used were of analytical grade.

2.2. Methods

2.2.1. Preparation of NPs and Physicochemical Characterization

PGZ-loaded PLGA-PEG NPs were developed by the solvent displacement method [35]. The formulation of PGZ-NPs consists of two phases: the first is composed of the drug, dimethyl sulfoxide (DMSO), and acetone (organic phase) while the second phase consists of Tw 80 (surfactant) and water (aqueous phase). After complete solubilization of both phases, the organic phase was added drop by drop into 10 mL of the aqueous phase. Afterwards, the NPs dispersion was concentrated to 10 mL under reduced pressure (Bücchi B-480, Flawil, Switzerland).

The NPs mean size (Zav) and polydispersity index (PI) were determined by photon correlation spectroscopy (PCS) using a ZetaSizer Nano ZS (Malvern Instruments, Madrid, Spain). Measurements were carried out in triplicate at angles of 180° in 10-mm diameter cells at 25 °C. The surface charge, or Zeta potential (ZP), was calculated from electrophoretic mobility. This parameter can give information about the possibility of particles aggregation [36]. The encapsulation efficiency (EE) of PGZ in the NPs was determined indirectly following Equation (1). The non-entrapped PGZ was separated using filtration/centrifugation (1:10 dilution) with Ultracell–100 K (Amicon® Ultra; Millipore Corporation, Billerica, MA, USA) centrifugal filter devices at 12,000 rpm for 15 min. PGZ was measured using a previously validated high performance liquid chromatographic (HPLC) method [15].

$$EE(\%) = \frac{Total\ amount\ of\ PGZ\ -\ Free\ amount\ of\ PGZ}{Total\ amount\ of\ PGZ} \cdot 100 \qquad (1)$$

2.2.2. Tissue Samples

Samples were extracted from pigs (male, weight 30–40 kg, n = 6) following a process supervised by veterinary officials in accordance with the Ethics Committee of Animal Experimentation at the University of Barcelona. The pigs were anesthetized with intramuscular administration of ketamine HCl (3 mg/kg), xylazine (2.5 mg/kg) and midazolam (0.17 mg/kg). Once sedated, Propofol (3 mg/kg) was administered through the auricular vein and they were subsequently intubated and maintained under anesthesia by isoflurane inhalation. In order to induce pig euthanasia, sodium pentobarbital (250 mg/kg) was administered through the auricular vein under deep anesthesia.

After the sacrifice, mucosal samples were surgically removed from buccal, sublingual, nasal, and intestinal tissues, preserved in Hank's balanced salt solution and refrigerated until delivery to laboratory for the initiation of experiments.

2.2.3. Transmucosal Ex Vivo Permeations

The study was performed in Franz diffusion cells using buccal and nasal mucosae (0.5 mm thick), sublingual mucosa (0.3 mm thick), and uncut intestinal mucosa. The tissues were used for experiments and placed between the receptor and donor compartments. An aliquot of 0.2 mL of PGZ-NPs at 1 mg/mL were placed in the donor compartment and the same volume of samples was extracted from the receptor compartment at established time intervals of 6 h and replaced with fresh receptor medium (Transcutol/water, 6:4 v/v) at 37 $\pm$ 0.5 °C under continuous stirring. The quantitative determination of permeated PGZ per unit area ($\mu g/cm^2$) in the different tissues was analyzed six times by the HPLC method [15]. Kinetic parameters were estimated using GraphPad Prism® 6.0 (GraphPad Software Inc., San Diego, CA, USA).

2.2.4. Biopharmaceutical Parameters

- Determination of PGZ extracted and recovered in the tissues

After finishing the experiment, the mucosae were extracted and used to determine the amount of PGZ retained (Qr, μg PGZ/g tissue/cm^2). The mucosae were cleaned with sodium lauryl sulphate solution (0.05%) and washed with distilled water. The permeation area was excised and weighed, then the PGZ retained was extracted with methanol (1 mL) under sonication for 20 min in an ultrasound bath. The amount of PGZ was analyzed by HPLC.

To analyze the percentage of PGZ recovered from the mucosae, 1 mL of PGZ solution (110 μg/mL) was added to the different mucosae (six replicates), and kept for 6 h at 37 $\pm$ 1 °C using a water bath.

A standard solution of 1 mL PGZ at 110 µg/mL was also kept at 37 ± 1 °C for the same period as a reference.

The PGZ retained from mucosae permeation and recovery samples was quantified using a validated HPLC method [15].

- Data analysis

The cumulative amount of PGZ (µg) permeated through mucosae was plotted as a function of time (h). The slope and intercept of the linear portion of the plot was derived by regression using GraphPad Prism®, 5.0 version software (GraphPad Software Inc., San Diego, CA, USA).

The flux values (J_{ss}, µg/min/cm^2) across the mucosae and the permeability coefficients (K_p) were calculated per unit surface area versus time plot. In this plot, the lag time (T_l, min) is the intercept with the x-axis (time), determined by linear regression analysis of the permeation data using GraphPad Prism® 5.01 (GraphPad Software Inc., San Diego, CA, USA). The flux values are demonstrated by Equation (2):

$$J_{ss} = \frac{Qt}{A} \cdot t \quad (2)$$

where Qt is the quantity of PGZ transferred across the mucosae into the receptor compartment (µg), A is the active cross-sectional area accessible for diffusion (cm^2), and t is the time of exposure (min).

The permeability coefficients (K_p, cm/min) were obtained by Equation (3):

$$K_p = \frac{J_{ss}}{C_0} \quad (3)$$

where J_{ss} is the flux calculated at the steady state and C_0 is the initial drug concentration in the donor compartment.

Parameters of permeation (cm) and diffusion (min^{-1}), P_1 and P_2, respectively, were estimated from Equations (4) and (5):

$$K_p = P_1 \cdot P_2 \quad (4)$$

$$T_l = \frac{1}{6} \cdot P_2 \quad (5)$$

The theoretical human steady-state plasma concentration (C_{ss}) of the drug, which predicted the potential systemic concentration achieved after mucosae administration, was obtained using Equation (6):

$$C_{ss} = J_{ss} \cdot \frac{A}{Clp} \quad (6)$$

where C_{ss} is the plasma steady-state concentration, J_{ss} the flux determined in this study, A the hypothetical area of application, and Clp the plasmatic clearance. The calculations were based on a maximum area of application of 20 cm^2 for buccal, 15 cm^2 for sublingual, and 150 cm^2 for nasal [37,38] mucosae, as well as a human Clp value of 2.26 L/h ± 1.22 [39] in order to ensure the local action of the formulation.

In addition, the mean transit time (MTT, day) of the drug in the mucosae was also obtained using Equation (7):

$$MTT = \left[\frac{V_1}{P_1 \cdot P_2 \cdot A_E}\right] + \left[\frac{1}{2 \cdot P_2}\right] \quad (7)$$

where V_1 (mL) is the volume of the donor compartment and A_E (cm^2) is the area of experimental mucosae samples.

2.2.5. Rheological Behavior

The PGZ-NPs were placed in glass vials with rubber tops and aluminum capsules, then stored at room temperature (23 ± 3 °C). Rheological properties were determined at t_0 = 24 h after NPs preparation using a rotational Haake RheoStress 1 rheometer (Thermo Fischer Scientific, Karlsruhe, Germany) connected to a temperature control Thermo Haake Phoenix II + Haake C25P and equipped with cone-plate geometry (0.105 mm gap) including a Haake C60/2Ti mobile cone (60 mm in diameter and 2° angle). The temperature was adjusted to 25 °C. PGZ-NPs were tested in two replicates, each undergoing a program consisting of a Three-Step Shear Profile: firstly, a ramp-up period from $0\ \text{s}^{-1}$ to $50\ \text{s}^{-1}$ over a 3-min span, followed by a constant shear rate period at $50\ \text{s}^{-1}$ for 1 min, and finally the ramp-down period from $50\ \text{s}^{-1}$ to $0\ \text{s}^{-1}$ for 3 min. The data from the flow curves ($\tau = (\dot{\gamma})$) were fitted to different mathematical models. The equations are summarized in Table 1.

Viscosity mean value at t_0 and 25 °C was determined from the constant shear stretch at $50\ \text{s}^{-1}$ of the viscosity curves ($\eta = (\dot{\gamma})$). The determination of the disturbance of the microstructure during the test or "apparent thixotropy" (Pa/s) was also evaluated.

Table 1. Mathematical models for regression analysis.

Flow Curve—Models: $\tau = f(\dot{\gamma})$	
Newton	$\tau = \eta \cdot \dot{\gamma}$
Bingham	$\tau = \tau_0 + (\eta_0 \cdot \dot{\gamma})$
Ostwald-de-Waele	$\tau = K \cdot \dot{\gamma}^n$
Herschel-Bulkley	$\tau = \tau_0 + K \cdot \dot{\gamma}^n$
Casson	$\tau = \sqrt[n]{\left(\tau_0^n + (\eta_0 \cdot \dot{\gamma})^n\right)}$
Cross	$\tau = \dot{\gamma} \cdot (\eta_\infty + (\eta_0 - \eta_\infty)/(1 + (\dot{\gamma}/\dot{\gamma}_0)^n))$

where τ is the shear stress (Pa), $\dot{\gamma}$ is the shear rate (1/s), η is the dynamic viscosity (Pa·s), τ_0 is the yield shear stress (Pa), η_0 is the zero shear rate viscosity, η_∞ is the infinity shear rate viscosity, n is the flow index, and K is the consistency index [40]. The mathematical model was selected on the basis of the correlation coefficient value (r).

2.2.6. Short-Term Stability

The PGZ-NPs were analyzed for their stability at 4 °C and 25 °C by light backscattering and transmission profiles using Turbiscan®Lab Formulaction (Toulouse, France). A glass measurement cell was filled with 20 mL of formulation. The radiation source was a pulsed near-infrared light and was received by transmission and backscattering detectors at angles of 90° and 4° from the incident beam, respectively. Data were analyzed once a month for 24 h at 1-h intervals over a period of three months.

2.2.7. Statistical Analysis

The statistical analysis of the permeation studies was made using GraphPad Prism® 6.0 (GraphPad Software Inc., San Diego, CA, USA). The values were expressed as averages ± SEM. The software packages Haake RheoWin®Job Manager V.3.3 and RheoWin®Data Manager V.3.3 (Thermo Electron Corporation, Karlsruhe, Germany) were used to carry out the testing and analysis of the obtained rheological data, respectively.

3. Results

3.1. Physicochemical Characterization

After previous factorial design, the PGZ-NPs showed a size around 160.0 ± 1.3 nm with PI values in the range of monodisperse systems (PI < 0.1) and high association efficiency (≈92%). Moreover, the ZP was −13.9 mV, which is indicative of the stability of these systems [41].

3.2. Ex Vivo Permeation Studies

Figure 1a shows the permeation profile of PGZ (µg) from NPs in buccal, sublingual, nasal, and intestinal mucosae. This revealed that the cumulative permeated amount of PGZ after 6 h of assay was higher in intestinal mucosa with a value of 15.40 µg, while buccal, sublingual, and nasal mucosae presented values of 5.06, 6.20, and 6.80 µg, respectively. The permeability parameters were calculated for all mucosae studied except intestinal mucosa because it did not show a linear stretch, which is necessary to calculate these parameters (Figure 1b).

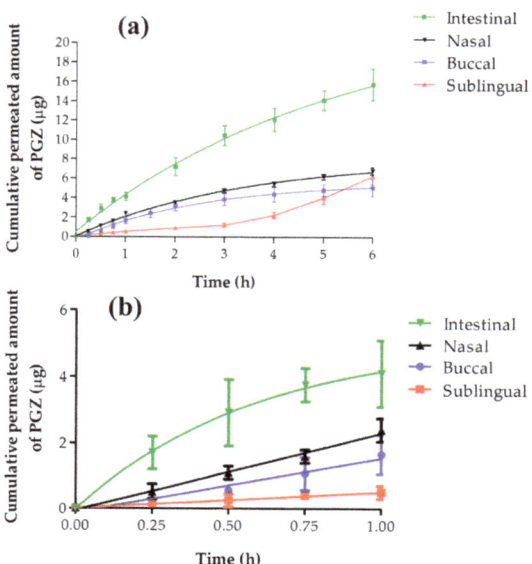

Figure 1. (a) Cumulative permeated amount of Pioglitazone (PGZ) within 6 h; (b) Cumulative permeated amount of PGZ within 1 h.

3.2.1. Retained Amount of PGZ

The NPs showed Significant Statistical Differences (SSD) ($p < 0.05$) in all tissues, except buccal between sublingual mucosa (Figure 2). The highest retained amounts were obtained by sublingual and buccal mucosa with median values of 158.45 and 132.66 (µg PGZ/g tissue/cm^2), respectively. The nasal mucosa presented values of 129.81 (µg PGZ/g tissue/cm^2). The intestinal mucosa showed a low retained amount of PGZ compared with the other mucosae. The percentage of recovery calculated experimentally for each tissue were: buccal 34.84%; sublingual 32.73%; nasal 37.52%; intestinal 14.87%.

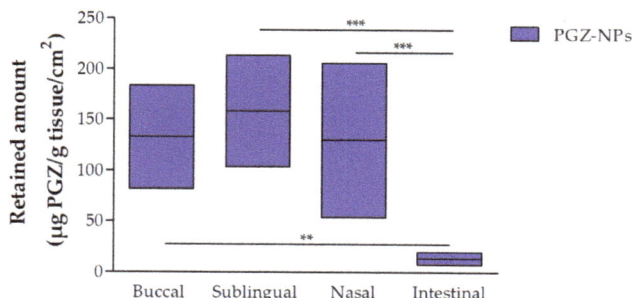

Figure 2. Retained amount of PGZ from nanoparticles (NPs) in different tissues. ($n = 6$). One-way analysis of variance (ANOVA) with Tukey's multiple comparison tests were performed to assess the statistical significance ($p < 0.05$).

3.2.2. Permeation and Predictions Parameters Data

Table 2 shows the permeation and prediction parameters of PGZ from NPs through different mucosae. It was observed that J_{ss} and K_p showed similar values between all studied mucosae without SSD ($p > 0.05$). Concerning Tl, sublingual mucosa showed a value of 175.60 min, followed by buccal and nasal mucosae with values of 41.21 and 3.0 min, respectively. These results revealed an SSD between nasal mucosa with respect to buccal and sublingual mucosa, suggesting that nasal administration makes possible the achievement of state of steady equilibrium in the shortest time. With respect to the other mucosae studied, nasal mucosa also showed an SSD with the lowest values of vehicle/tissue partition coefficient (P1) and the highest values of diffusion coefficient (P2) and C_{ss}.

Table 2. Permeations and prediction parameters of different tissues with PGZ-NPs.

Permeation and Prediction Parameters	Buccal [a]	Sublingual [b]	Nasal [c]
J_{ss} (µg/(min/cm^2)) × 10^2	4.28 (2.83–5.72)	5.19 (4.91–5.50)	5.19 (4.91–5.50)
K_p (cm/min) × 10^5	4.28 (2.83–5.72)	5.19 (4.91–5.50)	5.20 (4.92–5.50)
Tl (min)	41.21 (27.27–55.15)	175.60 [a] (174.30–179.50)	3.00 [a,b] (1.08–5.00)
P$_1$ (cm) × 10^4	93.74 (93.73–93.74)	547.37 [a] (514.35–592.73)	8.85 [a,b] (3.37–16.51)
P$_2$ (min^{-1})	0.004 (0.003–0.006)	0.0009 (0.0009–0.0009)	0.05 [a,b] (0.03–0.15)
Mean Transit Time, MTT (day)	5.80 (3.84–7.77)	4.54 (4.31–4.77)	4.17 [a] (3.95–4.41)
C_{ss} (µg/mL)	0.02 (0.01–0.03)	0.02 (0.02–0.02)	0.20 [a,b] (0.19–0.21)

[a,b,c] Results are expressed by median, minimum, and maximum ($n = 6$). One-way analysis of variance (ANOVA) with Tukey's multiple comparison tests were performed to assess the statistical significance between each mucosa with respect to PGZ-NPs at ($p < 0.05$).

The value of C_{ss} in the nasal mucosa was 10 times greater than the other mucosae studied, signifying that PGZ administered through this route would achieved greater concentrations of PGZ in the bloodstream (relative to the other tissues).

3.3. Rheological Study

Flow and viscosity curves are depicted in Figure 3. Table 3 displays the results obtained from the rheological characterization of PGZ-NPs. The flow curves indicated no thixotropic behavior in the system since the rheograms did not exhibit hysteresis loop. The mathematical model that provided the best overall match of experimental data based on the highest correlation coefficient of regression (r) was the Newton model. PGZ-NPs showed a viscosity of 1.110 mPa·s.

Table 3. Rheological properties of PGZ-NPs.

Rheologic Parameters	PGZ-NPs
Viscosity (mPa·s) at 50 s^{-1} and 25 °C	$1.110 \pm 2.362 \times 10^{-2}$
Flow behavior (best fitting model)	Newtonian Newton * ($r = 0.9993$)

*: After discarding the first and last data.

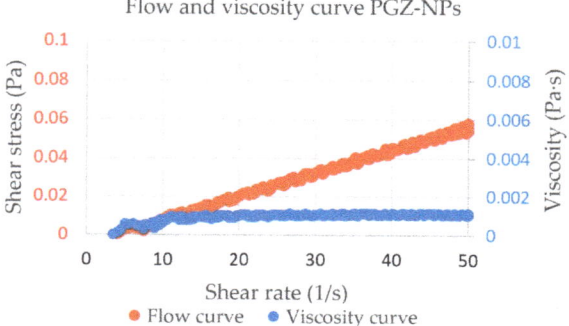

Figure 3. Rheograms obtained for the PGZ-NPs.

3.4. Short-Term Stability

Figure 4a,b show the backscattering profiles of PGZ-NPs at 4 °C and at 25 °C for three months. In both profiles it was observed that after the first month there was an increment of sedimentation and after the second month the samples became unstable with a difference of backscattering above 10%.

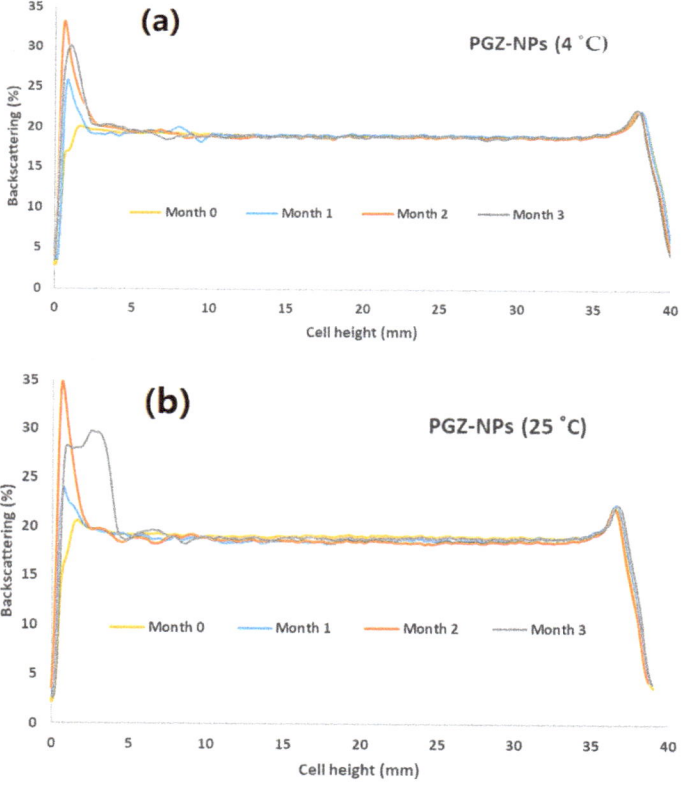

Figure 4. Stability of PGZ-NPs: (**a**) 4 °C and (**b**) 25 °C.

4. Discussion

Currently, AD remains incurable and the pharmacological options have notable disadvantages such as conventional dosage forms exclusively for oral administration, which then cause discomfort among geriatric patients who have difficulty swallowing; being limited to only treat the cognitive symptoms; first-pass metabolism; and ineffective ability to cross the blood-brain barrier (BBB) [42,43]. Recently, the anti-inflammatory and neuroprotective effects of PPAR-γ ligands coupled with the advantages of nanotechnology-based drug delivery systems have come to represent a breadth of new possibilities in the treatment of AD [5,44,45]. By taking into account the fact that PGZ metabolizes in the liver and has low solubility, which limits the absorption rate, it can be concluded that it is necessary to optimize the delivery of the therapeutic product to the brain by designing a more appropriate drug delivery system and determining the most effective administration route. The PGZ-loaded PLGA-PEG NPs obtained in this study represent a promising strategy to facilitate the delivery of drugs to the brain. The physicochemical evaluation of this formulation showed favorable properties for the penetration of the drug across the blood-brain barrier (BBB) and the delivery of the drug in a controlled and sustained manner. Such advantages include small size (160.0 ± 1.3 nm), high association efficiency (≈92%), and good stability [41,46]. In addition, NPs are generally advantageous because of their good biocompatibility, capacity to adjust drug release, and remarkable enhancement of efficacy and bioavailability [29,47,48]. The surface coating of PNPs with PEG provides an increase in circulation lifetime and an improvement of drug delivery across the BBB [49]. The ability of NPs to cross biological membranes is influenced by size, shape, NP composition, and surface properties. The exact mechanism by which NPs cross lipid bilayers remains unknown because of the complexity of both NPs and cell membranes. Nanotoxicity and cell plasma membrane disruptions are concerns of NP designers [50,51]. Hypotheses such as endocytosis, the formation of nanoscale membrane holes, or membrane translocation have been proposed. Some studies support the idea that NPs cross the cell membrane via adhesive or diffusive mechanisms [51]. Clearly, further studies are required in order to assure the success of biomedical applications of these delivery systems.

The ex vivo permeation studies of PGZ-loaded PLGA-PEG NPs through different mucosae (Figure 1a) revealed that intestinal mucosa had the highest amount of drug permeated at 6 h of the assay (15.40 µg) followed by nasal (6.80 µg), sublingual (6.20 µg), and buccal (5.06 µg) mucosa. The high permeability of this formulation in all mucosae is likely due to its nano-size structure and lipophilic nature, which confers larger specific surface area and has a permeation-enhancing effect [52]. Although the amount of PGZ permeated through the intestinal mucosa was higher, it is important to consider that this route has notable disadvantages in the drug delivery to the brain, including first-pass metabolism. Gastrointestinal drug degradation constitutes one of the causes of the poor bioavailability of therapeutic agents using this route [53].

The permeation and prediction parameters (Table 2) were calculated for all of the mucosae studied except for intestinal mucosa, because the permeation profile of this mucosa did not show a linear stretch necessary for the calculation of these parameters. The values of J_{ss} and K_p obtained for buccal, sublingual, and nasal mucosa were similar without SSD ($p > 0.05$). However, Tl for nasal mucosa (3 min) was significantly lower with respect to buccal (175.60 min) and sublingual mucosae (41.21 min), which indicates a rapid onset of action using the nasal route [54]. Moreover, the estimated vehicle/tissue partition coefficient (P_1) for nasal mucosa was lower compared with that of other mucosae, whereas the diffusion coefficient (P_2) and C_{ss} were higher, demonstrating that PGZ permeation is more favorable in this tissue and consequently that there is greater probability to deliver effective concentrations of PGZ at the site of action more quickly [55]. These results suggest that nasal mucosa represents an attractive and non-invasive method for drug delivery to the brain [56]. Nasal physiology and histology is characterized by high vascularization, large absorptive surface area, the avoidance of first-pass metabolism, and a porous and endothelial membrane, all of which provide important advantages to deliver drugs to the central nervous system (CNS) [57]. Furthermore, the nasal passage offers direct transport from the nasal cavity to the brain and is painless and uncomplicated for drug administration [58]. The correct formulation of the dosage form is essential for pharmacological therapy by intranasal administration with the aim of avoiding the elimination of the drug through nasal mucociliary clearance [45]. PGZ-loaded PLGA-PEG NPs as a drug delivery system provide several advantages such as rapid drug permeation, drug protection, and prolonged retention at the site of drug absorption for a suitable period of time [55,59].

The rheogram of PGZ-NPs (Figure 3) shows a linear relationship between the shear stress and the strain rate, which is characteristic of Newtonian behavior [60]. Considering the nasal mucosa as the best mucosa for drug administration, this rheology and the low viscosity obtained (about 1 mPa·s, similar to the water) are ideal for nasal spray application of the formulation [61].

For the stability assay, the PGZ-NPs showed incremental yet stable sedimentation up to the second month, after which the sample became unstable with a difference of backscattering exceeding 10% (Figure 4). This instability of particles is due to the aggregation phenomena and the limited stability of polymeric NPs in aqueous suspension is well known. These results indicate that improved long-term stability could be attained by the removal of water from the solution by lyophilization or a spray-drying technique [62,63].

5. Conclusions

The results obtained showed that PGZ-NPs have appropriate physicochemical characteristics to facilitate their permeability through different types of mucosa. According to the permeations and prediction parameters of these delivery systems, nasal mucosa constitutes the most convenient administration route to treat AD due to the enhanced drug permeation in this tissue, resulting in a greater likelihood of achieving effective concentrations of the drug at the site of action.

Acknowledgments: This work was supported by the Coordination for the Improvement of Higher Education Personnel (CAPES)—Brazil and Spanish Ministry of Science and Innovation (MAT2014-59134R). Marcelle Silva-Abreu also acknowledges her Ph.D. scholarship—CAPES, Brazil. The authors would like to thank the University of Barcelona for the financial support to cover the cost of open access publication. Thanks to María-José Fábrega for the design of the graphical abstract. Additionally, thanks to Jonathan Proctor for his review of the use of the English language.

Author Contributions: Marcelle Silva-Abreu carried out all the experiments, analyzed the data/results and wrote the paper; Lupe Carolina Espinoza analyzed the results and helped write the paper; Lyda Halbaut analyzed the rheological studies; Marta Espina examined the statistical analysis; María Luisa García corrected and analyzed the physicochemical characterization; and Ana Cristina Calpena conceived and designed all the experiments.

Conflicts of Interest: The authors declare no conflict of interest.

References

1. Alzheimer's Association. 2016 Alzheimer's disease facts and figures. *Alzheimer Dement. J. Alzheimer Assoc.* **2016**, *12*, 459–509. [CrossRef]
2. El Kadmiri, N.; Said, N.; Slassi, I.; El Moutawakil, B.; Nadifi, S. Biomarkers for Alzheimer Disease: Classical and Novel Candidates' Review. *Neuroscience* **2018**, *370*, 181–190. [CrossRef] [PubMed]
3. Wilkinson, D.; Schindler, R.; Schwam, E.; Waldemar, G.; Jones, R.W.; Gauthier, S.; Lopez, O.L.; Cummings, J.; Xu, Y.; Feldman, H.H. Effectiveness of donepezil in reducing clinical worsening in patients with mild-to-moderate alzheimer's disease. *Dement. Geriatr. Cogn. Disord.* **2009**, *28*, 244–251. [CrossRef] [PubMed]
4. Kumar, K.; Kumar, A.; Keegan, R.M.; Deshmukh, R. Recent advances in the neurobiology and neuropharmacology of Alzheimer's disease. *Biomed. Pharmacother.* **2018**, *98*, 297–307. [CrossRef] [PubMed]
5. Yao, L.; Li, K.; Zhang, L.; Yao, S.; Piao, Z.; Song, L. Influence of the Pro12Ala polymorphism of PPAR-γ on age at onset and sRAGE levels in Alzheimer's disease. *Brain Res.* **2009**, *1291*, 133–139. [CrossRef] [PubMed]
6. Combarros, O.; Rodriguez-Rodriguez, E.; Mateo, I.; Vazquez-Higuera, J.L.; Infante, J.; Berciano, J.; Sanchez-Juan, P. APOE dependent-association of PPAR-γ genetic variants with Alzheimer's disease risk. *Neurobiol. Aging* **2011**, *32*, 547.e1–547.e6. [CrossRef] [PubMed]

7. Radenkovic, M. Pioglitazone and Endothelial Dysfunction: Pleiotropic Effects and Possible Therapeutic Implications. *Sci. Pharm.* **2014**, *82*, 709–721. [CrossRef] [PubMed]
8. Suzuki, S.; Mori, Y.; Nagano, A.; Naiki-Ito, A.; Kato, H.; Nagayasu, Y.; Kobayashi, M.; Kuno, T.; Takahashi, S. Pioglitazone, a Peroxisome Proliferator-Activated Receptor γ Agonist, Suppresses Rat Prostate Carcinogenesis. *Int. J. Mol. Sci.* **2016**, *17*, 2071. [CrossRef] [PubMed]
9. Jia, C.; Huan, Y.; Liu, S.; Hou, S.; Sun, S.; Li, C.; Liu, Q.; Jiang, Q.; Wang, Y.; Shen, Z. Effect of Chronic Pioglitazone Treatment on Hepatic Gene Expression Profile in Obese C57BL/6J Mice. *Int. J. Mol. Sci.* **2015**, *16*, 12213–12229. [CrossRef] [PubMed]
10. Park, H.J.; Park, H.S.; Lee, J.U.; Bothwell, A.L.; Choi, J.M. Sex-Based Selectivity of PPARγ Regulation in Th1, Th2, and Th17 Differentiation. *Int. J. Mol. Sci.* **2016**, *17*, 1347. [CrossRef] [PubMed]
11. Tobiasova, Z.; Zhang, L.; Yi, T.; Qin, L.; Manes, T.D.; Kulkarni, S.; Lorber, M.I.; Rodriguez, F.C.; Choi, J.M.; Tellides, G.; et al. Peroxisome proliferator-activated receptor-γ agonists prevent in vivo remodeling of human artery induced by alloreactive T cells. *Circulation* **2011**, *124*, 196–205. [CrossRef] [PubMed]
12. Fakhfouri, G.; Ahmadiani, A.; Rahimian, R.; Grolla, A.A.; Moradi, F.; Haeri, A. WIN55212-2 attenuates amyloid-beta-induced neuroinflammation in rats through activation of cannabinoid receptors and PPAR-γ pathway. *Neuropharmacology* **2012**, *63*, 653–666. [CrossRef] [PubMed]
13. El-Zaher, A.A.; Elkady, E.F.; Elwy, H.M.; Saleh, M. Simultaneous spectrophotometric determination of glimepiride and pioglitazone in binary mixture and combined dosage form using chemometric-assisted techniques. *Spectrochim. Acta Part A Mol. Biomol. Spectrosc.* **2017**, *182*, 175–182. [CrossRef] [PubMed]
14. Klotz, L.; Burgdorf, S.; Dani, I.; Saijo, K.; Flossdorf, J.; Hucke, S.; Alferink, J.; Novak, N.; Beyer, M.; Mayer, G.; et al. The nuclear receptor PPARγ selectively inhibits Th17 differentiation in a T cell–intrinsic fashion and suppresses CNS autoimmunity. *J. Exp. Med.* **2009**, *206*, 2079–2089. [CrossRef] [PubMed]
15. Silva-Abreu, M.; Espinoza, L.C.; Rodriguez-Lagunas, M.J.; Fabrega, M.J.; Espina, M.; Garcia, M.L.; Calpena, A.C. Human Skin Permeation Studies with PPARγ Agonist to Improve Its Permeability and Efficacy in Inflammatory Processes. *Int. J. Mol. Sci.* **2017**, *18*, 2548. [CrossRef] [PubMed]
16. Heneka, M.T.; Sastre, M.; Dumitrescu-Ozimek, L.; Hanke, A.; Dewachter, I.; Kuiperi, C.; O'Banion, K.; Klockgether, T.; Van Leuven, F.; Landreth, G.E. Acute treatment with the PPARγ agonist pioglitazone and ibuprofen reduces glial inflammation and Aβ1–42 levels in APPV717I transgenic mice. *Brain* **2005**, *128*, 1442–1453. [CrossRef] [PubMed]
17. Sato, T.; Hanyu, H.; Hirao, K.; Kanetaka, H.; Sakurai, H.; Iwamoto, T. Efficacy of PPAR-γ agonist pioglitazone in mild Alzheimer disease. *Neurobiol. Aging* **2011**, *32*, 1626–1633. [CrossRef] [PubMed]
18. Hyma, P.; Abbulu, K. Formulation and characterisation of self-microemulsifying drug delivery system of pioglitazone. *Biomed. Prev. Nutr.* **2013**, *3*, 345–350. [CrossRef]
19. He, W.; Li, Y.; Zhang, R.; Wu, Z.; Yin, L. Gastro-floating bilayer tablets for the sustained release of metformin and immediate release of pioglitazone: Preparation and in vitro/in vivo evaluation. *Int. J. Pharm.* **2014**, *476*, 223–231. [CrossRef] [PubMed]
20. Ahad, A.; Al-Saleh, A.A.; Akhtar, N.; Al-Mohizea, A.M.; Al-Jenoobi, F.I. Transdermal delivery of antidiabetic drugs: Formulation and delivery strategies. *Drug Discov. Today* **2015**, *20*, 1217–1227. [CrossRef] [PubMed]
21. Jug, M.; Hafner, A.; Lovric, J.; Kregar, M.L.; Pepic, I.; Vanic, Z.; Cetina-Cizmek, B.; Filipovic-Grcic, J. An overview of in vitro dissolution/release methods for novel mucosal drug delivery systems. *J. Pharm. Biomed. Anal.* **2018**, *147*, 350–366. [CrossRef] [PubMed]
22. Fonseca-Santos, B.; Chorilli, M. An overview of polymeric dosage forms in buccal drug delivery: State of art, design of formulations and their in vivo performance evaluation. *Mater. Sci. Eng. C* **2017**. [CrossRef] [PubMed]
23. Fonseca-Santos, B.; Gremiao, M.P.; Chorilli, M. Nanotechnology-based drug delivery systems for the treatment of Alzheimer's disease. *Int. J. Nanomed.* **2015**, *10*, 4981–5003. [CrossRef] [PubMed]
24. Sosnik, A.; das Neves, J.; Sarmento, B. Mucoadhesive polymers in the design of nano-drug delivery systems for administration by non-parenteral routes: A review. *Prog. Polym. Sci.* **2014**, *39*, 2030–2075. [CrossRef]
25. Lee, G.H.; Lee, S.J.; Jeong, S.W.; Kim, H.C.; Park, G.Y.; Lee, S.G.; Choi, J.H. Antioxidative and antiinflammatory activities of quercetin-loaded silica nanoparticles. *Colloids Surf. B Biointerfaces* **2016**, *143*, 511–517. [CrossRef] [PubMed]
26. Desmet, E.; Van Gele, M.; Lambert, J. Topically applied lipid- and surfactant-based nanoparticles in the treatment of skin disorders. *Expert Opin. Drug Deliv.* **2016**, *14*, 109–122. [CrossRef] [PubMed]

27. Crucho, C.I.C.; Barros, M.T. Polymeric nanoparticles: A study on the preparation variables and characterization methods. *Mater. Sci. Eng. C Mater. Biol. Appl.* **2017**, *80*, 771–784. [CrossRef] [PubMed]
28. Jin, K.; Luo, Z.; Zhang, B.; Pang, Z. Biomimetic nanoparticles for inflammation targeting. *Acta Pharm. Sin. B* **2017**, *8*, 23–33. [CrossRef]
29. El-Say, K.M.; El-Sawy, H.S. Polymeric nanoparticles: Promising platform for drug delivery. *Int. J. Pharm.* **2017**, *528*, 675–691. [CrossRef] [PubMed]
30. Mansuri, S.; Kesharwani, P.; Jain, K.; Tekade, R.K.; Jain, N.K. Mucoadhesion: A promising approach in drug delivery system. *React. Funct. Polym.* **2016**, *100*, 151–172. [CrossRef]
31. Labarre, D. The Interactions between Blood and Polymeric Nanoparticles Depend on the Nature and Structure of the Hydrogel Covering the Surface. *Polymers* **2012**, *4*, 986–996. [CrossRef]
32. Shen, Z.; Nieh, M.-P.; Li, Y. Decorating Nanoparticle Surface for Targeted Drug Delivery: Opportunities and Challenges. *Polymers* **2016**, *8*, 83. [CrossRef]
33. Ozturk-Atar, K.; Eroglu, H.; Calis, S. Novel advances in targeted drug delivery. *J. Drug Target.* **2017**, 1–10. [CrossRef] [PubMed]
34. Lautenschlager, C.; Schmidt, C.; Fischer, D.; Stallmach, A. Drug delivery strategies in the therapy of inflammatory bowel disease. *Adv. Drug Deliv. Rev.* **2014**, *71*, 58–76. [CrossRef] [PubMed]
35. Fessi, H.; Puisieux, F.; Devissaguet, J.; Ammoury, N.; Benita, S. Nanocapsule formation by interfacial polymer deposition following solvent displacement. *Int. J. Pharm.* **1989**, *55*, R1–R4. [CrossRef]
36. Clogston, J.; Patri, A. Zeta potential measurement. In *Characterization of Nanoparticles Intended for Drug Delivery*; McNeil, S.E., Ed.; Humana Press: Totowa, NJ, USA, 2011; pp. 63–70.
37. Kapoor, M.; Cloyd, J.C.; Siegel, R.A. A review of intranasal formulations for the treatment of seizure emergencies. *J. Control. Release* **2016**, *237*, 147–159. [CrossRef] [PubMed]
38. Christrup, L.; Lundorff, L.; Werner, M. Novel formulations and routes of administration for opioids in the treatment of breakthrough pain. *Therapy* **2009**, *6*, 695–706. [CrossRef]
39. Wittayalertpanya, S.; Chompootaweep, S.; Thaworn, N. The Pharmacokinetics of Pioglitazone in Thai Healthy Subjects. *J. Med. Assoc. Thail.* **2006**, *89*, 2116–2122.
40. Schramm, G. *A Practical Approach to Rheology and Rheometry*, 2nd ed.; Gebrueder HAAKE: Karlsruhe, Germany, 1994.
41. Silva-Abreu, M.; Calpena, A.C.; Espina, M.; Silva, A.M.; Gimeno, A.; Egea, M.A.; Garcia, M.L. Optimization, Biopharmaceutical Profile and Therapeutic Efficacy of Pioglitazone-loaded PLGA-PEG Nanospheres as a Novel Strategy for Ocular Inflammatory Disorders. *Pharm. Res.* **2018**, *35*, 11. [CrossRef] [PubMed]
42. Sozio, P.; Cerasa, L.S.; Marinelli, L.; Di Stefano, A. Transdermal donepezil on the treatment of Alzheimer's disease. *Neuropsychiatr. Dis. Treat.* **2012**, *8*, 361–368. [CrossRef] [PubMed]
43. Ulep, M.G.; Saraon, S.K.; McLea, S. Alzheimer Disease. *J. Nurse Pract.* **2017**. [CrossRef]
44. Saraiva, C.; Praca, C.; Ferreira, R.; Santos, T.; Ferreira, L.; Bernardino, L. Nanoparticle-mediated brain drug delivery: Overcoming blood-brain barrier to treat neurodegenerative diseases. *J. Control. Release* **2016**, *235*, 34–47. [CrossRef] [PubMed]
45. Kumar, B.; Jalodia, K.; Kumar, P.; Gautam, H.K. Recent advances in nanoparticle-mediated drug delivery. *J. Drug Deliv. Sci. Technol.* **2017**, *41*, 260–268. [CrossRef]
46. Tapeinos, C.; Battaglini, M.; Ciofani, G. Advances in the design of solid lipid nanoparticles and nanostructured lipid carriers for targeting brain diseases. *J. Control. Release* **2017**, *264*, 306–332. [CrossRef] [PubMed]
47. Kreuter, J. Drug delivery to the central nervous system by polymeric nanoparticles: What do we know? *Adv. Drug Deliv. Rev.* **2014**, *71*, 2–14. [CrossRef] [PubMed]
48. Han, J.; Zhao, D.; Li, D.; Wang, X.; Jin, Z.; Zhao, K. Polymer-Based Nanomaterials and Applications for Vaccines and Drugs. *Polymers* **2018**, *10*, 31. [CrossRef]
49. Wen, M.M.; El-Salamouni, N.S.; El-Refaie, W.M.; Hazzah, H.A.; Ali, M.M.; Tosi, G.; Farid, R.M.; Blanco-Prieto, M.J.; Billa, N.; Hanafy, A.S. Nanotechnology-based drug delivery systems for Alzheimer's disease management: Technical, industrial, and clinical challenges. *J. Control. Release* **2017**, *245*, 95–107. [CrossRef] [PubMed]
50. Nakamura, H.; Watano, S. Direct Permeation of Nanoparticles across Cell Membrane: A Review. *KONA Powder Part. J.* **2018**, *35*, 49–65. [CrossRef]

51. Leroueil, P.R.; Hong, S.; Mecke, A.; Baker, J.R., Jr.; Orr, B.G.; Banaszak Holl, M.M. Nanoparticle interaction with biological membranes: Does nanotechnology present a Janus face? *Acc. Chem. Res.* **2007**, *40*, 335–342. [CrossRef] [PubMed]
52. Patel, R.R.; Chaurasia, S.; Khan, G.; Chaubey, P.; Kumar, N.; Mishra, B. Cromolyn sodium encapsulated PLGA nanoparticles: An attempt to improve intestinal permeation. *Int. J. Biol. Macromol.* **2016**, *83*, 249–258. [CrossRef] [PubMed]
53. Dunnhaupt, S.; Barthelmes, J.; Hombach, J.; Sakloetsakun, D.; Arkhipova, V.; Bernkop-Schnurch, A. Distribution of thiolated mucoadhesive nanoparticles on intestinal mucosa. *Int. J. Pharm.* **2011**, *408*, 191–199. [CrossRef] [PubMed]
54. Fortuna, A.; Alves, G.; Serralheiro, A.; Sousa, J.; Falcao, A. Intranasal delivery of systemic-acting drugs: Small-molecules and biomacromolecules. *Eur. J. Pharm. Biopharm.* **2014**, *88*, 8–27. [CrossRef] [PubMed]
55. Khan, A.R.; Liu, M.; Khan, M.W.; Zhai, G. Progress in brain targeting drug delivery system by nasal route. *J. Control. Release* **2017**, *268*, 364–389. [CrossRef] [PubMed]
56. Lochhead, J.J.; Thorne, R.G. Intranasal delivery of biologics to the central nervous system. *Adv. Drug Deliv. Rev.* **2012**, *64*, 614–628. [CrossRef] [PubMed]
57. Touitou, E.; Illum, L. Nasal drug delivery. *Drug Deliv. Transl. Res.* **2013**, *3*, 1–3. [CrossRef] [PubMed]
58. Pardeshi, C.V.; Belgamwar, V.S. Direct nose to brain drug delivery via integrated nerve pathways bypassing the blood-brain barrier: An excellent platform for brain targeting. *Expert Opin. Drug Deliv.* **2013**, *10*, 957–972. [CrossRef] [PubMed]
59. Mogoşanu, G.D.; Grumezescu, A.M.; Bejenaru, C.; Bejenaru, L.E. Polymeric protective agents for nanoparticles in drug delivery and targeting. *Int. J. Pharm.* **2016**, *510*, 419–429. [CrossRef] [PubMed]
60. Abdelhalim, M.A. The rheological properties of different GNPs. *Lipids Health Dis.* **2012**, *11*, 14. [CrossRef] [PubMed]
61. Fernandez-Campos, F.; Clares Naveros, B.; Lopez Serrano, O.; Alonso Merino, C.; Calpena Campmany, A.C. Evaluation of novel nystatin nanoemulsion for skin candidosis infections. *Mycoses* **2013**, *56*, 70–81. [CrossRef] [PubMed]
62. Abrego, G.; Alvarado, H.L.; Egea, M.A.; Gonzalez-Mira, E.; Calpena, A.C.; Garcia, M.L. Design of nanosuspensions and freeze-dried PLGA nanoparticles as a novel approach for ophthalmic delivery of pranoprofen. *J. Pharm. Sci.* **2014**, *103*, 3153–3164. [CrossRef] [PubMed]
63. Ramos Yacasi, G.R.; Garcia Lopez, M.L.; Espina Garcia, M.; Parra Coca, A.; Calpena Campmany, A.C. Influence of freeze-drying and γ-irradiation in preclinical studies of flurbiprofen polymeric nanoparticles for ocular delivery using d-(+)-trehalose and polyethylene glycol. *Int. J. Nanomed.* **2016**, *11*, 4093–4106. [CrossRef] [PubMed]

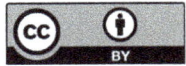

© 2018 by the authors. Licensee MDPI, Basel, Switzerland. This article is an open access article distributed under the terms and conditions of the Creative Commons Attribution (CC BY) license (http://creativecommons.org/licenses/by/4.0/).

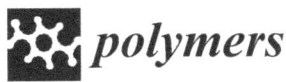

Article

Assessing Mucoadhesion in Polymer Gels: The Effect of Method Type and Instrument Variables

Jéssica Bassi da Silva [1], Sabrina Barbosa de Souza Ferreira [1], Adriano Valim Reis [1], Michael Thomas Cook [2] and Marcos Luciano Bruschi [1,*]

1 Laboratory of Research and Development of Drug Delivery Systems, Postgraduate Program in Pharmaceutical Sciences, Department of Pharmacy, State University of Maringa, Maringa, Parana CEP 87020-900, Brazil; jessicabassidasilva@gmail.com (J.B.d.S.); sbsferreira88@gmail.com (S.B.d.S.F.); avreis77@gmail.com (A.V.R.)
2 Research Centre in Topical Drug Delivery and Toxicology, Department of Pharmacy, Pharmacology and Postgraduate Medicine, University of Hertfordshire, Hatfield AL10 9AB, UK; m.cook5@herts.ac.uk
* Correspondence: mlbruschi@uem.br; Tel.: +55-44-3011-4870

Received: 8 January 2018; Accepted: 27 February 2018; Published: 1 March 2018

Abstract: The process of mucoadhesion has been widely studied using a wide variety of methods, which are influenced by instrumental variables and experiment design, making the comparison between the results of different studies difficult. The aim of this work was to standardize the conditions of the detachment test and the rheological methods of mucoadhesion assessment for semisolids, and introduce a texture profile analysis (TPA) method. A factorial design was developed to suggest standard conditions for performing the detachment force method. To evaluate the method, binary polymeric systems were prepared containing poloxamer 407 and Carbopol 971P®, Carbopol 974P®, or Noveon® Polycarbophil. The mucoadhesion of systems was evaluated, and the reproducibility of these measurements investigated. This detachment force method was demonstrated to be reproduceable, and gave different adhesion when mucin disk or ex vivo oral mucosa was used. The factorial design demonstrated that all evaluated parameters had an effect on measurements of mucoadhesive force, but the same was not observed for the work of adhesion. It was suggested that the work of adhesion is a more appropriate metric for evaluating mucoadhesion. Oscillatory rheology was more capable of investigating adhesive interactions than flow rheology. TPA method was demonstrated to be reproducible and can evaluate the adhesiveness interaction parameter. This investigation demonstrates the need for standardized methods to evaluate mucoadhesion and makes suggestions for a standard study design.

Keywords: pluronic f127; thermoresponsive polymers; thermogelling polymers; detachment force; rheology; texture profile analysis

1. Introduction

Mucosal surfaces cover the nasal, ocular, buccal, rectal, vaginal, and gastrointestinal areas among other parts of the body. Drugs may be administered to these sites for local effect, and their high permeability makes them attractive for systemic drug delivery. However, the natural clearance mechanisms from these sites limit residence time, decreasing drug absorption or duration of local effect [1]. In order to overcome these disadvantages, "mucoadhesive" systems have been developed, which adhere to mucosal membranes through a variety of attractive physicochemical interactions, enhancing retention, and thus the efficacy of medicines [2–5].

Mucoadhesive polymers are a group of materials employed in different pharmaceutical systems. They are defined as hydrophilic macromolecules, which contain numerous functional organic groups (i.e., carboxylic, hydroxyl, amide, and amine groups) able to establish interactions with mucosal membranes [6,7]. These polymers can be classified according to their interactions with the mucosa (covalent bonds or non-covalent intermolecular interactions). Non-covalent bonds believed to enhance mucoadhesion include hydrogen-bonding, hydrophobic interactions, and electrostatic interactions. Mucoadhesive polymers may be cationic, anionic, or non-ionic [8–10]. Anionic polymers, such as poly(acrylic acid) derivates, are believed to form hydrogen bonds below their pKa between their carboxylic groups and the hydroxyl groups of the mucus glycoprotein. It has also been suggested that ion-dipole interactions may occur when in the carboxylate form [9]. Moreover, poly(acrylic acid) derivates may be combined in solution with thermoresponsive polymers, like poloxamer 407 (P407), to enhance retention [11]. Thermoresponsive polymers transition from a liquid to a viscous gel above a critical temperature, allowing for passage through an applicator before thickening upon application to the body [11–13].

In vitro or ex vivo techniques are crucial in the performance testing of mucoadhesive drug delivery systems and are cost-effective in selecting efficient systems when compared with in vivo methods. These methods are able to evaluate mucoadhesive formulations, without using animal models, and may offer mechanistic understanding of mucoadhesion [14–17]. Numerous techniques have been developed to assess and understand the mucoadhesion of drug delivery systems. The development of new methods should be validated by comparison with a gold standard in vitro technique, or in vivo performance. New methods to investigate the mucoadhesive profile of semisolid polymer systems are typically developed in-house on bespoke equipment, and have not been through validation, which emphasizes the importance of standardized techniques [18–20]. Furthermore, each dosage form may require different experimental conditions and comparison may only be possible within dosage form types. The detachment force method (also known as the tensile method) is the most widely employed method to investigate adhesive interactions between a mucosal membrane (or other substrate) and a formulation. This method can be used for solid [19–21] and semisolid dosage forms [2,4,5,12,19,21–23] and it is known that instrumental parameters and experiment design influence test results. Other techniques, such as the rheological method, can result in different responses and interpretations depending on the analysis type used (flow or oscillatory) [19]. Therefore, it is very important to understand the variables of the method for mucoadhesion testing, considering that standardized methods have been required [1,3].

Therefore, this work aimed to investigate the importance of standardizing the conditions to perform the detachment force and the rheological methods for assessing mucoadhesion of semisolid systems, as well as for assessing mucoadhesive interactions by texture profile analysis.

2. Materials and Methods

2.1. Materials

Carbopol 971P® (C971P), Carbopol 974P® (C974P), and Noveon® Polycarbophil (PCB) were kindly donated by Lubrizol (Sao Paulo, Brazil). Triethanolamine, poloxamer 407 (P407), and mucin from porcine stomach (type II) were received from Sigma-Aldrich (Sao Paulo, Brazil). Porcine oral mucosa was sourced from a local slaughterhouse (Maringa, Brazil) and kept frozen at -20 °C. All reagents were used without further purification.

2.2. Preparation of Polymeric Systems

Monopolymeric formulations were prepared using P407 (15% or 20%, w/w) or C971P, C974P, and PCB (0.10%, 0.15%, 0.20%, 0.25%, or 0.50%, w/w). P407 solutions were prepared by dispersing the required amount of the polymer in purified water at 5 °C under mechanical stirring (500 rpm).

To prepare the poly(acrylic acid)-containing formulations, the required amount mass of the polymer was dispersed in purified water with mechanical stirring.

Binary polymeric blends were prepared by dispersion of C971P, C974P, or PCB (0.10%, 0.15%, 0.20%, 0.25%, or 0.50%, w/w) in purified water under mechanical stirring. The required amount of P407 (15% or 20%, w/w) was then added to the preparation. This mixture was maintained for 12 h at the temperature of 4 °C. After this period of time, the preparations were stirred, neutralized using triethanolamine, and refrigerated (4 °C) for at least 24 h before analysis.

2.3. Mucoadhesive Analysis by Detachment Force Evaluation

A TA-XTplus texture analyzer (Stable Micro Systems, Surrey, UK) was utilized to investigate the adhesive properties of the formulations [24]. Mucin disks were prepared by the compression of crude porcine mucin (200 mg) using a ring press with a 13-mm diameter die and a compression force of 10 tonnes, applied for 30 s. Moreover, pig buccal mucosa samples were obtained from pigs (white, young, and recent sacrificed) originated from a local slaughterhouse (authorized by the Brazilian Ministry of Agriculture for human consumption). They were cleaned with phosphate saline buffer (PSB), the cheek mucosa was gently removed, and the samples were prepared with the same diameter and area of the mucin disks (132.73 mm^2), using a surgical scalpel. Samples displaying wounds or bruises were not used. The mucosal substrate (disk or tissue) was then horizontally attached to the lower end of the probe (cylindrical, P/6), using double sided adhesive tape. Prior to testing, the disk or the mucosal tissue was hydrated by submersion in a 5% (w/v) aqueous solution of mucin or in PSB for 30 s, respectively. The excess surface liquid was withdrawn by gentle blotting. Samples of each formulation (5.0 g) were packed into shallow cylindrical vessels with 20 mm diameter, maintained at 37 °C, and placed under the probe, which was lowered at a speed of 1 mm/s until it reached the mucoadhesive hydrogel surface. Immediately, a downward force of 0.03 N was applied and the probe remained on the surface of the sample for 30 s; then the probe was withdrawn at a rate of 10.0 mm/s until complete detachment of the sample from the mucosal substrate. The Texture Exponent 32 software (Stable Micro Systems, Surrey, UK) was used to determine the force required for the detachment (F_{adh}) and the work of adhesion (W_{adh}) (the area under the force/distance curve). All measurements were performed with at least six replicates.

Mucin disks and porcine buccal mucosa were chosen as substrate models, due to the great use of them in the literature. Moreover, pigs have a greater similarity of anatomy, physiology, metabolism and histology than other animals when compared with humans [25,26]. Detachment force, the maximum force necessary to remove the sample from mucosal substrate, and work of adhesion, the area under the force-displacement curve, were evaluated by two-way analysis of variance (ANOVA), using Tukey post hoc test. The p-value < 0.05 was taken to denote significance.

To evaluate the effects of the instrumental parameters on the F_{adh} and W_{adh}, a polymeric system composed of 15% (w/w) P407 and 0.25% (w/w) PCB at 37 °C was also studied. A full factorial design $2^4 + 4C$ was created by Statistic 8.0® software (StatSoft Company, Tulsa, OK, USA). The influence of the variables: substrate (X_1), force (X_2), speed of upward probe (X_3) and time of substrate-sample contact (X_4) were investigated. Each factor was set at one of two levels, low (−) or high (+) (Table 1). Four central points were also used to evaluate the curvature and the errors related with isolated effects or the interaction between them.

Table 1. Matrix of factorial design $2^4 + 4C$ for binary polymeric systems composed of 15% (w/w) P407 and 0.25% (w/w) PCB, at 37 °C, and values for the low and high levels of each variable.

Standard Run	Independent Variables			
	X_1	X_2	X_3	X_4
1	A	−	−	−
2	B	−	−	−
3	A	+	−	−
4	B	+	−	−
5	A	−	+	−
6	B	−	+	−
7	A	+	+	−
8	B	+	+	−
9	A	−	−	+
10	B	−	−	+
11	A	+	−	+
12	B	+	−	+
13	A	−	+	+
14	B	−	+	+
15	A	+	+	+
16	B	+	+	+
17	A	0	0	0
18	B	0	0	0
19	A	0	0	0
20	B	0	0	0
Factor		−	0	+
X_1 Substrate	A: Mucin disk			B: Oral pig mucosal
X_2 Force (N)		0.03	0.065	0.10
X_3 Speed (mm/s)		1.00	5.50	10.0
X_4 Time (s)		30.0	75.0	120.0

2.4. Mucoadhesive Analysis Using Rheological Methods

2.4.1. Continuous Shear (Flow) Rheology

The increase in consistency index due to a synergism between mucin and polymer systems was measured using a modified version of the method described by Hassan and Gallo [27,28]. The polymeric blends previously prepared, 5% (w/w) mucin aqueous solution (prepared just before the measurements), and their mixture were evaluated. The mixtures were composed of the polymeric systems with 5% (w/w) mucin added under vigorous stirring for 15 min prior to analysis. Flow rheometry was performed using a controlled stress rheometer (MARS II, Haake Thermo Fisher Scientific Inc., Newington, Germany), equipped with parallel steel cone-plate geometry of 60 mm; separated by a fixed distance of 0.052 mm. Analysis was performed in flow mode at 37 ± 1 °C, over shear rates ranging from 0 to 2000 s^{-1}, increasing over a period of 150 s, and was maintained at the superior limit for 10 s and then decreased during the same period. At least six replicates of each sample were evaluated, and the upward flow curves were fitted using Power Law equation (Oswald-de-Waele) as shown below [2,27,29,30]:

$$\tau = k \cdot \gamma^n \tag{1}$$

where τ is the shear stress (Pa), k is the consistency index [$(Pa.s)^n$], γ is the rate of shear (s^{-1}), and n is the flow behavior index (dimensionless).

2.4.2. Oscillatory Rheology

Oscillatory measurements were performed at 37 ± 1 °C, using the same rheometer and geometry previously described, and in oscillation mode. Samples of each polymeric system, mucin aqueous solution 5% (w/w) and the polymeric systems with 5% (w/w) mucin were placed to the inferior plate, allowing for 1 min equilibration prior to testing. The linear viscoelastic region of each formulation was determined and a frequency sweep was performed from 0.1 to 10.0 Hz. The elastic modulus (G'), viscous modulus (G''), dynamic viscosity (η'), and the loss tangent (tan δ) were calculated using RheoWin 4.10.0000 (Haake) software (Thermo Fisher Scientific Inc., Newington, Germany). All measurements were performed in at least six replicates [29]. Calculation of the interaction parameter for the polymeric systems (P407/C971P, P407/C974P, and P407/PCB) with mucin was determined by the difference between the storage (elastic) modulus of the mixture, and the theoretical value of the storage modulus obtained by summation of the individual parts [29,31], at an oscillatory frequency of 10.0 Hz as demonstrated in the equation.

$$\Delta G' = G'_{\text{mixture}} - (G'_{\text{mucin}} + G'_{\text{polymeric system}}) \tag{2}$$

2.5. Texture Profile Analysis

The texture profile analysis (TPA) of polymeric blends, 5% (w/w) mucin aqueous solution and the mixture of both were performed using a TA-XTplus Texture Analyzer (Stable Micro Systems; Surrey, UK) in TPA mode, at 37 °C, to evaluate adhesive interactions. Bottles containing 16 g of formulations were submitted to a double compression by an analytical probe (10 mm diameter). The two times of compression (at 2 mm/s) were performed on the sample, with a predefined depth (15 mm). A delay period of 15 s was permitted between the end of the first compression and the beginning of the second. From the force-time and force-distance plot, the mechanical properties were obtained, namely: hardness (maximum force obtained during the first compression), compressibility (the work required to deform the sample during the first pass of the probe), adhesiveness (work required to overcome the attractive forces between the surfaces of the probe and the formulation), elasticity (ability to stretch and return to its original size and shape), and cohesiveness (work spent to unite the surface of the sample and the surface of the probe) [2,29]. All analysis was performed in at least five replicates. The interaction parameter of these variables was calculated by the difference between the values observed for the mixture (polymeric blend with 5% (w/w) mucin) and the sum of the individual contributions of polymeric system and mucin solution.

2.6. Statistical Analysis

The responses obtained were statistically compared using two-way analysis of variance (ANOVA). In all cases, individual differences between means were identified using Tukey's test. Moreover, significant differences were accepted when p <0.05 for all methods [32].

3. Results and Discussion

3.1. Polymeric Systems

Previously characterized binary polymer blends [23,30,33,34] were selected to evaluate the robustness of the mucoadhesive methods. These systems, composed of P407 and poly(acrylic acid) derivatives possess different rheological and mechanical properties. These polymers contribute in a unique way to the formulation properties. With a temperature increase, P407 increases the viscosity of the system and the other decreases it (C971P, C974P, or PCB). Although other polymers as natural polymers (i.e., gelatin and agar) and synthetic polymers (i.e., poly(vinylpyrrolidone) and poly(vinyl alcohol)) were already widely used to investigate the mucoadhesion process, the selected thermorresponsive blends, besides being very well characterized as a complex system, can be a challenge for different mucoadhesion analyses [23,30,33,34]. The carbomers C971P and C974P are mucoadhesive polymers crosslinked with allyl-ethers of pentaerythritol, displaying a concentration ranging from 56% to 68% of carboxylic groups in the chain. However, C974P displays a higher crosslinking degree than C971P. PCB is also a high-molecular-weight polymer of polyacrylic acid, cross-linked with divinylglycol or polyalkenyl ethers, displaying a large number of carboxylic groups (COOH) on the molecular chain, and known by its strong mucoadhesive properties [23,30,34]. The P407 monopolymeric formulation displays higher consistency at body temperatures than the blends containing the same amount of this thermogelling polymer [12,23,35]. Rheological, texture, and mucoadhesion studies have been performed to select the most suitable mucoadhesive semi-solid systems of each blend in previous studies (Table 2).

Table 2. Mucoadhesive profile (using porcine mucin disk), gelation temperature, and rheological interaction parameter of the selected formulations containing poloxamer 407 (P407) and Cabopol 971P® (C971P), Carbopol 974P® (C974P), or Noveon® Polycarbophil (PCB).

Systems	Polymer Amount (%, w/w)	Mucoadhesive Force (N)	Gelation Temperature (°C)	Interaction Parameter (Pa)
P407/C971P [a]	20/0.20	0.352 ± 0.04	27.88 ± 0.06	1944.73 ± 381.93
P407/C974P [b]	15/0.25	0.231 ± 0.03	36.04 ± 0.06	2509.33 ± 215.85
P407/PCB [c]	15/0.15	0.237 ± 0.01	36.42 ± 0.02	1927.03 ± 93.85

[a] [34]; [b] [30]; [c] [23].

The interaction parameter evaluates the adhesive interaction between polymers and can select optimal formulations for pharmaceutical and biomedical application [29,30]. The gelation temperature and adhesiveness are also important for performance testing of thermogelling systems to ensure that they solidify on application and are retained on the mucosa. The P407/C971P (20/0.20%, w/w), P407/C974P (15/0.25%, w/w), and P407/PCB (15/0.25%, w/w) system were selected based on previously-published information [23,30,34]. A gelation temperature range near the body temperature, between 25 and 37 °C, is considered appropriate for pharmaceutical systems [2,13].

Methods for analyzing the performance (e.g., mucoadhesion) should be investigated for accuracy, precision, specificity, linearity, and range [36]. In this work, some of these characteristics (precision by repeatability and robustness) were studied to evaluate the importance of standardizing the conditions of method. The robustness of an analytical method is defined by ICH guidelines as a measurement of resistance against small variations of the analytical parameter. Thus, it is possible to verify the robustness of the method by demonstrating its reliability during the normal use [36]. In this study, the methods to investigate the mucoadhesive characteristic were kept constant and the semi-solid formulations were changed to consider the formulations as a parameter or independent variable. Even known the temperature is not the same at 37 °C for different routes, and diseases are able to change the body temperature (e.g., fever), 37 °C was kept through the studied methods. Since most mucosal routes demonstrate this mean temperature. In addition, the selected thermoresponsive systems maintain their physicochemical profile with small variation of temperature (30–38 °C) and gel in this temperature range.

3.2. Analysis of the Detachment Force

The detachment force is an in vitro method widely used to analyze the mucoadhesive properties of the most dosage forms. By this method, it is possible to measure the W_{adh}, which is based on the area under a force-distance curve obtained during the detachment process, as well as the F_{adh}, defined as the maximum force to separate an adhesive surface from a mucous substrate [1,3,30,35,37]. There is not a standard methodology to this determination [37,38], so not only the choice of the technique, but also the choice of membrane (mucus or other mucosal types) and instrument parameters are critical to investigate the mucoadhesive properties of drug delivery systems. The limited use of the human mucosa means that ex vivo animal models are required, but these require validation and an understanding of intra-species variability. Moreover, the process of mucus/mucosa preparation can modify the physicochemical properties and results in an altered structure when compared to a fresh mucosa [37,38]. To begin this process, a standardization of this method using mucin disks and oral porcine mucosa for the three semi-solid systems was proposed.

The results of the detachment force method (Figure 1 and Table S1) demonstrate the reproducibility of the method with a coefficient of variation (or relative standard deviation), lower than 5% for mucin disks and lower than 12% for porcine oral mucosa, with the variation believed to be a result of the mucosa's natural variability [33,39,40]. Previous studies have demonstrated differences among mucin from different sites. Likewise, the variability between individuals and mucosa thickness may also affect results on ex vivo mucosa [16,37,41]. In a previous investigation using mucin disks, polymeric blends containing P407/C971P, P407/C974P, or P407/PCB showed the same values of the mucoadhesion force, when compared by this method, supporting its reliability between laboratories [23,30,34].

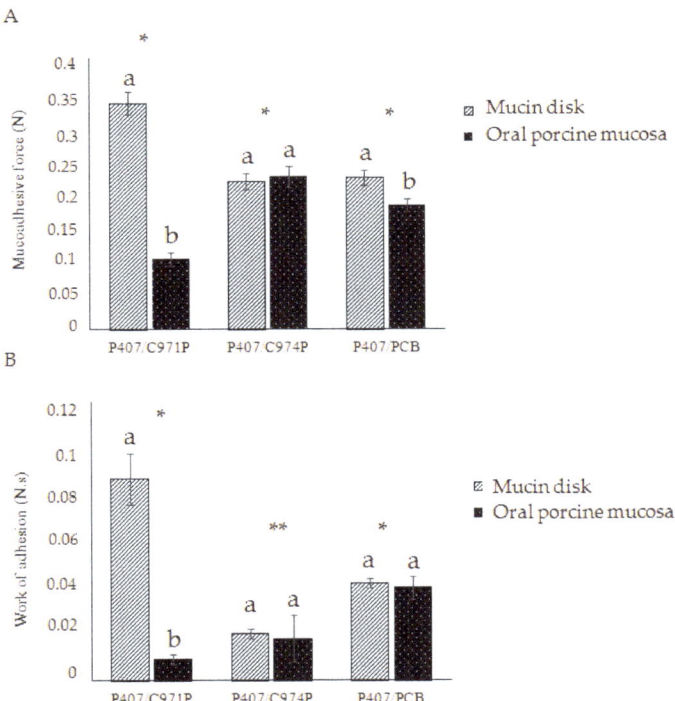

Figure 1. Mucoadhesive force F_{adh} (**A**) and work of adhesion W_{adh} (**B**) of the polymeric blends containing P407 and C971P, C974P, or PCB, obtained by detachment force method using porcine mucin disks or oral porcine mucosa as substrates. The symbols (* and **) and the letters (a and b) represent the significant difference ($p < 0.05$) among the polymeric systems and the substrates, respectively.

The P407/C971P formulation demonstrated the greatest mucoadhesive strength on mucin disks, with the rank order P407/C971P > P407/PCB > P407/C974P. Binary polymeric systems composed of P407 and poly(acrylic acid) derivatives have the availability of the carboxylic groups present in the mucoadhesive polymer decreased. It is believed that interactions between P407 and the mucoadhesive polymer reduces the possibility of interaction between the poly(acrylic acid) derivate and the mucin. However, C971P has higher carboxyl concentration, when compared with C974P and PCB, which allows the P407/C971P system to interact with mucin groups even with the P407 interaction [2,33,34,39,42,43]. Moreover, P407/C971P demonstrated in TPA analysis higher values of hardness, cohesiveness, and compressibility, which contribute with the higher values of mucoadhesion observed with mucin disk. Using porcine buccal mucosa as a substrate gave a different rank-order of mucoadhesion: P407/C974P > P407/PCB > P407/C971P. The PCB with an intermediate amount of free carboxyl groups had in the two cases, also the intermediate mucoadhesive force. Furthermore, C974P, a more cross-linked material with a lower amount of hydroxyl groups, demonstrated similar results using mucin disk and animal mucosa. It is believed that the polymer has greater attractive forces among its polymeric chains, which can be also observed ahead by the high cohesiveness value, in TPA analysis. Creating a more cohesive system, with reduced mucin interaction, macroscopic differences were not observed with the substrate variation [19,23,44].

The discrepant answers observed between the results obtained with the two substrates for the P407/C971P system can suggest this formulation uses hydration to establish adhesive bonds between mucin and polymeric blend [1,40,45]. The C971P polymer exhibits lower cross-linking degree allowing higher swelling in presence of water. Therefore, in a low-hydration surface, such as the mucin disk, this system does not swell and displays a greater response than in high hydrated surface as the animal mucosa [43]. The water concentration also influences the tensile strength method [42], and a super hydration state of some polymers can reduce their mucoadhesive performance [43,46–48]. Thus, the selection of the mucosal surface needs to consider the composition and consistency of the formulation analyzed, where the most consistent systems (with high mechanical resistance) have better response using mucin disks.

To compare in vitro and in vivo tests, the same condition of analysis should be used [17]. However, using the same parameters, significant differences were observed between analyses performed with isolated mucin and ex vivo mucosa, particularly in the P407/C971P system. Furthermore, the W_{adh} response, related to elasticity and plasticity, demonstrated a significant difference between the three polymeric systems. On the other hand, for the F_{adh} response, significant difference was not found between the binary blends ($p > 0.05$). Therefore, the W_{adh} is suggested as a better response for the detachment force method and, when calculated as an N·mm unit, it can be converted to Joules, showing the energy dispending at the separation process of the adhesive surfaces.

In order to optimize this method, the responses of the P407/PCB polymeric blend were evaluated (Table 3) under the variation of the instrumental parameters in a factorial design.

Table 3. Response values of the mucoadhesive force (N) and the work adhesion (N·mm) of the binary polymeric system containing 15% (w/w) P407 and 0.25% (w/w) PCB, at 37 °C, using porcine mucin disks (A) or porcine oral mucosa (B). Each value represents the mean of at least three replicates. In all cases, the coefficient of variation of replicate analyses was less than 12%.

Experiment	Factors				Adhesive Force (N)	Work (N·mm)
	Substrate	Applied Force (N)	Velocity (mm/s)	Time (s)		
1	A	0.03	1.00	30	0.133	0.131
2	B	0.03	1.00	30	0.121	0.081
3	A	0.10	1.00	30	0.189	0.829
4	B	0.10	1.00	30	0.128	0.110
5	A	0.03	10.0	30	0.169	0.313
6	B	0.03	10.0	30	0.255	0.110
7	A	0.10	10.0	30	0.329	0.927
8	B	0.10	10.0	30	0.223	0.405
9	A	0.03	1.00	120	0.138	0.259
10	B	0.03	1.00	120	0.120	0.055
11	A	0.10	1.00	120	0.365	0.740
12	B	0.10	1.00	120	0.110	0.083
13	A	0.03	10.0	120	0.200	0.469
14	B	0.03	10.0	120	0.115	0.245
15	A	0.10	10.0	120	1.247	1.033
16	B	0.10	10.0	120	0.303	0.383
17 (C)	A	0.065	5.50	75	0.191	0.548
18 (C)	B	0.065	5.50	75	0.157	0.125
19 (C)	A	0.065	5.50	75	0.236	0.715
20 (C)	B	0.065	5.50	75	0.169	0.242

The Pareto diagrams (Figure 2) shows the estimated effect of each factor and their interactions. A factor and an interaction are considered to influence the response only if the estimated effect is significant, i.e., $p < 0.05$. It was found that variation of substrate, force, probe velocity rate, and contact time influenced the F_{adh}. Applied force had the highest positive influence, and the substrate had a negative influence on this response of mucoadhesive force. For the W_{adh}, only the contact time and some interactions demonstrated positive influence on the response. Speed and the change of the substrate from mucin disk to animal mucosa had the greatest negative contribution.

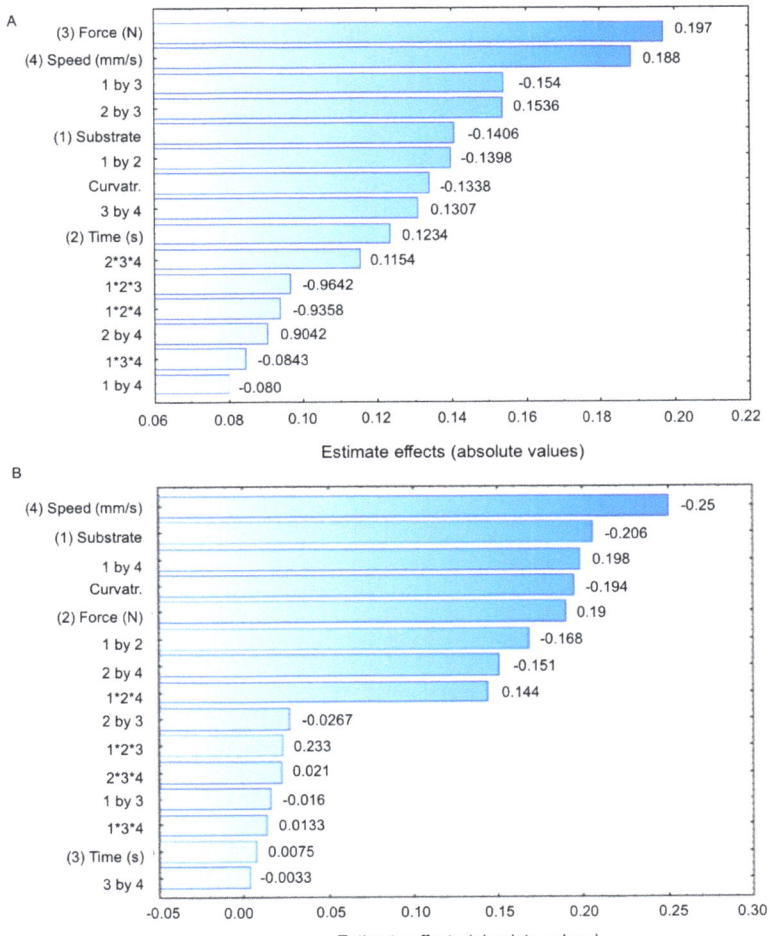

Figure 2. Pareto diagrams with the estimate effect of the parameters about the mucoadhesive force F_{adh} (**A**) and work adhesion W_{adh} (**B**) for the binary polymeric system composed of 15% (w/w) P407 and 0.25% (w/w) PCB, at 37 °C, and their interactions.

The surface response plots (Figure 3) demonstrate that the largest F_{adh} was obtained using the mucin disk, 0.1 N of contact force, 120 s of contact time, and a speed of 10 mm/s. On the other hand, for the W_{adh} (Figure 4), the highest value was observed using mucin disk, 0.1 N, 1 mm/s, which was time independent. The surface was adjusted to the experimental data by multiple adjusted correlation coefficient values R^2_{adj}. Thus, through the regression analysis, it was observed that 93.98% of the variation in the F_{adh} response is explained with this model ($R^2_{adj} = 0.9398$). Moreover, 96.08% of the variation in the W_{adh} response is explained with this model ($R^2_{adj} = 0.9608$). Therefore, the method can estimate the F_{adh} and the W_{adh} according to these parameters.

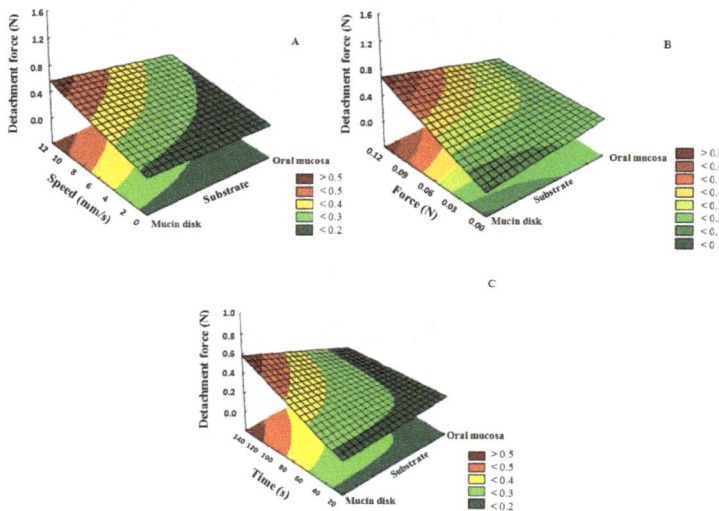

Figure 3. Response surface plots of the detachment force (F_{adh}) using mucin disk or oral mucosa influenced by some factors: (**A**) speed of probe ascent (mm/s); (**B**) applied force (N); (**C**) analysis time (s).

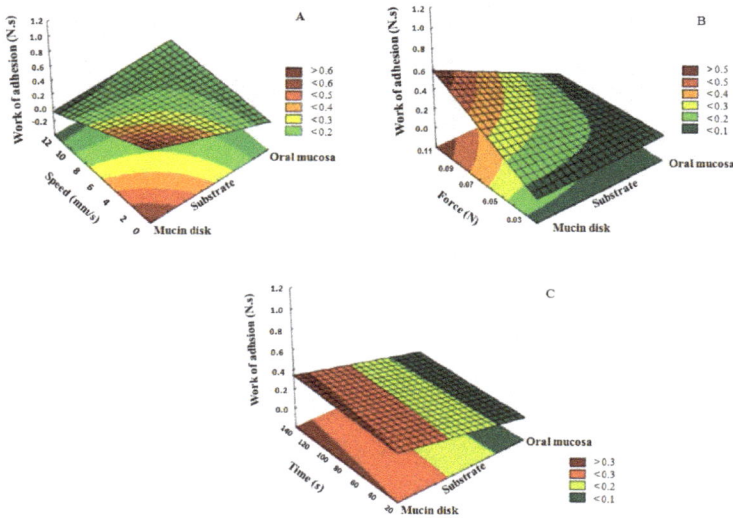

Figure 4. Response surface graphs of the work adhesion (W_{adh}) using mucin disk or oral mucosa influenced by some factors: (**A**) speed of probe ascent (mm/s); (**B**) applied force (N); (**C**) analysis time (s).

Additionally, the desirability of the method was evaluated for both responses, which represents the combination of factors required to obtain a better response [49]. Figure 5 shows the desirability response for the F_{adh} results, which is 85% of the maximum value experimentally obtained (1.147 N).

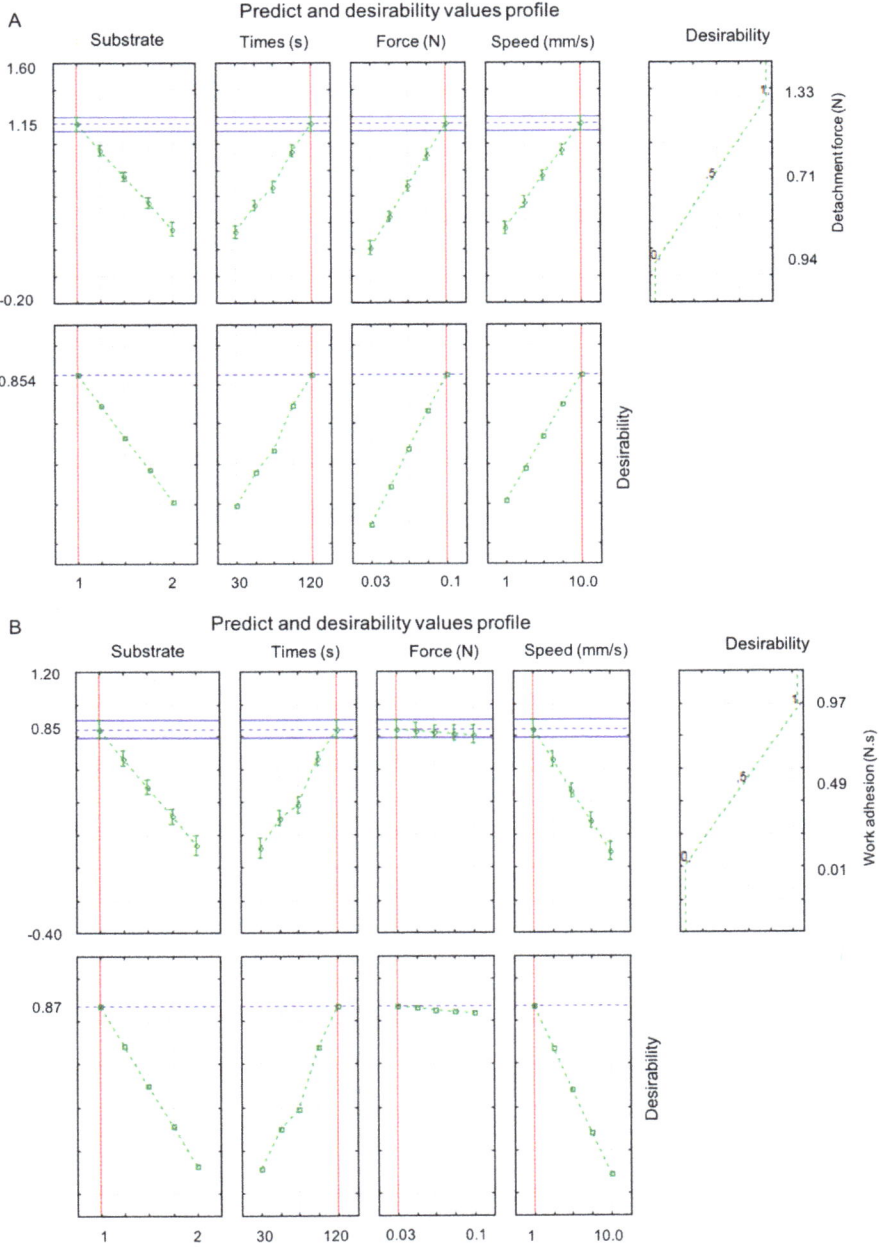

Figure 5. Profile of prediction and desirability values of the detachment force (**A**) and work adhesion (**B**) related to the substrate, time (s), applied force (N), and speed of probe ascent (mm/s).

About the W_{adh} (Figure 5B), the desirability was at 92% of the maximum experimental value (1.019 N.mm). Moreover, the substrate variation from the mucin disk to the animal mucosa reduced both results for the studied semi-solid formulation. It was also observed that the F_{adh} increases when changing the levels from minimum to maximum for time, force, and speed parameters. Prior studies had demonstrated the increase of contact time between formulation and substrate surface increases the interaction between mucin and polymer chains; thus, higher values of adhesion are obtained [43,50]. About the W_{adh}, changing the levels from minimum to maximal for force and speed parameters, the response is greater as well. On the other hand, the time was not relevant to this answer. The statistical analysis suggests that it is not possible to compare results present in the literature, which use different substrates and parameters, for the tensile strength method. Thus, it is clear the necessity of standardization of this method, to have real comparisons among mucoadhesive profiles of different formulations and polymeric systems.

The desirability cannot show the proximity to real values, which characterizes a limitation of the in vitro methods. Nevertheless, this analysis allows a standardization of this method using both responses, since the higher value is obtained using these parameters. Therefore, for semi-solid formulations containing P407 and poly(acrylic) derivative, it can be suggested that the use of mucin disk, a force of 0.1 N, 120 s of contact time, and 10 mm/s probe speed will obtain better F_{adh} measurement. Using a mucin disk, 0.1 N of force, 30 s of contact time, and a probe speed of 10 mm/s can be used to obtain a better W_{adh} response.

Therefore, with the information obtained, it will be possible in future studies to select and validate the best conditions to perform comparisons.

3.3. Rheological Methods

Rheological analysis represents an in vitro model which can predict the in vivo behavior of adhesive formulations and also investigate their structural interactions. The mucoadhesion process is a phenomenon which combines different interaction types and the rheological method is used to evaluate these interactions between mucin and polymeric system [3,16,18,51]. The mucoadhesion process is characterized when the rheological response of a polymer-mucin mixture is higher than the isolated contributions, giving rise to an "interaction parameter" [8,20,28,47].

There are different ways to use the rheological analysis in studying mucoadhesion. It can be performed by consistency measurement over a range of shear rates or by monitoring the viscoelastic properties [27]. Whilst rheology is preferred as a secondary technique, it is often used to measure changes in viscosity or elastic behavior [2,8,23,40,47]. However, a lack of understanding about the meaning of the interaction parameter further confounds the great variability of results in the literature. Therefore, a standardization of the interpretation of results from the rheological analysis was proposed for the three semi-solid systems using the continuous shear analyses to evaluate the mucoadhesive properties (Table 4).

Table 4. Values of the consistency index (k) for polymeric blends containing poloxamer 407 (P407) and Carbopol 971P® (C971P), Carbopol 974P® (C974P), or Noveon® Polycarbophil (PCB)[a] at 37 °C. Each value represents the mean (±standard deviation) of at least six replicates.

Formulation	k (Pa.s) of Polymeric System	k (Pa.s) of Mixture	Interaction Parameter (Pa.s)
P407/C 971P	43,143.33 ± 470.78	227.70 ± 9.74	−42,915.67
P407/C974P	139.40 ± 6.01	107.60 ± 2.84	−31.83
P407/PCB	60.96 ± 3.31	97.63 ± 2.07	36.64
Mucin solution	0.033 ± 0.001		

The addition of mucin to the polymeric system demonstrates reduced consistency of the P407/C971P and P407/C974P systems, with a positive interaction parameter for the PCB-containing system. Consistency is a measure of internal friction and the presence of mucin appears to reduce interaction within the formulation. Comparing with the data in Figure 1A, it can be seen that P407/C971P had the greatest force of adhesion, and a very large, negative, interaction parameter. It is suggested that a negative parameter for the consistency index could be a result of interaction between mucin and mucoadhesive polymer, which reduces bridging of poloxamer micelles in the formulation, lowering the overall consistency. It is also possible that the mucin glycoproteins affect the micellization behavior in an unpredictable manner. On the other hand, the P407/PCB polymeric system mixed with mucin exhibited a consistency index greater than the mucin and polymeric systems isolated. This is evidence of a strong interaction between the polymers and mucin, forming a highly cohesive system.

As already described in the literature, there are disadvantages in the use of flow rheometry as a method to evaluate mucoadhesive properties. The continuous shear analysis is a destructive test, then the mucin–polymer interactions can be disrupted, and it is not often possible to observe the mucoadhesion phenomenon [8,29,40,47]. This study exposes the limitations of the continuous flow rheological method to evaluate the mucoadhesive profile of semi-solid systems, and it is best used to understand mechanistic aspects.

For oscillatory rheology, the synergism between polymer and mucin is employed to evaluate mucoadhesion. This technique has advantageous characteristics, such as being a non-destructive method which simulates the formulation behavior during application. Recently, Jones and co-workers [52] reinforced the correlation between viscoelasticity and mucoadhesion, using linear regression [8]. The adhesive interactions in the polymeric blends were observed by the elastic modulus (G') analysis of the mixture as a function of frequency. When the G' of the mixture is higher than the isolated polymer and mucin contributions, $\Delta G' > 0$, rheological synergism occurs [2,29,53]. The observed and calculated values of G' moduli were obtained at 10.0 Hz, since in this oscillatory frequency the systems are forced at higher oscillatory intensity.

The elastic, or "storage" modulus measures the storage and recovered energy at each deformation cycle, reflecting the solid component of a viscoelastic material [47]. The elastic modulus will demonstrate higher values if a sample is predominantly elastic, i.e., highly structured. In contrast, the loss modulus (G'') demonstrates the lost energy at each cycle, and will be higher when the sample is predominantly viscous. The frequency sweep at the linear viscoelastic region allows the three-dimensional structure of the sample to be preserved throughout analysis. The type of cross-linked structure can be revealed in the oscillations, where a small effort is exerted at each frequency. The oscillatory analysis allows the differentiation of the physical entanglements and secondary bonds, since in low frequencies the polymeric physical entanglements can be separated, while, secondary bonds remain fixed [46,47]. The results are displayed in Table 5.

Table 5. Values of the elastic modulus (G') for polymeric blends containing poloxamer 407 (P407) and Carbopol 971P® (C971P), Carbopol 974P® (C974P), or Noveon® Polycarbophil (PCB)[a] at 37 °C. Each value represents the mean (±standard deviation) of at least six replicates.

Formulation	G' (Pa) Polymeric System	G' (Pa) Mixture	Interaction Parameter (Pa)
P407/C971P	16,646.00 ± 612.97	15,368.17 ± 865.56	−1305.68
P407/C974P	3246.00 ± 227.49	5528.83 ± 320.13	2254.99
P407/PCB	2660.00 ± 85.46	4826.50 ± 279.20	2138.65
Mucin	27.85 ± 2.74		

The viscoelastic response of the systems suggests the entanglement and secondary bonds (hydrogen bonds) between mucoadhesive polymers and mucus glycoproteins for the P407/C974P and P407/PCB binary systems, since the establishment of secondary bonds results in the increase of the elasticity into the formulations. Furthermore, the difference observed on the rheological interaction parameter of the three formulations can be attributed to the structural differences of these polymers [46,54].

Formulations which show high viscosity have demonstrated to suffer low clearance and, consequently, they remain longer at the action site [55]. However, despite having higher viscosity, the P407/C971P platform displayed rheological antagonism, demonstrating that the addition of mucin did not increase overall interaction in the system. Edsman & Hägerström had already demonstrated positive values (rheological synergism) for low concentrations of cross-linking polymers, while high concentration of them results in negative values. In this sense, the evaluation of the G' gives positive values for weakly hydrogels and strongly cross-linked hydrogels will demonstrate a negative interaction parameter [20].

The system composed of P407 and C971P has the higher polymeric concentration when compared with the P407/C974P and P407/PCB formulations. Large concentrations of the polymers into the mixture added mucin, as well as the high viscosity of this system reduces the availability of the solvent, which makes the interpenetration of the polymer and mucin chains difficult, since them flexibility and mobility are reduced [47,56].

Oscillatory rheometry is a valid and sensitive method to evaluate interactions in polymer-mucin mixtures, and although the P407/C974P and P407/PCB formulations had demonstrated similar answers between these methods, a direct comparison with the standard tensile method was not possible. Moreover, it was observed that the results depend more on the polymer concentration than of the polymers chemical structure, since P407/C974P and P407/PCB systems exhibited similar results. In this way, to use the oscillatory rheology as a method to evaluate the mucoadhesive profile of semi-solid formulations, a prior cohesiveness analyses must be done.

3.4. Texture Profile Analysis

TPA is a quick and common analytical methodology. It can be used for the mechanical characterization of semi-solid pharmaceutical dosage forms and aid understanding of structure. The results of this analysis allow easy identification of the physicochemical interactions among the components of the formulations and also allow prediction of the behavior of these systems under different analytical conditions, and during use in pharmaceuticals. The values obtained by this technique are: hardness, elasticity, adhesiveness, cohesiveness, and compressibility [57,58].

The development of pharmaceutical dosage forms for topical application requires formation of a target profile. These formulations need to be easily removed from the packing to have good spreadability, bio/mucoadhesion, and adequate viscosity in order to facilitate retention and thus patient compliance with the treatment. Moreover, for mucoadhesive systems the resistance to the natural defense processes needs to be considered [34,40,57,58].

To be easily applied, a semi-solid needs to demonstrate low values for hardness and compressibility, since these values indicate how easy it is to remove the formulation from the packing, as well as the spreadability and removal of the product at the desirable site. However, very low values of them can impair the retention of the formulation. Ideally, semi-solid systems must demonstrate high values of adhesion to ensure retention. In addition, high values of elasticity aid retention, because the systems have a tendency to return to their structure. On the other hand, high values to the cohesiveness parameter are also desirable [2,23,29,57–60].

In order to obtain pharmaceutical systems with acceptable mechanical characteristics, ensuring in vivo retention and therapeutic efficiency, the texture profile properties of the formulations must be studied. As previously mentioned, the chosen systems have already demonstrated themselves to be favorable pharmaceutical systems, about the TPA properties [23,30,34]. In addition to studying mechanical properties, it may be used to evaluate the mucoadhesion profile of semi-solid systems by the analysis of the polymer-mucin interaction.

Comparing the results of polymeric systems with and without mucin (Table 6) there was a decrease in the hardness, compressibility and adhesiveness. The cohesiveness had increased values for two of the three systems, and the elasticity was unaltered. The P407/C971P system demonstrated higher values of hardness, compressibility and adhesiveness than P407/C974P and P407/PCB, probably because its polymeric concentration is also greater. In this sense, this formulation displayed also superior hardness, compressibility and adhesiveness responses. However, the decrease of this parameter after mucin addition was more significant, since the C971P presents a lower degree of crosslinking; therefore, it has a greater number of free carboxyl groups for interaction with the mucin, which promotes a more intense disintegration of this blend when compared with those containing other adhesive polymers (C974P and PCB). Similar to rheological analysis, it appears that polymer–mucin interactions may not provide constructive synergism in these systems.

The absence of change in the elasticity of the systems, even with the mucin addition, reflects the results obtained in the oscillatory rheology where the viscoelastic property was retained. Furthermore, the decrease of hardness and compressibility in the added mucin systems agrees with the flow rheology and demonstrates the loss of internal friction in these systems after mucin addition. The cohesiveness of the P407/C974P blend with mucin was superior to the two other blends. Probably, it is due to the C974P chemical structure, since it is a poly(acrylic acid) derivative with a higher degree of cross-linking, providing a more cohesive system, and the increase of the attractive force in the formulation is more dramatic.

The interaction parameters of the responses obtained by TPA were calculated between the polymeric blends and mucin solution (Figure 6); this is an important value to investigate the mucoadhesive profile of the semi-solid preparations. All polymer blends showed a negative interaction parameter, i.e., the mixture with mucin in all the cases obtained lower values when compared with the pure polymeric systems. In this way, the results suggest the interaction between mucoadhesive polymer and mucin, which promotes mechanical changes.

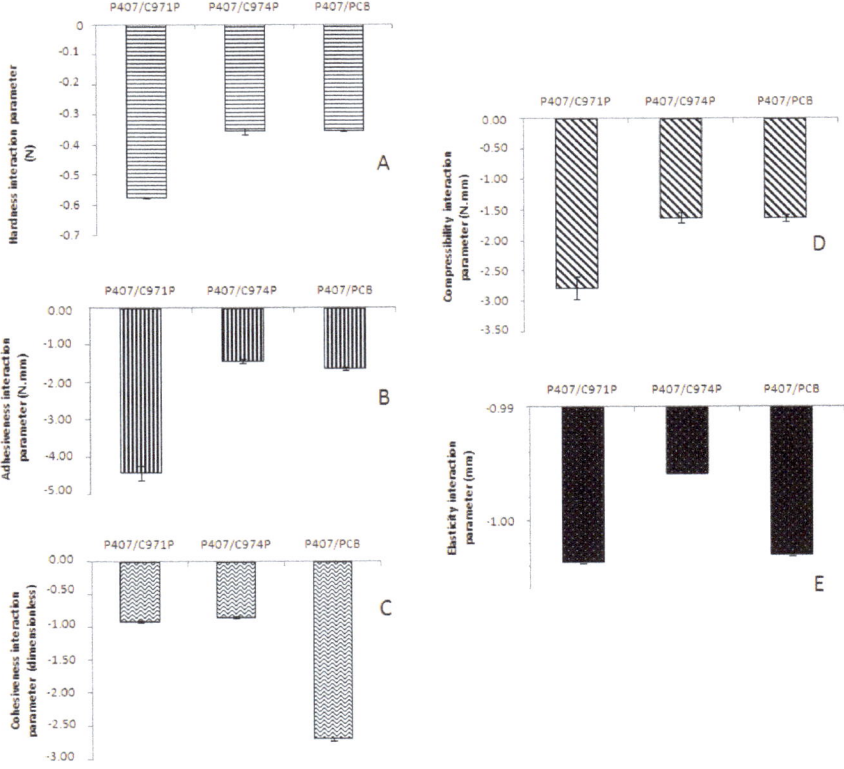

Figure 6. Mechanical properties obtained by texture profile analysis (TPA) of the polymeric systems containing poloxamer 407 (P407), mucin and Carbopol 971P® (C971P), Carbopol 974P® (C974P) or Noveon® Polycarbophil (PCB) and of pure mucin solution: (**A**) hardness, (**B**) adhesiveness, (**C**) cohesiveness, (**D**) compressibility, (**E**) elasticity.

The adhesiveness interaction parameter is a result of interaction between the formulation and polycarbonate probe. Therefore, negative values for mucoadhesive formulations are expected. Considering a higher adhesive polymer-mucin interaction, there are fewer free carboxyl groups to interact with the probe, and the adhesiveness of the mixture on the probe is lower when compared with the mixture with added mucin. Thus, as a new way to measure mucoadhesive properties of semi-solid systems, the analysis of the adhesiveness interaction parameter can be simple and accessible with fast execution. Moreover, a correlation was observed between this method and the tensile strength method using the mucin disks, since the adhesive profile of the three evaluated systems demonstrated a similar ranking evaluation.

Table 6. Mechanical results obtained by texture profile analysis from the binary polymeric formulations composed of poloxamer 407 (P407) and Carbopol 971P® (C971P), Carbopol 974P® (C974P), or Noveon® Polycarbophil (PCB) with or in the absence of mucin. Each value represents the mean (±standard deviation) of at least six replicates.

System	TPA Results				
	Hardness (N)	Compressibility (N·mm)	Adhesiveness (N·mm)	Elasticity (mm)	Cohesiveness (Dimensionless)
P407/C971P	1.48 ± 0.04	6.74 ± 0.29	7.65 ± 0.45	1.00 ± 0.01	0.87 ± 0.01
P407/C971P + mucin	0.95 ± 0.01	4.06 ± 0.18	3.32 ± 0.19	1.00 ± 0.00	0.92 ± 0.01
P407/C974P	0.64 ± 0.03	2.99 ± 0.12	2.53 ± 0.12	1.00 ± 0.01	0.91 ± 0.01
P407/C974P + mucin	0.34 ± 0.00	1.48 ± 0.08	1.20 ± 0.05	1.00 ± 0.00	1.02 ± 0.01
P407/PCB	0.56 ± 0.02	2.66 ± 0.10	2.46 ± 0.06	1.00 ± 0.00	0.92 ± 0.01
P407/PCB + mucin	0.26 ± 0.01	1.14 ± 0.06	0.93 ± 0.05	1.00 ± 0.01	0.91 ± 0.02

4. Conclusions

This study utilized the tensile strength method with porcine mucin disks and porcine oral (cheek) mucosa, flow and oscillatory rheometry, as well as texture profile analysis, to evaluate the mucoadhesive performance of the three polymeric systems composed of poloxamer 407 and poly(acrylic acid) derivatives. It was also possible to investigate these methods to understand the parameters which can influence experimental results, highlighting the need for standardization. The reproducibility of the methods for these semi-solid formulations was also shown. The tensile strength method demonstrated differences when comparing the mucin disk and oral ex vivo mucosa. The factorial design displayed that all evaluated parameters have an effect in the F_{adh}; but the same was not observed for W_{adh}, for which most interactions did not influence response. W_{adh} was suggested as a more appropriate metric for evaluating mucoadhesion. The oscillatory rheology was more capable of showing adhesive interactions than continuous flow rheology. However, each rheological analysis needs to be associated with complementary analyses. Furthermore, the texture profile analysis method with the mucin addition was shown to be reproducible by the evaluation of the adhesiveness interaction parameter. In this sense, each one of the methods has an important place within the evaluation of mucoadhesion of semi-solid pharmaceutical systems, but it is very important to understand the importance and influence of the conditions of analysis on experimental results. There is a clear need for standardized methods to evaluate mucoadhesive properties of semisolid drug delivery systems.

Supplementary Materials: The following are available online at http://www.mdpi.com/2073-4360/10/3/254/s1, Table S1: Mucoadhesive force determined by the tensile method, on mucin disk or porcine oral mucosa, using polymeric blends containing poloxamer 407 (P407) and Carbopol 971P® (C971P), Carbopol 974P® (C974P), or Noveon® Polycarbophil (PCB).

Acknowledgments: The authors would like to thank CAPES (Higher-Education Education Personnel Improvement Coordination), CNPq (National Counsel of Technological and Scientific Development), and FINEP (Financier of Studies and Projects) of Brazil for financial assistance.

Author Contributions: M.L.B., J.B.d.S., and S.B.d.S.F. conceived, designed, and performed the experiments; J.B.d.S., S.B.d.S.F., A.V.R., M.T.C., and M.L.B. analyzed the data; J.B.d.S., M.L.B., and M.T.C. wrote the paper.

Conflicts of Interest: The authors declare no conflict of interest.

References

1. Bassi da Silva, J.; de Souza Ferreira, S.B.; de Freitas, O.; Bruschi, M.L. A critical review about methodologies for the analysis of mucoadhesive properties of drug delivery systems. *Drug Dev. Ind. Pharm.* **2017**, *9045*, 1–67. [CrossRef] [PubMed]
2. Bruschi, M.L.; Jones, D.S.; Panzeri, H.; Gremião, M.P.D.; de Freitas, O.; Lara, E.H.G. Semisolid Systems Containing Propolis for the Treatment of Periodontal Disease: In Vitro Realease Kinetics, Syringeability, Rheological, Textural and Mucoadhesive Properties. *J. Pharm. Sci.* **2007**, *99*, 4215–4227. [CrossRef] [PubMed]
3. Cook, M.T.; Khutoryanskiy, V.V. Mucoadhesion and mucosa-mimetic materials—A mini-review. *Int. J. Pharm.* **2015**, *495*, 991–998. [CrossRef] [PubMed]
4. Borghi-Pangoni, F.B.; Junqueira, M.V.; de Souza Ferreira, S.B.; Silva, L.L.; Rabello, B.R.; Caetano, W.; Diniz, A.; Bruschi, M.L. Screening and In Vitro Evaluation of Mucoadhesive Thermoresponsive System Containing Methylene Blue for Local Photodynamic Therapy of Colorectal Cancer. *Pharm. Res.* **2015**. [CrossRef] [PubMed]
5. Nho, Y.-C.; Park, J.-S.; Lim, Y.-M. Preparation of Poly(acrylic acid) Hydrogel by Radiation Crosslinking and Its Application for Mucoadhesives. *Polymers (Basel)* **2014**, *6*, 890–898. [CrossRef]
6. Lejoyeux, F.; Ponchel, G.; Wouessidjewe, D.; Peppas, N.A.; Duchêne, D. Bioadhesive tablets influence of the testing medium composition on bioadhesion. *Drug Dev. Ind. Pharm.* **1989**, *15*, 2037–2048. [CrossRef]
7. Almeida, H.; Amaral, M.H.; Lobão, P.; Lobo, J.M.S. In situ gelling systems: A strategy to improve the bioavailability of ophthalmic pharmaceutical formulations. *Drug Discov. Today* **2014**, *19*, 400–412. [CrossRef] [PubMed]
8. Mansuri, S.; Kesharwani, P.; Jain, K.; Tekade, R.K.; Jain, N.K. Mucoadhesion: A promising approach in drug delivery system. *React. Funct. Polym.* **2016**, *100*, 151–172. [CrossRef]
9. Peppas, N.A.; Huang, Y. Nanoscale technology of mucoadhesive interactions. *Adv. Drug Deliv. Rev.* **2004**, *56*, 1675–1687. [CrossRef] [PubMed]
10. Woertz, C.; Preis, M.; Breitkreutz, J.; Kleinebudde, P. Assessment of test methods evaluating mucoadhesive polymers and dosage forms : An overview. *Eur. J. Pharm. Biopharm.* **2013**, *85*, 843–853. [CrossRef] [PubMed]
11. Karolewicz, B. A review of polymers as multifunctional excipients in drug dosage form technology. *Saudi Pharm. J.* **2015**. [CrossRef] [PubMed]
12. Junqueira, M.V.; Borghi-Pangoni, F.B.; de Souza Ferreira, S.B.; Bruschi, M.L. Evaluation of the methylene blue addition in binary polymeric systems composed by poloxamer 407 and Carbopol 934P using quality by design: Rheological, textural, and mucoadhesive analysis. *Drug Dev. Ind. Pharm.* **2016**, *9045*, 1–41. [CrossRef] [PubMed]
13. Yun Chang, J.; Oh, Y.K.; Soo Kong, H.; Jung Kim, E.; Deuk Jang, D.; Taek Nam, K.; Kim, C.K. Prolonged antifungal effects of clotrimazole-containing mucoadhesive thermosensitive gels on vaginitis. *J. Control. Release* **2002**, *82*, 39–50. [CrossRef]
14. Accili, D.; Menghi, G.; Bonacucina, G.; Di Martino, P.; Palmieri, G.F. Mucoadhesion dependence of pharmaceutical polymers on mucosa characteristics. *Eur. J. Pharm. Sci.* **2004**, *22*, 225–234. [CrossRef] [PubMed]
15. Reineke, J.; Cho, D.Y.; Dingle, Y.L.; Cheifetz, P.; Laulicht, B.; Lavin, D.; Furtado, S.; Mathiowitz, E. Can bioadhesive nanoparticles allow for more effective particle uptake from the small intestine? *J. Control. Release* **2013**, *170*, 477–484. [CrossRef] [PubMed]
16. Vetchý, D.; Landová, H.; Gajdziok, J.; Dolezel, P.; Danek, Z.; Stembírek, J. Determination of dependencies among in vitro and in vivo properties of prepared mucoadhesive buccal films using multivariate data analysis. *Eur. J. Pharm. Biopharm.* **2014**, *86*, 498–506. [CrossRef] [PubMed]
17. Laulicht, B.; Cheifetz, P.; Tripathi, A.; Mathiowitz, E. Are in vivo gastric bioadhesive forces accurately reflected by in vitro experiments? *J. Control. Release* **2009**, *134*, 103–110. [CrossRef] [PubMed]
18. Eshel-Green, T.; Bianco-Peled, H. Mucoadhesive acrylated block copolymers micelles for the delivery of hydrophobic drugs. *Colloids Surf. B Biointerfaces* **2016**, *139*, 42–51. [CrossRef] [PubMed]
19. Hägerström, H.; Edsman, K. Interpretation of mucoadhesive properties of polymer. *J. Pharm. Pharmacol.* **2001**, *53*, 1589–1599. [CrossRef]
20. Hägerström, H.; Edsman, K. Limitations of the rheological mucoadhesion method: The effect of the choice of conditions and the rheological synergism parameter. *Eur. J. Pharm. Sci.* **2003**, *18*, 349–357. [CrossRef]

21. Pund, S.; Joshi, A.; Vasu, K.; Nivsarkar, M.; Shishoo, C. Gastroretentive delivery of rifampicin: In vitro mucoadhesion and in vivo gamma scintigraphy. *Int. J. Pharm.* **2011**, *411*, 106–112. [CrossRef] [PubMed]
22. Bromberg, L.; Temchenko, M.; Alakhov, V.; Hatton, T.A. Bioadhesive properties and rheology of polyether-modified poly(acrylic acid) hydrogels. *Int. J. Pharm.* **2004**, *282*, 45–60. [CrossRef] [PubMed]
23. De Souza Ferreira, S.B.; Bassi da Silva, J.; Borghi-Pangoni, F.B.; Junqueira, M.V.; Bruschi, M.L. Linear correlation between rheological, mucoadhesive and textural properties of thermoresponsive polymer blends for biomedical applications. *J. Mech. Behav. Biomed. Mater.* **2017**, *68*, 265–275. [CrossRef] [PubMed]
24. Otero-Espinar, F.J.; Delgado-Charro, B.; Anguiano-Igea, S.; Blanco-Mendez, J. Use of tensile test in the study of the bioadhesive and swelling properties of polymers. In *Data Adquisition and Measurement Techniques*; Muñoz-Ruiz, A., Vromans, H., Eds.; Interpharm Press Inc.: Buffalo Grove, IL, USA, 1998; pp. 295–342.
25. Aka-Any-Grah, A.; Bouchemal, K.; Koffi, A.; Agnely, F.; Zhang, M.; Djabourov, M.; Ponchel, G. Formulation of mucoadhesive vaginal hydrogels insensitive to dilution with vaginal fluids. *Eur. J. Pharm. Biopharm.* **2010**, *76*, 296–303. [CrossRef] [PubMed]
26. Varum, F.J.O.; Veiga, F.; Sousa, J.S.; Basit, A.W. Mucoadhesive platforms for targeted delivery to the colon. *Int. J. Pharm.* **2011**, *420*, 11–19. [CrossRef] [PubMed]
27. Ivarsson, D.; Wahlgren, M. Comparison of in vitro methods of measuring mucoadhesion: Ellipsometry, tensile strength and rheological measurements. *Colloids Surf. B Biointerfaces* **2012**, *92*, 353–359. [CrossRef] [PubMed]
28. Hassan, E.E.; Gallo, J.M. A Simple Rheological Method for the in Vitro Assessment of Mucin-Polymer Bioadhesive Bond Strength. *Pharm. Res.* **1990**, *7*, 491–495. [CrossRef] [PubMed]
29. Jones, D.S.; Bruschi, M.L.; de Freitas, O.; Gremião, M.P.D.; Lara, E.H.G.; Andrews, G.P. Rheological, mechanical and mucoadhesive properties of thermoresponsive, bioadhesive binary mixtures composed of poloxamer 407 and carbopol 974P designed as platforms for implantable drug delivery systems for use in the oral cavity. *Int. J. Pharm.* **2009**, *372*, 49–58. [CrossRef] [PubMed]
30. De Souza Ferreira, S.B.; Bassi da Silva, J.; Junqueira, M.V.; Borghi-Pangoni, F.B.; Guttierres, R.; Bruschi, M.L. The importance of the relationship between mechanical analyses and rheometry of mucoadhesive thermoresponsive polymeric materials for biomedical applications. *J. Mech. Behav. Biomed. Mater.* **2017**, *74*, 142–153. [CrossRef] [PubMed]
31. Hemphill, T.; Campos, W.; Pilehvari, A. Yield-power law model more accurately predicts mud rheology. *Oil Gas J.* **1993**, *91*, 45–50.
32. Jones, D.S. *Pharmaceutical Statistics*; Pharmaceutical Press: London, UK, 2002.
33. Zhu, Z.; Zhai, Y.; Zhang, N.; Leng, D.; Ding, P. The development of polycarbophil as a bioadhesive material in pharmacy. *Asian J. Pharm. Sci.* **2013**, *8*, 218–227. [CrossRef]
34. De Souza Ferreira, S.B.; Moço, T.D.; Borghi-Pangoni, F.B.; Junqueira, M.V.; Bruschi, M.L. Rheological, mucoadhesive and textural properties of thermoresponsive polymer blends for biomedical applications. *J. Mech. Behav. Biomed. Mater.* **2015**, *55*, 164–178. [CrossRef] [PubMed]
35. Bassi da Silva, J.; Khutoryanskiy, V.V.; Bruschi, M.L.; Cook, M.T. A mucosa-mimetic material for the mucoadhesion testing of thermogelling semi-solids. *Int. J. Pharm.* **2017**, *528*, 586–594. [CrossRef] [PubMed]
36. Ich Topic Q2 (R1). Validation of Analytical Procedures: Text and methodology. *Int. Conf. Harmon.* **2005**, 1–17. Available online: http://www.ich.org/fileadmin/Public_Web_Site/ICH_Products/Guidelines/Quality/Q2_R1/Step4/Q2_R1__Guideline.pdf (accessed on 7 January 2018).
37. Nair, A.B.; Kumria, R.; Harsha, S.; Attimarad, M.; Al-Dhubiab, B.E.; Alhaider, I.A. In vitro techniques to evaluate buccal films. *J. Control. Release* **2013**, *166*, 10–21. [CrossRef] [PubMed]
38. Nep, E.I.; Conway, B.R. Grewia gum 2: Mucoadhesive properties of compacts and gels. *Trop. J. Pharm. Res.* **2011**, *10*, 393–401. [CrossRef]
39. Tang, X.; Wang, C. Study on the physical properties of bioadhesive polymers. *Chin. Pharm. J.* **2005**, *40*, 361–364.
40. Carvalho, F.C.; Bruschi, M.L.; Evangelista, R.C.; Gremião, M.P.D. Mucoadhesive drug delivery systems. *Braz. J. Pharm. Sci.* **2010**, *46*, 1–18. [CrossRef]
41. Deacon, M.P.; Davis, S.S.; White, R.J.; Nordman, H.; Carlstedt, I.; Errington, N.; Rowe, A.J.; Harding, S.E. Are chitosan–mucin interactions specific to different regions of the stomach? Velocity ultracentrifugation offers a clue. *Carbohydr. Polym.* **1999**, *38*, 235–238. [CrossRef]

42. Leung, S.S.; Robinson, J.R. In the last decade, bioadhesive polymers/co- polymers have received considerable attention for controlled drug delivery. *J. Control. Release* **1988**, *5*, 223–231.
43. Blanco-Fuente, H.; Vila-Dorrío, B.; Anguiano-Igea, S.; Otero-Espinar, F.J.; Blanco-Méndez, J. Tanned leather: A good model for determining hydrogels bioadhesion. *Int. J. Pharm.* **1996**, *138*, 103–112. [CrossRef]
44. Lejoyeux, F.; Ponchel, G.; Duchene, D. Influence of some technological parameters on the bioadhesive characteristics of polyacrilic acid matrices. *STP Pharma* **1989**, *5*, 893–898.
45. Haugstad, K.E.; Håti, A.G.; Nordgård, C.T.; Adl, P.S.; Maurstad, G.; Sletmoen, M.; Draget, K.I.; Dias, R.S.; Stokke, B.T. Direct determination of chitosan-mucin interactions using a single-molecule strategy: Comparison to alginate-mucin interactions. *Polymers (Basel)* **2015**, *7*, 161–185. [CrossRef]
46. Madsen, F.; Eberth, K.; Smart, J.D. A rheological examination of the mucoadhesive/mucus interaction: The effect of mucoadhesive type and concentration. *J. Control. Release* **1998**, *50*, 167–178. [CrossRef]
47. Callens, C.; Ceulemans, J.; Ludwig, A.; Foreman, P.; Remon, J.P. Rheological study on mucoadhesivity of some nasal powder formulations. *Eur. J. Pharm. Biopharm.* **2003**, *55*, 323–328. [CrossRef]
48. Saiano, F.; Pitarresi, G.; Cavallaro, G.; Licciardi, M.; Giammona, G. Evaluation of mucoadhesive properties of α,β-poly(N-hydroxyethyl)-DL-aspartamide and α,β-poly(aspartylhydrazide) using ATR–FTIR spectroscopy. *Polymer (Guildf)* **2002**, *43*, 6281–6286. [CrossRef]
49. Yang, P.; Chen, H.; Liu, Y.-W. Application of response surface methodology and desirability approach to investigate and optimize the jet pump in a thermoacoustic Stirling heat engine. *Appl. Therm. Eng.* **2017**, *127*, 1005–1014. [CrossRef]
50. Jones, D.S.; Woolfson, A.D.; Brown, A.F. Textural, viscoelastic and mucoadhesive properties of pharmaceutical gels composed of cellulose polymers. *Int. J. Pharm.* **1997**, *151*, 223–233. [CrossRef]
51. Khutoryanskiy, V.V. Advances in Mucoadhesion and Mucoadhesive Polymers. *Macromol. Biosci.* **2011**, *11*, 748–764. [CrossRef] [PubMed]
52. Jones, D.S.; Laverty, T.P.; Morris, C.; Andrews, G.P. Statistical modelling of the rheological and mucoadhesive properties of aqueous poly(methylvinylether-*co*-maleic acid) networks: Redefining biomedical applications and the relationship between viscoelasticity and mucoadhesion. *Colloids Surf. B. Biointerfaces* **2016**, *144*, 125–134. [CrossRef] [PubMed]
53. Andrews, G.P.; Jones, D.S. Rheological characterization of bioadhesive binary polymeric systems designed as platforms for drug delivery implants. *Biomacromolecules* **2006**, *7*, 899–906. [CrossRef] [PubMed]
54. Hägerström, H. Polymer Gels as Pharmaceutical Dosage Forms: Rheological Performance and Physicochemical Interactions at the Gel-Mucus Interface for Formulations Intended for Mucosal Drug Delivery. Ph.D. Thesis, Faculty of Pharmacy, Uppsala University, Uppsala, Sweden, 2003.
55. Illum, L.; Farraj, N.F.; Fisher, A.N.; Gill, I.; Miglietta, M.; Benedetti, L.M. Hyaluronic acid ester microspheres as a nasal delivery system for insulin. *J. Control. Release* **1994**, *29*, 133–141. [CrossRef]
56. Lee, J.W.; Park, J.H.; Robinson, J.R. Bioadhesive dosage forms: The next generation. *J. Pharm. Sci.* **2000**, *89*, 850–866. [CrossRef]
57. Jones, D.S.; Woolfson, A.D.; Djokic, J. Texture profile analysis of bioadhesive polymeric semisolids: Mechanical characterization and investigation of interactions between formulation components. *J. Appl. Polym. Sci.* **1996**, *61*, 2229–2234. [CrossRef]
58. Baloglu, E.; Karavana, S.Y.; Senyigit, Z.A.; Guneri, T. Rheological and mechanical properties of poloxamer mixtures as a mucoadhesive gel base. *Pharm. Dev. Technol.* **2011**, *16*, 627–636. [CrossRef] [PubMed]
59. Tugcu-Demiröz, F.; Acartürk, F.; Erdoğan, D. Development of long-acting bioadhesive vaginal gels of oxybutynin: Formulation, in vitro and in vivo evaluations. *Int. J. Pharm.* **2013**, *457*, 25–39. [CrossRef] [PubMed]
60. Gratieri, T.; Gelfuso, G.M.; Rocha, E.M.; Sarmento, V.H.; de Freitas, O.; Lopez, R.F.V. A poloxamer/chitosan in situ forming gel with prolonged retention time for ocular delivery. *Eur. J. Pharm. Biopharm.* **2010**, *75*, 186–193. [CrossRef] [PubMed]

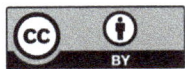

© 2018 by the authors. Licensee MDPI, Basel, Switzerland. This article is an open access article distributed under the terms and conditions of the Creative Commons Attribution (CC BY) license (http://creativecommons.org/licenses/by/4.0/).

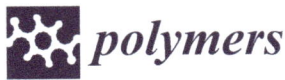

Article

Formulation of Carbopol®/Poly(2-ethyl-2-oxazoline)s Mucoadhesive Tablets for Buccal Delivery of Hydrocortisone

Leire Ruiz-Rubio [1,*], María Luz Alonso [2], Leyre Pérez-Álvarez [1], Rosa Maria Alonso [2], Jose Luis Vilas [1] and Vitaliy V. Khutoryanskiy [3,*]

1. Macromolecular Chemistry Group (LABQUIMAC), Department of Physical Chemistry, Faculty of Science and Technology, University of the Basque Country, UPV/EHU, Barrio Sarriena, s/n, 48940 Leioa, Spain; leyre.perez@ehu.eus (L.P.-Á.); joseluis.vilas@ehu.es (J.L.V.)
2. Analytical Chemistry Department, Faculty of Science and Technology, University of the Basque Country, UPV/EHU, Barrio Sarriena, s/n, 48940 Leioa, Spain; marialuz.alonso@ehu.eus (M.L.A.); rosamaria.alonso@ehu.eus (R.M.A.)
3. School of Pharmacy, University of Reading, Whiteknights, P.O. Box 224, Reading RG6 6AD, UK
* Correspondence: leire.ruiz@ehu.eus (L.R.-R.); v.khutoryanskiy@reading.ac.uk (V.V.K.); Tel.: +34-946017972 (L.R.-R.); +44-1183786119 (V.V.K.)

Received: 25 December 2017; Accepted: 7 February 2018; Published: 11 February 2018

Abstract: Poly(2-ethyl-2-oxazoline) has become an excellent alternative to the use of poly(ethylene glycol) in pharmaceutical formulations due to its valuable physicochemical and biological properties. This work presents a formulation of poorly-water soluble drug, hydrocortisone, using interpolymer complexes and physical blends of poly(2-ethyl-2-oxazoline)s and two Carbopols® (Carbopol 974 and Carbopol 971) for oromucosal administration. The swelling, hydrocortisone release and mucoadhesive properties of a series of tablet formulations obtained by combination of different Carbopols with poly(2-ethyl-2-oxazoline)s of different molecular weights have been evaluated in vitro.

Keywords: poly(2-ethyl-2-oxazoline); Carbopol®; mucoadhesion; interpolymer complexes

1. Introduction

The development of dosage forms containing poorly-water soluble drugs remains a challenging task for formulation science. Several approaches have been reported to improve the solubility and transport of lipophilic drugs, including particle size reduction, preparation of solid dispersions, microemulsions or complexation with various pharmaceutical excipients [1–3]. Polyethylene glycols (PEGs) have been widely used to formulate poorly-water soluble drugs [4] and in other pharmaceutical applications [5]. However, lately some unfavorable effects related to PEG use have emerged, such as adverse side effects in the body, or unexpected changes in the pharmacokinetics [6]. In addition, some cases of hypersensitivity and laxative effect when using PEG in oral dosage forms have been reported [6,7]. Consequently, various synthetic and natural hydrophilic polymers have been considered as potential alternatives to PEG. In the last years, poly(2-oxazoline)s (POZs) have been highlighted as promising polymers and studies have been focused on the use of these polymers for biomedical applications [8–10]. The main advantages of POZs include: they are easy to synthesize; they do not form peroxides; and they are stable at room temperature and in water. They could be easily cleared from the body and are not excessively hydroscopic [11–13]. On the contrary, PEG can be accumulated in some organs and form vacuoles due to its desiccant nature [14,15]. In addition, poly(2-oxazoline)s are highly versatile materials with a capability to form functional materials and structures depending on the nature of the pending side chain used. These various structures have received increased interest in the use of these polymers in the last years [10,12,13].

Oral delivery of drugs remains the most popular route for medicine administration. Some aspects such as control and ease of administration by the patient, rapid removal in case of toxic effects, limited local enzymatic activity, low irritation problems, high versatility for local or systemic release systems increased the interest in these dosage forms [16,17]. One of the more effective strategies is to deliver drugs in the oral cavity through the adhesion of dosage forms to the buccal mucosa. These dosage forms could be used for the treatment of some conditions directly in the oral cavity and also could be used for systemic drug delivery [18,19]. Among the various dosage forms explored for buccal administration, tablets are still the most commonly used, because of several advantages they offer. Mucoadhesive polymers have a crucial role in tablet formulations due to their ability to adhere to specific regions of the mucosal surface and prolonged residence time of the formulation. Carbomers, usually named Carbopols, are weakly cross-linked polymers of acrylic acid with excellent mucoadhesive properties, being extensively used in a dosage forms design. The presence of high amounts of carboxylic groups in their structure allows water absorption and their high swelling degree. These carboxylic groups are dissociated in a basic environment (pK_a around 6), and cause chain repulsion, polymer swelling and formation of gels.

However, it is often difficult to control the drug release from Carbopol® based matrixes and their pH sensitivity could complicate the correlation between the in vitro and in vivo drug release [20,21]. Several approaches have been reported to use hydrogen-bonded interpolymer complexes based on Carbopols® and non-ionic polymers to develop dosage forms capable of overcoming these disadvantages [22].

The aim of this work is to develop a formulation for poorly-water soluble drug, hydrocortisone, based on poly(2-ethyl-2-oxazoline)s and Carbopols® for buccal delivery. The lack of mucoadhesion of poly(2-ethyl-2-oxazoline)s was improved by forming interpolymer complexes with Carbopols that present excellent adhesion to oral mucosa. In this work, we evaluated swelling, hydrocortisone release and mucoadhesive properties of a series of tablet formulations based on different Carbopols® and poly(2-ethyl-2-oxazoline)s of different molecular weights in vitro.

2. Materials and Methods

2.1. Reagents and Solutions

Poly(2-ethyl-2-oxazoline)s (50, 200, and 500 kDa; named as 50, 200 and 500 in the text, respectively) and hydrocortisone (HC) were purchased from Sigma-Aldrich Irvine, UK) and Carbopol 974 (highly cross-linked, 28,400–39,400 cP) and Carbopol 971 (moderately cross-linked, 4000–11,000 cP) were obtained from Lubrizol (Hazelwood, UK). HPLC grade acetonitrile (ACN) was purchased from Teknokroma (Barcelona, Spain). Sodium chloride, calcium chloride, potassium chloride, sodium hydrogen carbonate and potassium dihydrogen phosphate were obtained from Merck (Darmstadt, Germany) and used for preparation of artificial saliva fluids. A Milli-Q water purification system from Millipore (Bedford, MA, USA) was used. The drug hydrocortisone and internal standard dexamethasone (DXM) were purchased from Sigma-Aldrich (St Louis, MO, USA). Standard stock solutions of drug and internal standard were prepared in acetonitrile at a concentration of 1000 mg/L. Working solutions were prepared by dilution from stock solutions with the mix of excipients and polymers used in the pharmaceutical formulation of tablets (magnesium state, poly(2-ethyl-2-oxazoline) and Carbopols 974 and Carbopol 971) in artificial saliva.

2.2. Complex Formation

Interpolymer complexes were prepared by mixing separate 0.1 wt % polymer solutions in deionized water. Solutions were mixed to give different unit molar ratios of the polymer components. The complexation between Carbopol and POZ was evaluated in water without adjusting pH and also at pH 2 (which was adjusted by addition of 0.1 mol/L HCl). The obtained interpolymer complexes were left for 2 days in the media, and then they were separated, washed twice with the solvent and freeze-dried in a Heto PowerDry LL3000 Freeze Dryer (Thermo Scientific, Loughborough, UK) for at least two days. The composition with the maximum concentration yield was selected for the tablet formulation.

Infrared spectra of the interpolymer complexes and pure components were recorded using Nicolet Nexus FTIR spectrophotometer Thermo Scientific, Loughborough, UK) in KBr pellets, at a resolution of 4 cm^{-1} and 32 scans. Glass transition temperatures (T_g) were determined using Mettler-Toledo Differential Scanning Calorimeter, DSC 822^e (Gießen, Germany), heating from 20 to 180 °C at 20 °C·min^{-1}, and the T_g was taken as the mid-point of the curve inflection.

2.3. Tablet Formulation and Preparation

Three different tablet formulations were prepared in this study: (1) physical mixtures of pure polymers, Carbopols and poly(2-ethyl-2-oxazoline)s at 50/50 *w/w*; (2) interpolymer complexes of Carbopols/Poly(2-ethyl-2-oxazoline)s at 50/50 *w/w* prepared in water; and (3) interpolymer complexes of Carbopols/POZ at 50/50 *w/w* prepared at pH 2. Polymer mixture or interpolymer complex powders were mixed with hydrocortisone (5 *w/w* %) and magnesium stearate (2.5 *w/w* % as a lubricant) in a Willy A Bachofen AG Maschinenfabrik mixer (Muttenz, Switzerland). The powders were compressed into tablets using a Riva Minipress (Hampshire, UK), single punch tablet press (Riva, Hampshire, UK) filled manually and press settings selected to preserve similar tablet strength between batches. An average weight of the tablets was 50 ± 1 mg and the average diameter of tablets was 6 ± 0.3 mm.

2.4. Mucoadhesion of the Tablets

The mucoadhesive properties of the tablets were analyzed using a TA.XT Plus Texture Analyser (Stable Micro System, Surrey, UK). Freshly isolated porcine buccal mucosal tissues taken from female Great White pigs were obtained from local abattoir. Before each test, the tissue was equilibrated at 37 ± 0.5 °C in a solution simulating saliva (0.43 g NaCl, 0.22 g CaCl$_2$, 0.75 g KCl, 0.20 g NaHCO$_3$ and 0.9 g KH$_2$PO$_4$ dissolved in 1 L of deionized water, pH 6.75) [23]. The tablets were manually attached to the texture analyzer probe by using double-sided adhesive tape. The porcine tissue was set on the mucoadhesion rig and moisturized with artificial saliva. The tablets were put in contact with the mucosa for 1 min with a downward force of 0.1 N. Then, the probe was withdrawn from the tissue at a 1 mm·s^{-1}. Each experiment was repeated at least three times, the detachment force and the total work of adhesion, calculated from the area under the detachment curve, were measured. Mucoadhesion results were analyzed using one way, non-paired ANOVA (analysis of variance) with Tukey test.

2.5. Swelling Behavior

The swelling properties of the tablets were studied in a simulated saliva. The test was performed using metallic mesh baskets (2 cm diameter, 3 cm height) placed inside glass vials (3.5 cm in diameter and 6 cm in height). The tablets were weighed and placed into the metallic baskets. The initial weight of the samples and the weight of each basket used (after being immersed into the medium were used for the test and wiped always in the same manner) were accurately recorded. The tablets were kept in excess of medium for 3 days and weighed regularly, by weighing the baskets with the tablet samples inside. The weights of the baskets were taken into consideration to calculate the weight of the swollen samples. The swelling ratio (*SR*) of the tablets was calculated using the following equation (Equation (1)) [24]:

$$SR = \frac{W_s - W_i}{W_i} \quad (1)$$

where W_i is the initial tablet weight and W_s is the weight of the sample after additional swelling, respectively.

2.6. Hydrocortisone Release from the Tablets

2.6.1. Instruments and Chromatographic Conditions

For the analysis of hydrocortisone released from the tablets, 2690 high performance liquid chromatography equipment (HPLC) and a 484 diode array detector (DAD) (Waters, Milford, MA, USA) were used. A Sartorius CP224S Scale (Goettegen, Germany) was used with a precision of ±0.0001. The pH measurements were performed on a GLP22 Crison pH meter (Barcelona, Spain). Dissolution tests were carried out at 37 °C in a USP dissolution apparatus II (paddle) using a Sotax AT 7smart Dissolution Tester (Nordring, Switzerland) in accordance with the US and European Pharmacopeia with paddle method.

Chromatographic separation was achieved on a C-18 (50 mm × 4.6 mm, 3.5 µm) Waters XBridge column (Waters Corporation, Milford, MA, USA), using an isocratic mode with a 77:23 (H_2O:acetonitrile) mobile phase at a flow rate of 0.6 mL/min. A sample aliquot of 10 µL was injected into the column at 30 °C and the working wavelength was 245 nm [24–27].

2.6.2. Dissolution Tests

An in vitro drug release study from tablets, to simulate the physiological conditions at the buccal mucosa level, was carried out. The dissolution profiles of the tablet samples were obtained in 500 mL of simulated saliva (pH 6.75). The paddle rotational speed was set at 100 rpm at a constant temperature bath of 37.0 ± 0.5 °C. The dissolution experiment was initiated by placing the sample in the dissolution vessel. Sample aliquots of 5 mL were withdrawn at specific intervals (0, 1, 3, 5, 24, 48, and 72 h) replaced with an equal volume of fresh medium. The aliquots were filtered through a 0.45 µm PTFE filter prior to the injection in the HPLC system (Method validation in the Supplementary Materials, Figure S1) [24,28].

3. Results and Discussion

3.1. Fabrication of Poly(2-ethyl-2-oxazoline)/Carbopol Interpolymer Complexes

The cooperative interaction between poly(2-ethyl-2-oxazoline)s and Carbopols leads to the formation of a gel like precipitate, being a white powder when it is dried. This precipitate is an interpolymer complex formed due to hydrogen bonding between carboxylic groups of Carbopol and amide groups of poly(2-oxazoline). The yield of different interpolymer complexes formed for each combination of the 974 and 971 Carbopols with POZ of different molecular weights have been studied both in water (final pH 5) and at pH 2 (Figure 1). Since Carbopol 974 is a more cross-linked sample presenting a higher viscosity than Carbopol 971 (weakly cross-linked), variations on the swelling and release properties could be expected. In addition, poly(2-ethyl-2-oxazoline) samples used in this study have three molecular weights (50, 200, and 500 kDa) that could also affect the yield of complexation. However, the maximum yield for all evaluated systems was obtained around 50/50 w/w feed composition independent of the molecular weights, so this feed composition was selected for production of interpolymer complexes used for tablet formulation.

The formation of interpolymer complexes between the complementary polymers was confirmed by FTIR spectra and by differential scanning calorimetry (DSC) (Figure 2). The FTIR bands of the carbonyl region are shown, where Carbopol present a carboxyl stretching band corresponding to its self-association is located at 1709 cm^{-1} and a stretching band of amide I of POZ at 1643 cm^{-1}. In the interpolymer complex, a shift of the C=O bands could be observed to 1732 cm^{-1}, while the amide I band shifts to 1625 cm^{-1}. These bands are related to hydrogen bond formation between the carboxyl groups of Carbopol and the amide groups of poly(2-ethyl-2-oxazoline) [29–32]. Figure 2b shows the DSC thermograms of Carbopol 974, POZ 500 and their interpolymer complex formed in water. Carbopol 974 presents a T_g at 132 °C, whereas the T_g of poly(2-ethyl-2-oxazoline) 500 is located at 63 °C. The interpolymer complexes of these polymers formed in water present an intermediate glass transition of 124 °C, similar to the changes observed in other interpolymer complexes formed via hydrogen bonding [33–35].

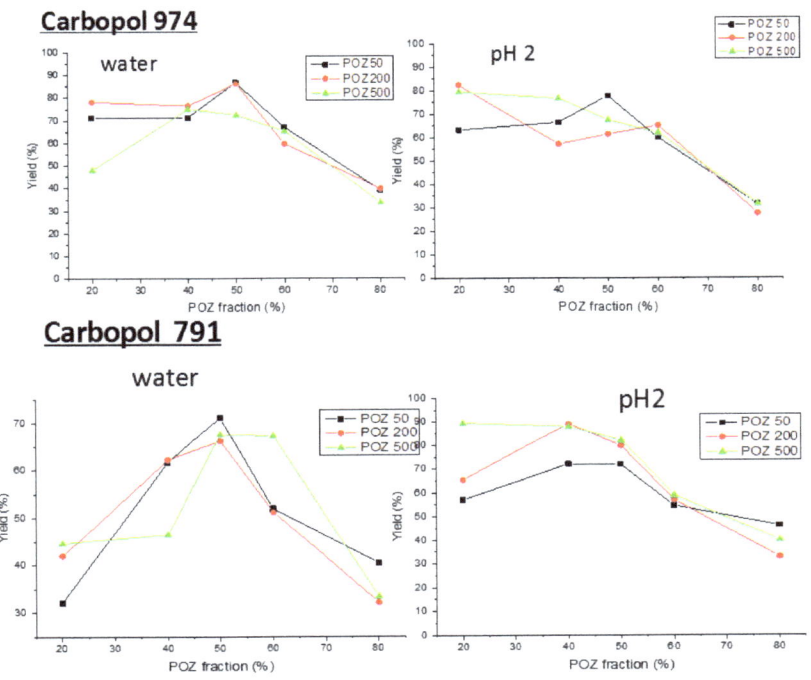

Figure 1. Yields of interpolymer complexes (wt %) for different Carbopol/poly(2-ethyl-2-oxazoline) systems in water and at pH 2.

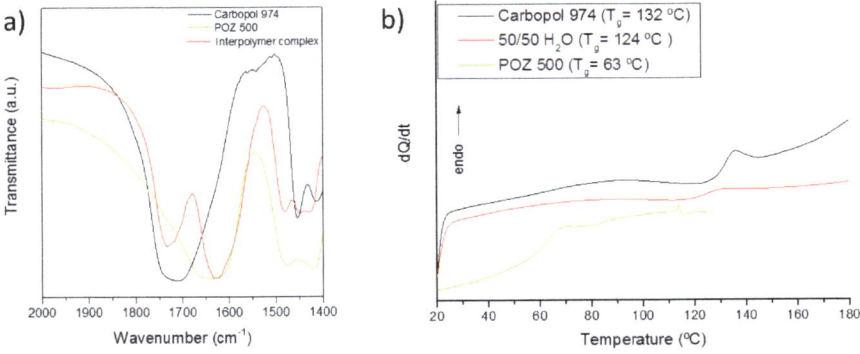

Figure 2. Analysis of Carbopol 974/poly(2-ethyl-2-oxazoline) 500 complex, and pure components by: (**a**) FTIR; and (**b**) DSC.

3.2. Mucoadhesion Studies

The mucoadhesion is an important property in the development of drug delivery systems for buccal, nasal or ocular administration. Several hydrophilic polymers containing functional groups capable to form hydrogen bonds, such as carboxylic acids, have good adhesion properties [36–39].

Different methods can be used to evaluate the adhesion of polymers to a mucosal tissue. One of the most common methods used to analyze the mucoadhesion of solid dosage forms is based on the measurement of the so-called detachment force. The force of detachment and the total work of adhesion are used by many researchers to evaluate the mucoadhesive properties of solid dosage forms [36]. In the present work, the maximum detachment force and the total work of adhesion for Carbopol/poly(2-ethyl-oxazoline) tablets to mucosal tissue were determined (Figure 3). The data generated in these experiments indicated that there is a linear correlation between the maximal detachment force and the total work of adhesion in almost all of the samples.

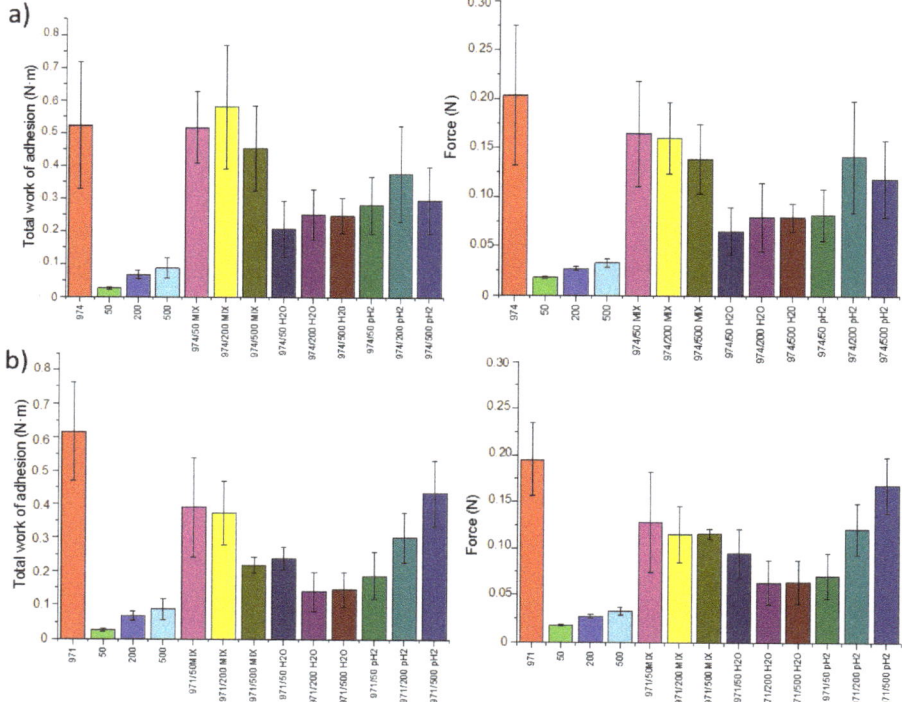

Figure 3. The total work of adhesion (**left**) and detachment force (**right**) on porcine buccal tissues at 37 °C for: (**a**) Carbopol 974/poly(2-ethyl-2-oxazoline) tablets; and (**b**) Carbopol 971/poly(2-ethyl-oxazoline) tablets.

Overall, pure poly(2-ethyl-2-oxazoline)s exhibit poor mucoadhesive properties, with their total work of adhesion being between 0.018 and 0.032 N·m, increasing slightly with increase in the polymer molecular weight. Some increase in the adhesiveness of poly(2-ethyl-2-oxazoline)s with larger molecular weight could be related to improved ability of larger macromolecules to entangle with mucin biomacromolecules. On the contrary, Carbopols exhibit excellent mucoadhesive properties due to the ability of their carboxylic groups to form strong hydrogen bonds with the oligosaccharide chains present in the mucin [40,41]. This physical interaction promotes strong adhesion of the tablets to mucosal tissue; the values of the force of detachment for tablets prepared from pure Carbopol 974 and Carbopol 971 are 0.20 ± 0.04 and 0.18 ± 0.04 N, respectively. The total work of adhesion values for Carbopol 974 and Carbopol 971 are also quite high: 0.52 ± 0.19 and 0.62 ± 0.15 N·m, respectively.

Physical mixtures of Carbopols and poly(2-ethyl-2-oxazoline)s (50/50 *w/w*) were prepared and their mucoadhesive properties were evaluated. The values of the detachment forces and the total work of adhesion of physical mixtures are greater than those recorded for pure POZ tablets. However, these mixtures are heterogeneous, since there is no interaction between the components, and the tablet erosion (analyzed in the following section) was greater than in the rest of the formulations. Usually, interpolymer complexes present intermediate properties of polymer components, as it has been shown for the T_g. Since interpolymer complexes present enhanced stability and resistance to erosion due to polymer-polymer interactions, an improvement in POZ mucoadhesion and stability by the complexation with Carbopols could be expected. Figure 3 shows an improvement in mucoadhesive properties of POZs after complexation with Carbopols regardless of their molecular weight. With respect to the pH of the medium during complexation process, it is noteworthy that when the main excipient of the tablet is the interpolymer complexes obtained in water, they present inferior mucoadhesion than that of the physical mixture. However, when the interpolymer complexes are obtained in acidic media (pH fix to 2), the adhesion of the tablets increases, being similar to the ones obtained for physical mixtures. This fact indicates a diminished mucoadhesion for complexes prepared in the swollen state of Carbopol polymer at neutral pH due to stronger interaction between complementary polymers. Thus, interpolymer complexation leads to materials with high mucoadhesive properties similar to those of physical mixtures but homogeneous and presenting slower erosion.

In the systems based on Carbopol 974, the dosage forms prepared with physical mixtures and interpolymer complexes at pH 2 were not significantly different from pure Carbopol 974 ($p > 0.05$) independently of POZ molecular weight. However, the tablets based on Carbopol 971 complexes with POZ were significantly different from pure Carbopol 971 ($p < 0.05$), except for the interpolymer complexes formed by high molecular weight POZ 500 at pH 2, which present a mucoadhesion similar to that of the physical mixtures ($p > 0.05$). In this case, the molecular weight of poly(2-ethyl-2-oxazoline)s complexed with Carbopol 971 seem to linearly increase their mucoadhesion at pH 2. The lower cross-linking of the Carbopol varies the influence of the molecular weight of POZ on the ionization of the network and the access to carboxylic groups capable to interact with the mucin. Similar phenomenon was also observed in the swelling studies.

3.3. Swelling Studies

The swelling behavior of the formulated tablets is a crucial factor since it directly affects the polymer solubility and the drug release process when tablets are located in the mouth. The polymer swelling improves the consolidation of the tablets on the mucosal tissue increasing the mobility of the molecules and facilitating the penetration and release of the drug in the mucus layer. The swelling behavior of the tablets in an ion-containing solution (simulating the saliva) was monitored for three days. Figure 4 shows the variation of the swelling degree of Carbopols and poly(2-ethyl-2-oxazoline)s. The difference between the components could be observed; Carbopols present greater swelling capability, whereas poly(2-ethyl-2-oxazoline) presents poorer swelling, <5 g/g. Figure 5 shows the swelling degree and the photographs of the erosion of the tablets of the prepared Carbopols/poly(2-ethyl-2-oxazoline)s complexes taken at regular time intervals. Physical mixtures showed erosion during the first 3 h of swelling, while interpolymer complexes remain stable until 24–48 h and no erosion was observed for complexes of Carbopol 971 formed at neutral pH during the first 71 h (Figure 5). These results show greater erosion of the tablets with weaker interpolymer interactions, and suggest enhanced Carbopol/POZ interaction leads to stable tablets, for the mentioned sample, as will be corroborated and explained below.

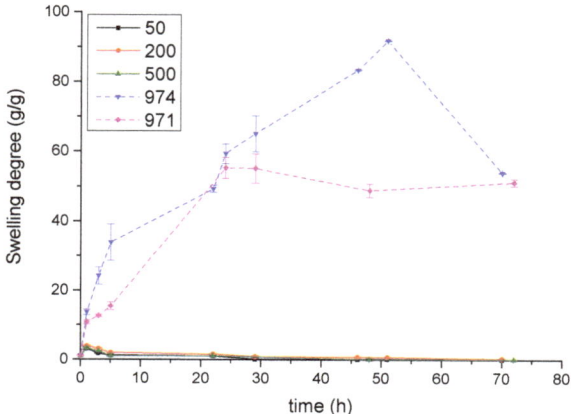

Figure 4. Swelling degree of pure polymers in simulated saliva.

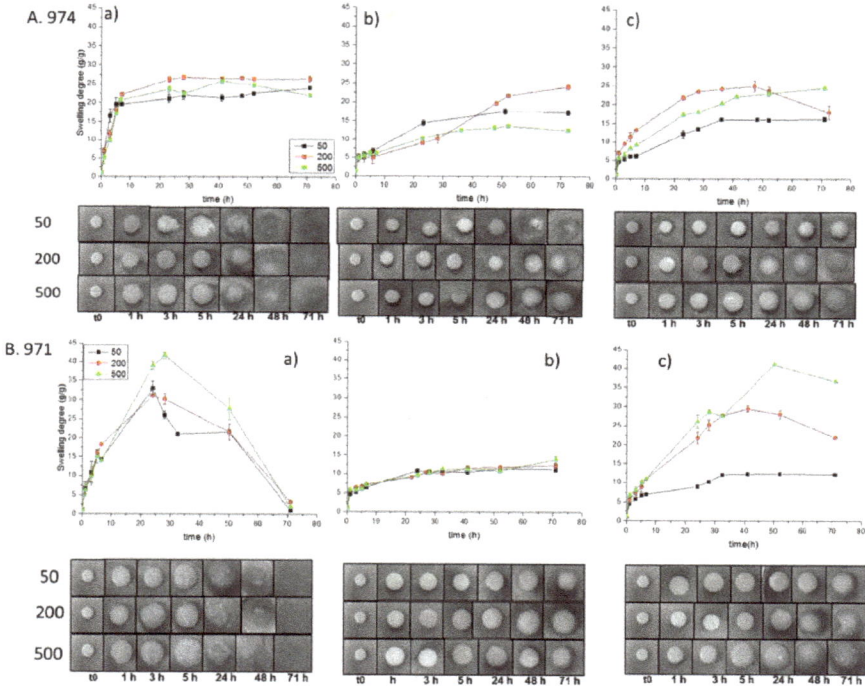

Figure 5. Swelling degree and photographs of the tablets of Carbopols/Poly(2-ethyl-2-oxazoline)s in saliva at 37 °C at regular time intervals: (**a**) physical mixture; (**b**) interpolymer complexes formed in water; and (**c**) interpolymer complexes formed at pH 2 (A Carbopol 974; and B. Carbopol 971).

The cross-linking density of Carbopols seems to have more influence on the swelling capability than the presence of poly(2-ethyl-2-oxazoline). Comparison of Figure 5A,B shows that tablets based on Carbopol 971 exhibit greater swelling degree than 974, being more prominent for tablet physical mixtures and interpolymer complexes formed at pH 2. This is in accordance with the more crosslinked structure of Carbopol 974 in comparison with Carbopol 971. Surprisingly, Carbopol 971 complexed with POZs under neutral pH conditions displayed a limited swelling for all the cases. This behavior can be ascribed to the H-bonding with POZs, which is more prominent when complexation is carried out with open and swollen Carbopol networks leading to a better interaction with POZs, that is the case for moderately cross-linked Carbopol 971 at neutral pH, when ionization of their carboxylic groups promotes maximum swelling of pure polyacid network.

As can be observed in Figure 5A, for more crosslinked Carbopol 974, physical mixtures and interpolymer complexes regardless of the solution pH used during the complexation, displayed a similar swelling uptake around 20%, what it takes to conclude that Carbopol structure limits swelling regardless the presence of POZ. Thus, it seems that the greater cross-linking of used polyacid network, which restricts Carbopol swelling, limits Carbopol/POZ interaction and consequently their influence on their complexes swelling. However, the effect of those restricted H-bonding could be observed on a retardation effect in those tablets formed by interpolymer complexes, which was more pronounced for complexes formed in water at pH 5, corroborating the above described role of Carbopol swelling in H-bonding interaction with POZs.

Analyzing the swelling of tablets containing POZ samples of different molecular weights, a different effect according to employed Carbopol structure and pH of the medium could be observed. In this sense, it could be observed that tablets with restricted swelling, because of stronger Carbopol/POZ interactions, did not show any dependence of their swelling on POZ molecular weight. Certainly, these limiting interactions result from an open network state during complexation, which facilitates POZ diffusion into Carbopol network. Thus, the behavior of tablets based on interpolymer complexes of Carbopol 971 in water should be particularly noted, which corresponds to the sample with the most swollen Carbopol prior to the complexation. All of them present very similar swelling degree, less than 10%, independent of POZ molecular weights and lower than the other cases, because POZ macromolecules penetration within polyacid network is favored for all the studied molecular weights (Figure 5B(b)). However, when Carbopol 971 network is collapsed as a consequence of a lower ionization degree at pH = 2, only POZ macromolecules with the lowest molecular weight can get inside Carbopol network promoting swelling restricting interactions (Figure 5B(c)). Similar effect was observed for Carbopol 974/POZs tablets, in which molecular weight of POZ did not show any clear effect on the swelling of the tablets when complexes were prepared in water (Figure 5B(b)). That is, in the swollen state of Carbopol, but limited swelling was found for the lowest molecular weight when complexes were formed at pH = 2 (Figure 5B(c)).

3.4. Dissolution Test

The release of hydrocortisone from the tablets was evaluated under sink conditions at pH 6.75. Figure 6 shows the dissolution profiles from the tablets based on Carbopol 974 and Carbopol 971 as well as their complexes and physical mixtures with POZ (enlarged release profiles of the first 10 h are shown in Figure S2). A direct correlation between the swelling of interpolymer complexes samples and HC release was observed. Hydrocortisone released faster from the tablets composed of a physical mixture of the polymer components than when interpolymer complexes were used. However, this is even more pronounced for the complexes formed by Carbopol 971, which can be explained according to their swelling behavior resulting from an enhanced complexation with POZ. Besides, it can be observed that there is no variation in the release profile from pure Carbopol 974 to physical mixtures of Carbopol 974 and POZs. These results are related to the wettability and the swelling degree of the tablets, since similar results were obtained in the swelling studies, and indicate that the main driving effect for this behavior is related to Carbopol 974. When using Carbopol 974 interpolymer complexes, the release rate slightly decreased compared to the physical mixtures and to pure Carbopol 974. However, highest decrease was measured for complexes that displayed lowest swelling. As was expected, Carbopol 971 complexes, for which Carbopol/POZs interaction were favored, showed lower swelling, HC release was slower and total HC released content was lower.

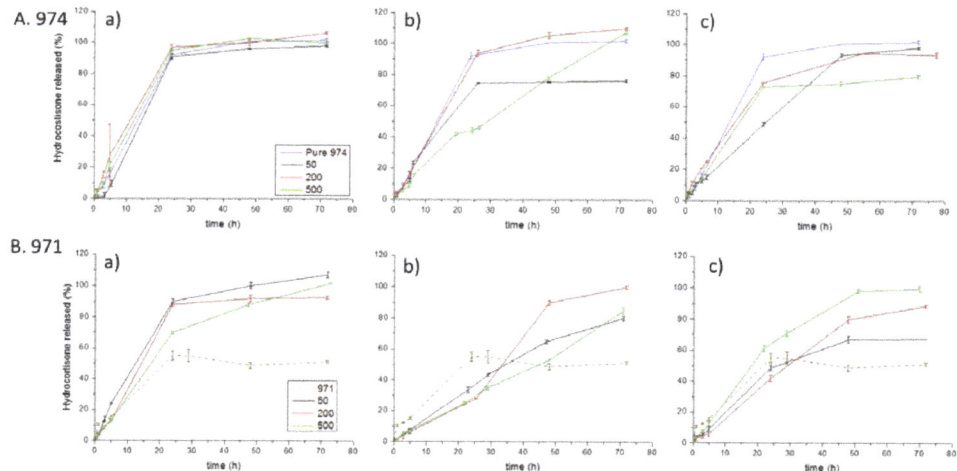

Figure 6. Release profiles of hydrocortisone from the tablets composed of poly(2-ethyl-2-oxazoline)s/Carbopols in simulated saliva at 37 °C: (**a**) physical mixture; (**b**) interpolymer complexes formed in water; and (**c**) interpolymer complexes formed at pH 2. (A Carbopol 974; and B. Carbopol 971).

The nature of interpolymer complexes, seems not only to change the swelling degree, but also varies the release profile of HC from the tablets. By analyzing Figure 6, a linear drug release could be observed in the beginning of the swelling process.

Hydrocortisone release from the tablets based on interpolymer complexes formed in water using weaker cross-linked Carbopol 971 displays a linear character in almost all the studied systems with slight variations between the different molecular weight of POZ. Similar observations were reported by Park et al. [21] in their study of theophylline release from chitosan/Carbopol 971, where at pH 6.8 the molecular weight of chitosan did not show any influence on the drug release, resulting in linear release profiles. These linear release profiles have been ascribed in previous studies to poorly-water soluble nature of the drugs used (similar to hydrocortisone), which tend to partition into less polar material (POZ in our case) [20,42].

4. Conclusions

In this work, the tablet formulations for buccal delivery of a poorly-water soluble drug, hydrocortisone, were developed based on poly(2-ethyl-oxazoline)s and Carbopols. The mucoadhesive properties of poly(2-ethyl-oxazoline)s have improved by their complexation/mixing with Carbopols. Swelling, erosion and hydrocortisone release for different tablet formulations using interpolymer complexes as main excipient have been evaluated. The tables formed from interpolymer complexes obtained in water present better swelling and release properties. The study suggests that Carbopol/poly(2-ethyl-oxazoline) tablets could present an adequate swelling and hydrocortisone release to be used in applications in which a prolonged release is required such as periodontitis disease.

Supplementary Materials: The following are available online at http://www.mdpi.com/2073-4360/10/2/175/s1, Figure S1: Chromatogram of HC and DXM solutions at a concentration of 1 mg/L of HC and DXM, Figure S2: Release profiles, first 10 hours, of hydrocortisone from the tablets composed of poly(2-ethyl-2-oxazoline)s/Carbopols in simulated saliva at 37 °C: (a) physical mixture, (b) interpolymer complexes in water and (c) interpolymer complexes at pH 2.

Acknowledgments: Authors thank the Basque Country Government for financial support (Ayudas para apoyar las actividades de los grupos de investigación del sistema universitario vasco, IT718-13 y FRONTIERS (ELKARTEK)).

Author Contributions: Leire Ruiz-Rubio designed and accomplished the experiments, including the preparation of the materials, mucoadhesive studies, and DSC and FTIR characterization. Swelling and HPLC measurements were performed by María Luz Alonso and Rosa María Alonso. Data analysis was conducted by Leyre Pérez-Álvarez and Leire Ruiz-Rubio. José Luis Vilas-Vilela and Vitaliy Khutoryanskiy evaluated the results.

Conflicts of Interest: The authors declare no conflict of interest.

References

1. Stegemann, S.; Leveiller, F.; Franchi, D.; de Jong, H.; Lindén, H. When poor solubility becomes an issue: From early stage to proof of concept. *Eur. J. Pharm. Sci.* **2007**, *31*, 249–261. [CrossRef] [PubMed]
2. Khadka, P.; Ro, J.; Kim, H.; Kim, I.; Kim, J.T.; Kim, H.; Cho, J.M.; Yun, G.; Lee, J. Pharmaceutical particle technologies: An approach to improve drug solubility, dissolution and bioavailability. *Asian J. Pharm. Sci.* **2014**, *9*, 304–316. [CrossRef]
3. Kalepu, S.; Nekkanti, V. Insoluble drug delivery strategies: Review of recent advances and business prospects. *Acta Pharm. Sin. B* **2015**, *5*, 442–453. [CrossRef] [PubMed]
4. Schulze, J.D.R.; Waddington, W.A.; Ell, P.J.; Parsons, G.E.; Coffin, M.D.; Basit, A.W. Concentration-Dependent Effects of Polyethylene Glycol 400 on Gastrointestinal Transit and Drug Absorption. *Pharm. Res.* **2003**, *20*, 1984–1988. [CrossRef] [PubMed]
5. Harris, J.M.; Dust, J.M.; McGill, R.A.; Harris, P.A.; Edgell, M.J.; Sedaghat-Herati, R.M.; Karr, L.J.; Donnelly, D.L. New Polyethylene Glycols for Biomedical Applications. In *Water-Soluble Polymers*; ACS Symposium Series; American Chemical Society: Washington, DC, USA, 1991; Volume 467, pp. 27–418. ISBN 0-8412-2101-4.
6. Knop, K.; Hoogenboom, R.; Fischer, D.; Schubert, U.S. Poly(ethylene glycol) in drug delivery: Pros and cons as well as potential alternatives. *Angew. Chem. Int. Ed.* **2010**, *49*, 6288–6308. [CrossRef] [PubMed]
7. Schuman, E.; Balsam, P.E. Probable anaphylactic reaction to polyethylene glycol electrolyte lavage solution. *Gastrointest. Endosc.* **1991**, *37*, 411. [CrossRef]
8. De Koker, S.; Hoogenboom, R.; De Geest, B.G. Polymeric multilayer capsules for drug delivery. *Chem. Soc. Rev.* **2012**, *41*, 2867. [CrossRef] [PubMed]
9. Bender, J.C.M.E.; Hoogenboom, R.; Van, V.P.A.A. Drug Delivery System Comprising Polyoxazoline and a Bioactive Agent. U.S. Patent 8,642,080 B2, 28 June 2010.
10. Hoogenboom, R. Poly(2-oxazoline)s: A polymer class with numerous potential applications. *Angew. Chem.* **2009**, *48*, 7978–7994. [CrossRef] [PubMed]
11. Mero, A.; Pasut, G.; Via, L.D.; Fijten, M.W.M.; Schubert, U.S.; Hoogenboom, R.; Veronese, F.M. Synthesis and characterization of poly(2-ethyl 2-oxazoline)-conjugates with proteins and drugs: Suitable alternatives to PEG-conjugates? *J. Control. Release* **2008**, *125*, 87–95. [CrossRef] [PubMed]
12. Barz, M.; Luxenhofer, R.; Zentel, R.; Vicent, M.J. Overcoming the PEG-addiction: Well-defined alternatives to PEG, from structure-property relationships to better defined therapeutics. *Polym. Chem.* **2011**, 1900–1918. [CrossRef]
13. Adams, N.; Schubert, U.S. Poly(2-oxazolines) in biological and biomedical application context. *Adv. Drug Deliv. Rev.* **2007**, *59*, 1504–1520. [CrossRef] [PubMed]
14. Yamaoka, T.; Tabata, Y.; Ikada, Y. Distribution and tissue uptaken of poly(ethylene glycol) with different molecular weights after intravenous administration to mice. *J. Pharma Sci.* **1994**, *83*, 601–606. [CrossRef]
15. Longley, B.L.; Zhao, H.; Lozanguiez, Y.L.; Conover, C.D. Biodistribution and excretion of radiolabeled 40 kDa polyethylene glycol following intravenous administration in mice. *J. Pharma. Sci.* **2013**, *102*, 2362–2370. [CrossRef] [PubMed]
16. Nokhodchi, A.; Raja, S.; Patel, P.; Asare-Addo, K. The role of oral controlled release matrix tablets in drug delivery systems. *BioImpacts* **2012**, *2*, 175–187. [CrossRef] [PubMed]
17. Stilhano, R.S.; Madrigal, J.L.; Wong, K.; Williams, P.A.; Martin, P.K.M.; Yamaguchi, F.S.M.; Samoto, V.Y.; Han, S.W.; Silva, E.A. Injectable alginate hydrogel for enhanced spatiotemporal control of lentivector delivery in murine skeletal muscle. *J. Control. Release* **2016**, *237*, 42–49. [CrossRef] [PubMed]
18. Carvalho, F.; Bruschi, M.; Evangelista, R.; Gremiao, M. Mucoadhesive drug delivery systems. *Brazilian J. Pharm. Sci.* **2010**, *46*, 1–17. [CrossRef]
19. Pinto, J.F. Site-specific drug delivery systems within the gastro-intestinal tract: From the mouth to the colon. *Int. J. Pharm.* **2010**, *395*, 44–52. [CrossRef] [PubMed]

20. Singla, A.K.; Chawla, M.; Singh, A. Potential Applications of Carbomer in Oral Mucoadhesive Controlled Drug Delivery System: A Review. *Drug Dev. Ind. Pharm.* **2000**, *26*, 913–924. [CrossRef] [PubMed]
21. Park, S.H.; Chun, M.K.; Choi, H.K. Preparation of an extended-release matrix tablet using chitosan/Carbopol interpolymer complex. *Int. J. Pharm.* **2008**, *347*, 39–44. [CrossRef] [PubMed]
22. Khutoryanskiy, V.V. Hydrogen-bonded interpolymer complexes as materials for pharmaceutical applications. *Int. J. Pharm.* **2007**, *334*, 15–26. [CrossRef] [PubMed]
23. Madsen, K.D.; Sander, C.; Baldursdottir, S.; Pedersen, A.M.L.; Jacobsen, J. Development of an ex vivo retention model simulating bioadhesion in the oral cavity using human saliva and physiologically relevant irrigation media. *Int. J. Pharm.* **2013**, *448*, 373–381. [CrossRef] [PubMed]
24. Mura, P.; Cirri, M.; Mennini, N.; Casella, G.; Maestrelli, F. Polymeric mucoadhesive tablets for topical or systemic buccal delivery of clonazepam: Effect of cyclodextrin complexation. *Carbohydr. Polym.* **2016**, *152*, 755–763. [CrossRef] [PubMed]
25. Hájková, R.; Solich, P.; Dvořák, J.; Šicha, J. Simultaneous determination of methylparaben, propylparaben, hydrocortisone acetate and its degradation products in a topical cream by RP-HPLC. *J. Pharm. Biomed. Anal.* **2003**, *32*, 921–927. [CrossRef]
26. De Palo, E.F.; Antonelli, G.; Benetazzo, A.; Prearo, M.; Gatti, R. Human saliva cortisone and cortisol simultaneous analysis using reverse phase HPLC technique. *Clin. Chim. Acta* **2009**, *405*, 60–65. [CrossRef] [PubMed]
27. Pendela, M.; Kahsay, G.; Baekelandt, I.; Van Schepdael, A.; Adams, E. Simultaneous determination of lidocaine hydrochloride, hydrocortisone and nystatin in a pharmaceutical preparation by RP-LC. *J. Pharm. Biomed. Anal.* **2011**, *56*, 641–644. [CrossRef] [PubMed]
28. Moribe, K.; Makishima, T.; Higashi, K.; Liu, N.; Limwikrant, W.; Ding, W.; Masuda, M.; Shimizu, T.; Yamamoto, K. Encapsulation of poorly water-soluble drugs into organic nanotubes for improving drug dissolution. *Int. J. Pharm.* **2014**, *469*, 190–196. [CrossRef] [PubMed]
29. Ruiz-Rubio, L.; Laza, J.M.; Pérez, L. Polymer–polymer complexes of poly(N-isopropylacrylamide) and poly (N,N-diethylacrylamide) with poly(carboxylic acids): A comparative study. *Colloid Polym. Sci.* **2014**, *292*, 423–430. [CrossRef]
30. Hamou, A.S.H.; Djadoun, S. Interpolymer complexes of poly(N,N-dimethylacrylamide/poly(styrene-co-acrylic acid): Thermal stability and FTIR analysis. *Macromol. Symp.* **2011**, *303*, 114–122. [CrossRef]
31. He, Y.; Zhu, B.; Inove, Y. Hydrogen bonds in polymer blends. *Prog. Polym. Sci.* **2004**, *29*, 1021–1151. [CrossRef]
32. Daniliuc, L.; David, C. Intermolecular interactions in blends of poly(vinyl alcohol) with poly(acrylic acid): 2. Correlation between the states of sorbed water and the interactions in homopolymers and their blends. *Polymer* **1996**, *37*, 5219–5227. [CrossRef]
33. Khutoryanskiy, V.V.; Dubolazov, A.V.; Nurkeeva, Z.S.; Mun, G.A. pH effects in the complex formation and blending of poly(acrylic acid) with poly(ethylene oxide). *Langmuir* **2004**, *20*, 3785–3790. [CrossRef] [PubMed]
34. Bayramgil, N.P. Therml degradation of [poly(N-vinylimidazole)-polyacrylic acid] interpolymer complexes. *Polym. Degrad. Stab.* **2008**, *93*, 1504–1509. [CrossRef]
35. Ruiz-Rubio, L.; Álvarez, V.; Lizundia, E.; Vilas, J.L.; Rodriguez, M.; León, L.M. Influence of α-methyl substitutions on interpolymer complexes formation between poly(meth)acrylic acids and poly(N-isopropyl(meth)acrylamide)s. *Colloid Polym. Sci.* **2015**, *293*, 1447–1455. [CrossRef]
36. Khutoryanskiy, V.V. Advances in mucoadhesion and mucoadhesive polymers. *Macromol. Biosci.* **2011**, *11*, 748–764. [CrossRef] [PubMed]
37. Khutoryanskaya, O.V.; Morrison, P.W.J.; Seilkhanov, S.K.; Mussin, M.N.; Ozhmukhametova, E.K.; Rakhypbekov, T.K.; Khutoryanskiy, V.V. Hydrogen-bonded complexes and blends of poly(acrylic acid) and methylcellulose: Nanoparticles and mucoadhesive films for ocular delivery of riboflavin. *Macromol. Biosci.* **2014**, *14*, 225–234. [CrossRef] [PubMed]
38. Singh, M.; Tiwary, A.K.; Kaur, G. Investigations on interpolymer complexes of cationic guar gum and xanthan gum for formulation of bioadhesive films. *Res. Pharm. Sci.* **2010**, *5*, 79–87. [CrossRef] [PubMed]
39. Salamat-Miller, N.; Chittchang, M.; Johnston, T.P. The use of mucoadhesive polymers in buccal drug delivery. *Adv. Drug Deliv. Rev.* **2005**, *57*, 1666–1691. [CrossRef] [PubMed]

40. Patel, M.M.; Smart, J.D.; Nevell, T.G.; Ewen, R.J.; Eaton, P.J.; Tsibouklis, J. Mucin/poly(acrylic acid) interactions: A spectroscopic investigation of mucoadhesion. *Biomacromolecules* **2003**, *4*, 1184–1190. [CrossRef] [PubMed]
41. Russo, E.; Selmin, F.; Baldassari, S.; Gennari, C.G.M.; Caviglioli, G.; Cilurzo, F.; Minghetti, P.; Parodi, B. A focus on mucoadhesive polymers and their application in buccal dosage forms. *J. Drug Deliv. Sci. Technol.* **2016**, *32*, 113–125. [CrossRef]
42. Lee, M.H.; Chun, M.K.; Choi, H.K. Preparation of Carbopol/chitosan interpolymer complex as a controlled release tablet matrix; Effect of complex formation medium on drug release characteristics. *Arch. Pharm. Res.* **2008**, *31*, 932–937. [CrossRef] [PubMed]

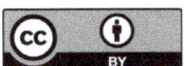

© 2018 by the authors. Licensee MDPI, Basel, Switzerland. This article is an open access article distributed under the terms and conditions of the Creative Commons Attribution (CC BY) license (http://creativecommons.org/licenses/by/4.0/).

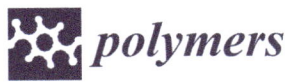

Article

Production and Characterization of a Clotrimazole Liposphere Gel for Candidiasis Treatment

Elisabetta Esposito [1,*], Maddalena Sguizzato [1], Christian Bories [2], Claudio Nastruzzi [1] and Rita Cortesi [1]

[1] Department of Life Sciences and Biotechnology, University of Ferrara, I-44121 Ferrara, Italy; maddalena.sguizzato@student.unife.it (M.S.); nas@unife.it (C.N.); crt@unife.it (R.C.)
[2] Antiparasitic Chemotherapy-CNRS 8076, Faculty of Pharmacy, F-92296 Chatenay-Malabry CEDEX, France; christian.bories@orange.fr
* Correspondence: ese@unife.it; Tel.: +39-0532-455259

Received: 12 January 2018; Accepted: 6 February 2018; Published: 8 February 2018

Abstract: This study describes the design and characterization of a liposphere gel containing clotrimazole for the treatment of *Candida albicans*. Lipospheres were produced by the melt-dispersion technique, using a lipid phase constituted of stearic triglyceride in a mixture with caprylic/capric triglyceride or an alkyl lactate derivative. The latter component was added to improve the action of clotrimazole against candida. The liposphere morphology and dimensional distribution were evaluated by scanning electron microscopy. Clotrimazole release kinetics was investigated by an in vitro dialysis method. An anticandidal activity study was conducted on the lipospheres. To obtain formulations with suitable viscosity for vaginal application, the lipospheres were added to a xanthan gum gel. The rheological properties, spreadability, leakage, and adhesion of the liposphere gel were investigated. Clotrimazole encapsulation was always over 85% w/w. The anticandidal study demonstrated that the encapsulation of clotrimazole in lipospheres increased its activity against *Candida albicans*, especially in the presence of the alkyl lactate derivative in the liposphere matrix. A dialysis method demonstrated that clotrimazole was slowly released from the liposphere gel and that the alkyl lactate derivative further controlled clotrimazole release. Adhesion and leakage tests indicated a prolonged adhesion of the liposphere gel, suggesting its suitability for vaginal application.

Keywords: clotrimazole; liposphere; alkyl lactate; xanthan gum; *Candida albicans*; mucoadhesion

1. Introduction

Candida albicans is a fungus that can locate in different host mucosal surfaces, standing as both a member of the normal microflora (yeast form) and a potential opportunistic pathogen (pseudohyphal form) [1,2]. The potential of *Candida albicans* to colonize various mucosal surfaces highly depends on the presence or absence of members of the normal bacterial microflora. Particularly, the fatty acid environment produced by the host and bacterial microflora can influence and regulate the germination of *Candida albicans* on mucosal surfaces [3–5]. The proliferation of *Candida albicans* can generate symptomatic infections, such as vulvovaginal candidiasis, experienced at least once by 75% of women and repeatedly by 6–9% of women [6].

Since a local treatment is the first line of choice in cases of acute vaginal yeast infection, a variety of topical preparations are on the market, mainly containing azole fungistatic agents such as ketoconazole, miconazole, and clotrimazole (CLO) [7]. However, the vaginal administration of these drugs as creams, gels, ovules, and pessaries is often related to some drawbacks, such as leakage of the formulation and low residence time in the vaginal cavity [8].

To solve this problem, a bioadhesive formulation should be able to increase the residence time of the dosage form and to enhance its local bioavailability [9,10]. In addition, the inclusion of the antifungal agent into a solid microparticulate system could control its residence time and delivery.

Among microparticulate systems, liposheres (LS) represent an interesting choice. LS are microparticles with a solid matrix constituted of lipids, such as triglycerides or fatty acid derivatives, with a mean diameter ranging between 0.2 and 500 µm, where drug molecules can be solubilized or dispersed [11–13]. Being constituted of lipids, LS possess attractive properties such as biocompatibility and the capacity to increase the entrapment and bioavailability of poorly water-soluble drug. LS are characterized by good physical stability, low-cost components, ease of preparation and of scaling-up. Because of their properties, LS have been proposed for the delivery of many drugs (e.g., antiinflammatory, antimalarial, antiepilepsy, hypoglycemic, vasodilator, antibiotics, anticancer agents, and vaccines) by oral, cutaneous, subcutaneous, or intramuscular administration [11–17]. Nonetheless, to our knowledge, LS have never been proposed for vaginal administration. On the basis of this last consideration, in the present investigation, LS were especially designed for CLO delivery on vaginal mucosa to treat *Candida albicans* infection. CLO is widely employed to treat fungal infections topically, indeed oral administration of this active compound is not convenient because of its short half-life and side effects [18]. Since CLO is poorly water-soluble, it requires a proper vehicle to rise the right levels of topical absorption [19]. The lipidic phase of LS was based on stearic triglyceride, a solid lipid commonly employed in foods, and caprylic/capric triglyceride (TRIC) or the lactic acid derivative C_{12}-C_{13} alkyl lactate (AL). These liquid auxiliary components have been employed in mixture with stearic triglyceride (TRIST) to possibly modulate and disorganize the solid LS microstructure. Indeed, it has been demonstrated that structured lipid carriers based on mixtures of solid and liquid lipids can encapsulate considerable amounts of drug, controlling its release and expulsion [20,21]. In addition, AL was chosen because of the peculiar antimicrobial activity of lactic acid derivatives, which can exert antifungal effect on the basis of their ability to reduce the pH of the milieu [22]. To obtain adhesive formulations with suitable viscosity for vaginal application, LS were added to a gel constituted of xanthan gum, an anionic polysaccharide [23]. Since polysaccharides are defined as polymeric carbohydrates, xanthan gum can be considered as a natural polymer or a biopolymer [24–26]. This polymer is naturally produced by *Xanthomonas campestris* by fermentation to stick the bacteria to the leaves of cabbage-like plants. In chilly water, xanthan gum hydrates rapidly, producing weak gels with shear–thinning properties. Noteworthily, its natural origin assures biocompatibility and biodegradability. Therefore, xanthan gum is widely employed in food products as well as in pharmaceutics as a thickener, stabilizer, and emulsifier. Moreover, it has been recently investigated for the fabrication of matrices with specialized drug release characteristics [25,26]. On the basis of the potential of LS and xanthan gum, in the present study, the association of these components has been proposed to produce a new vaginal delivery system.

2. Materials and Methods

2.1. Materials

The copolymer poly(ethylene oxide) (a)–poly(propylene oxide) (b) (a = 80, b = 27) (poloxamer 188) was a gift of BASF ChemTrade GmbH (Burgbernheim, Germany). Caprylic/capric triglycerides, Miglyol 812 N, (TRIC), was a gift of Cremer Oleo Division (Witten, Germany). C_{12}-C_{13} alkyl lactate, Cosmacol ELI (AL), was from Sasol (Milan, Italy). Stearic triglyceride (TRIST), xanthan gum, clotrimazole (CLO), agar, and all other reagents and HPLC solvents were purchased from Sigma-Aldrich, Merck (Darmstadt, Germany).

2.2. Methods

2.2.1. Liposphere Production

LS were produced by the melt-dispersion technique [11,12]. Briefly, 1 g of TRIST or a lipidic mixture (reported in Table 1), in the absence or in the presence of 20 mg of CLO, was melted at 75 °C and emulsified with 150 mL of an aqueous phase containing poloxamer 188 (5%, w/w).

Table 1. Liposphere (LS) composition.

Formulation	Composition (% w/w)			
	Tristearin (TRIST)	Caprylic/Capric Triglyceride (TRIC)	Alkyl Lactate (AL)	Clotrimazole (CLO)
LS_{TRIST}	100.00	-	-	-
$LS_{TRIST/TRIC}$	70.00	30.00	-	-
$LS_{TRIST/AL30}$	70.00	-	30.00	-
$LS_{TRIST/AL15}$	85.00	-	15.00	-
$LS_{TRIST/AL10}$	90.00	-	10.00	-
$LS_{TRIST/AL1}$	99.00	-	1.00	-
LS_{TRIST}-CLO	98.04	-	-	1.96
$LS_{TRIST/TRIC}$-CLO	68.69	29.35	-	1.96
$LS_{TRIST/AL30}$-CLO	68.69	29.35	-	1.96
$LS_{TRIST/AL15}$-CLO	83.34	-	14.70	1.96
$LS_{TRIST/AL10}$-CLO	88.24	-	9.80	1.96
$LS_{TRIST/AL1}$-CLO	97.06	-	0.98	1.96

The emulsion was stirred for 1 h at 2000 r.p.m. using a mechanical stirrer Eurostar Digital (IKA Labortechnik, Staufen, Germany) equipped with a three-blade rotor impeller with a diameter of 55 mm. The milky formulation was then rapidly cooled to about 20 °C under stirring in an ice bath, yielding a uniform dispersion of LS. The obtained LS were then washed with water and isolated by filtration through a paper filter. LS were left to dry overnight at 25 °C and weighed.

LS yield was calculated as follows [11]:

$$\% \text{ Yield} = \text{LS weight} \times 100/\text{Total weight of lipids employed for LS preparation} \qquad (1)$$

2.2.2. LS Morphological and Dimensional Analysis

The morphology of LS was evaluated by variable-pressure scanning electron microscopy (VPSEM) (Zeiss Evo 40XPV, Carl Zeiss AG, Oberkochen, Germany). Briefly, 10 mg of LS were directly put on a stub without any recoat and observed under variable pressure [27]. To analyze the internal morphology, dried LS were sectioned with a long stainless steel blade, under a binocular microscope. LS size distributions were determined measuring at least 300 LS/sample.

2.2.3. CLO Content of LS

The amount of encapsulated CLO per mg of dry LS was determined by disgregating 50 mg of LS in 5 mL of ethanol under stirring (300 r.p.m.) at 60 °C for 2 h.

The samples were filtered (nylon membrane filters, 0.2 μm pore size, Merck Millipore, Milan, Italy) and analyzed by high-performance liquid chromatography (HPLC) for CLO content, as previously reported [19]. HPLC determinations were performed using a two-plungers alternative pump (Jasco, Tokyo, Japan), an UV-detector operating at 210 nm, and a 7125 Rheodyne injection valve with a 50 μL loop. The samples were loaded on a stainless steel C-18 reverse-phase column (15 × 0.46 cm) packed with 5 μm particles (Hypersil BDS, Alltech, Fresno, CA, USA).

The elution was performed with a mobile phase containing methanol/water 80:20 v/v at a flow rate of 0.8 mL/min. The retention time of CLO was 6.8 min.

CLO encapsulation efficiency (EE) was calculated as follows [11]:

$$EE = \text{amount of CLO detected by HPLC} \times 100/\text{total amount of CLO employed} \qquad (2)$$

All data were the mean of four determinations on different batches of the same type of LS.

2.2.4. Anticandidal Activity Study

The antifungal activity was studied against *Candida albicans* (ATCC 10231). The experiment was performed based on the standardized protocol M27-A2, CLSI. Mother cultures of *C. albicans* strain were set up starting from 1.5 mL aliquots of a liquid nitrogen-stored inoculum put in 250 mL sterile flasks containing 98.5 mL of liquid YEPD medium (yeast extract 0.5%, bactopeptone 1%, glucose 2%; Oxoid, Thermo Fisher Diagnostics, Dardilly Cedex, France), placed at 37 °C on an orbital shaker (110 r.p.m.). The inocula were performed after growth (48 h/35 °C) on Sabouraud dextrose agar. The colonies were suspended in 0.85% sterile saline and this suspension was homogenized in a vortex mixer for 15 s; after that, the cell density was determined in a spectrophotometer, and the transmittance (λ = 530 nm) was adjusted to match the standard 0.5 on the McFarland scale (1×10^6 to 5×10^6 yeast/mL). Subsequently, a 1:50 dilution in RPMI 1640-MOPS-buffered medium was performed, resulting in a final concentration of $1.5 \pm 1.0 \times 10^3$ yeasts/mL.

The microdilution technique [28,29] was performed in 96-wells polystyrene sterile plates; the culture medium was RPMI1640-MOPS-buffered broth. The tested samples were: LS_{TRIST}-CLO, $LS_{TRIST/AL1}$-CLO, LS_{TRIST}, $LS_{TRIST/AL1}$, and CLO methanolic solution. Namely, 25 mg of the dry formulation was weighed and suspended in 200 µL of the culture medium in the first well, then two-fold serial dilutions were performed in wells from 1 to 10. For CLO methanolic solution, 100 µL of a CLO solution twice as concentrated as the desired final solution was diluted with 100 µL of culture medium in the first well.

To each well of the microdilution plate, 100 µL of the standardized inoculum was added. The experiments were run in triplicate. The plates were incubated at 35 °C for 48 h, afterwards 10 µL of 0.5% 2,3,5-triphenyltetrazolium chloride and 10 µL containing menadione 1 mM were added to all wells [21], and the plates were then reincubated at 35 °C for 120 min. After addition of 0.1 mL of acid isopropanol (isopropanol/HCl 1 N, 95:5, v/v), the plates were placed on a shaker for 5 min to dissolve the formazan crystals. The measurements were performed with a microplate reader at 550 nm, and the minimal inhibitory concentration (MIC) was determined. The statistical analysis was conducted by *t*-Student test.

2.2.5. Gel Production

A weighed amount of xanthan gum (0.5% w/w) was gradually added to citrate buffer 5 mM, pH 4 (prepared by dissolving citric acid monohydrate and trisodium citrate dihydrate in distilled water) and then mixed for 15 min [9]. The gel was left to stand at 25 °C overnight for complete swelling, afterwards LS (5% w/w), CLO (0.1% w/w), or AL (0.05% w/w) were alternatively added and manually mixed until homogeneous dispersion (gel names and compositions are reported in Table 2). Particularly for the preparation of Gel LS_{TRIST}-CLO and Gel $LS_{TRIST/AL1}$-CLO, LS_{TRIST}-CLO and $LS_{TRIST/AL1}$-CLO were respectively added into the xanthan gum gel, while Gel-CLO and Gel$_{AL1}$-CLO, employed as controls, were obtained by directly adding free CLO and AL into the xanthan gum gel.

Table 2. Gel composition.

Formulation	Gel Components (% w/w)				
	Tristearin	Alkyl Lactate	Clotrimazole	Xanthan Gum	Water
Gel LS$_{TRIST}$-CLO	4.902	-	0.098	0.500	94.500
Gel LS$_{TRIST/AL1}$-CLO	4.853	0.049	0.098	0.500	94.500
Gel-CLO	-	-	0.098	0.500	99.402
Gel$_{AL1}$-CLO	-	0.049	0.098	0.500	99.353

LS acronyms are reported in Table 1.

2.2.6. Viscosity Test

The rheology measurements were performed on Gel$_{AL1}$-CLO and Gel LS$_{TRIST/AL1}$-CLO by a Viscolead ADV, Fungilab viscometer (Fungilab, Barcelona, Spain). The gels were poured into a 250 mL beaker, where they were tested at 25 °C. The spindle was immersed to its immersion mark in the different areas of the beaker, for each trial. The viscosity was measured at different speeds, comprised between 1 and 100 r.p.m.

2.2.7. Spreadability Test

The spreading capacity of Gel$_{AL1}$-CLO and Gel LS$_{TRIST/AL1}$-CLO was evaluated. Namely, after 48 h from preparation, an amount of gel (100 mg) was placed on a Petri dish (3 cm diameter) and pressed by another glass dish with a 500 g mass. The time taken for the gel to fill the entire dish was measured.

The following equation was used for this purpose:

$$S = m \times l/t \quad (3)$$

in which S is the spreadability of the gel formulation, m is the weight (g) tied on the upper plate, l is the diameter (cm) of the glass plates, and t is the time (s) taken for the gel to fill the entire diameter [30]. The spreadability test was performed three times, and the mean values ± standard deviations were calculated.

2.2.8. Gel Leakage and Adhesion Test

To test leakage and adhesion of the formulations, citrate buffer pH 4.5 and simulated vaginal fluid (SVF) were prepared [9]. Briefly, to prepare SVF pH 4.5, NaCl, KOH, Ca(OH)$_2$, bovine serum albumin, lactic acid, acetic acid, glycerol, urea, and glucose were dissolved in distilled water [9]. Agar (1.5% w/w) was added to the citrate buffer or SVF and stirred at 95 °C until solubilization. The gels obtained after cooling were then cut to obtain rectangular agar slide.

The gels LS$_{TRIST/AL1}$-CLO and Gel$_{AL1}$-CLO were colored for the leakage test by dissolving rhodamine (0.05% w/w) in the gels before adding LS$_{TRIST/AL1}$-CLO or AL and CLO. For the leakage test, 50 mg of colored gels or 2.5 mg of dry LS$_{TRIST/AL1}$-CLO were placed onto one end of a citrate buffer or SVF agar slide. The agar slide was vertically put at an angle of 90° on one of the inner walls of a transparent box, maintained at 37 °C ± 1 °C. The running distance of the gel along the slide was measured 1 and 10 min after the formulation placement. Gel leakage was measured three times, and the mean values ± standard deviations were calculated.

For the adhesion test, 200 mg of Gel$_{AL1}$-CLO and Gel LS$_{TRIST/AL1}$-CLO, or 10 mg of dry LS$_{TRIST/AL1}$-CLO were placed at the center of citrate buffer and SVF agar slides. The agar slides were respectively immersed in 10 mL of citrate buffer or SVF at 37 °C ± 1 °C for 2 h. The gel or LS residence times on the slides (adhesion time) were visually compared [31]. The tests were performed three times.

2.2.9. In Vitro CLO Release Studies

The in vitro release studies were performed by dialysis on CLO alternatively included in $LS_{TRIST/AL1}$-CLO, LS_{TRIST}-CLO, Gel $LS_{TRIST/AL1}$-CLO, Gel LS_{TRIST}-CLO, and Gel_{AL1}-CLO [11].

Briefly, 200 mg of LS or 4 g of gel were placed into a dialysis tube (molecular weight cut-off 10,000–12,000; Medi Cell International, London, UK), then put into 40 mL of a receiving phase constituted of SVF/ethanol (80:20, v/v), and shaken in a horizontal shaker (MS1, Minishaker, IKA) at 175 r.p.m. at 37 °C. In addition, the release kinetics of free CLO were investigated, placing in dialysis tubes 2 mg of CLO dispersed in 4 mL of distilled water or in 4 g of xanthan gum gel. Samples of receiving phase were withdrawn at regular time intervals and analyzed by HPLC, as described above. Fresh receiving phase was added to maintain a constant volume. The CLO concentrations were determined six times in independent experiments, and the mean values ± standard deviations were calculated.

The experimental data obtained by the release experiments were fitted to the following semiempirical equations, respectively describing Fickian dissolutive (4) and diffusion (5) release mechanisms [32,33]

$$M_t/M\infty = K_{Diss}\, t^{0.5} + c \quad (4)$$

$$1 - M_t/M\infty = e^{-K_{diff}\, t} + c \quad (5)$$

where $M_t/M\infty$ is the drug fraction released at the time t, ($M\infty$ is the total drug content of the analyzed amount of LS), and K and c are coefficients calculated by plotting the linear forms of the indicated equations. The release data represented by the percentages of released drug (0–8 h) were used to produce theoretical release curves.

3. Results

3.1. Liposphere Production and Characterization

A preformulation study was performed to investigate the effect of the lipid composition on LS produced by the melt-dispersion technique [11,12,34]. Particularly, an LS matrix was constituted of sole TRIST or of TRIST in mixture with the liquid auxiliary components TRIC and AL (Table 1). Generally, the yields ranged between 80% and 97% w/w (Table 3).

Table 3. Liposphere mean diameter, yield, and clotrimazole encapsulation efficiency.

Formulation	Mean Diameter (μm)	Yield (%) [a]	CLO EE (%) [b]
LS_{TRIST}	50 ± 28	92.0 ± 1	-
$LS_{TRIST/TRIC}$	6.3 ± 8	88.3 ± 2	-
$LS_{TRIST/AL30}$	n.d. *	80.0 ± 1	-
$LS_{TRIST/AL15}$	n.d. *	86.0 ± 2	-
$LS_{TRIST/AL10}$	n.d. *	89.7 ± 3	-
$LS_{TRIST/AL1}$	54.2 ± 30	93.3 ± 2	-
LS_{TRIST}-CLO	55.2 ± 10	87.0 ± 8	85 ± 7
$LS_{TRIST/AL10}$-CLO	48.2 ± 7	88.2 ± 5	98 ± 2
$LS_{TRIST/AL1}$-CLO	63.4 ± 9	97.8 ± 2	90 ± 8

[a] LS weight × 100/total weight of lipids employed for LS preparation; [b] amount of CLO detected by HPLC × 100/total amount of CLO employed; * not determined; LS acronyms are reported in Table 1.

VPSEM enabled to observe LS characterized by a spheroidal shape, with mean diameters comprised between 6 and 75 µm, and aggregates of LS (Figure 1).

Namely, LS$_{TRIST}$ were spherical, with a 50 µm mean diameter, as shown in Table 3 and Figure 1A. The presence of TRIC (30% w/w) in mixture with TRIST (LS$_{TRIST/TRIC}$) maintained the LS spherical shape (Figure 1B) and involved a decrease of the LS mean diameter (Table 3). In contrast, the addition of AL (30%, 15%, and 10% w/w) to TRIST resulted in the formation of collapsed and aggregated LS, with mean diameters difficult to measure (Figure 1C–E, Table 3). A lower amount of AL (1% w/w) (LS$_{TRIST/AL1}$) resulted, instead, in spherical LS with a 54 µm mean diameter and few aggregates (Figure 1F, Table 3).

LS constituted of TRIST or TRIST/AL mixture (AL 1% and 10% w/w) were produced in the presence of CLO. The shape and mean diameters of LS$_{TRIST}$-CLO and LS$_{TRIST/AL1}$-CLO were almost unaffected by CLO (Figure 2A,C,D, Table 3), showing a spherical shape and mean diameters around 50 µm, while LS$_{TRIST/AL10}$-CLO were in large part aggregated (Figure 2B). LS$_{TRIST}$-CLO and LS$_{TRIST/AL1}$-CLO were characterized by a matrix-type structure, as it can be observed in Figure S1A,B showing sections of LS obtained by cutting the samples before VPSEM observation. Namely, the inner structure of LS$_{TRIST}$-CLO and LS$_{TRIST/AL1}$-CLO did not show a core–shell organization, suggesting that CLO is probably uniformly dispersed throughout the entire LS.

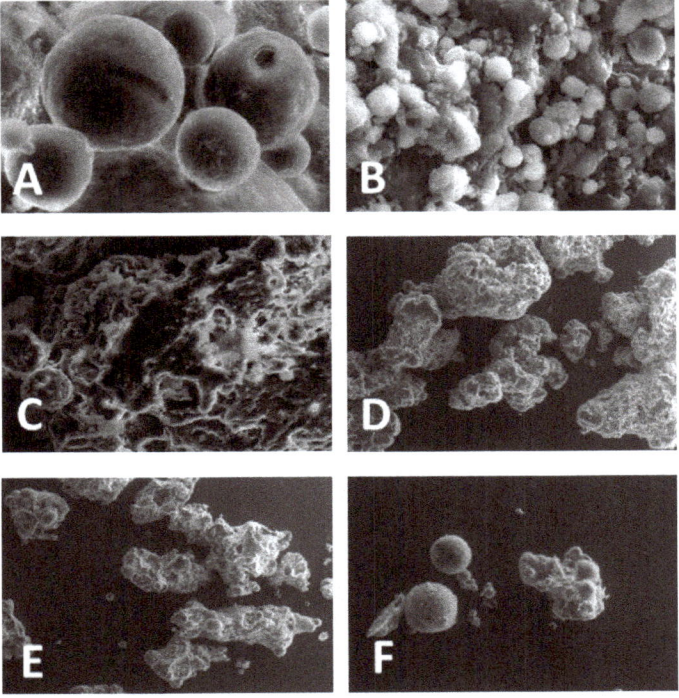

Figure 1. Variable-pressure scanning electron microscopy images (VPSEM) of LS$_{TRIST}$ (**A**), LS$_{TRIST/TRIC}$ (**B**), LS$_{TRIST/AL30}$ (**C**), LS$_{TRIST/AL15}$ (**D**), LS$_{TRIST/AL10}$ (**E**), and LS$_{TRIST/AL1}$ (**F**). Bar represents 20 µm in panels (**A**,**B**), and 50 µm in panels (**C**–**F**). LS acronyms are reported in Table 1.

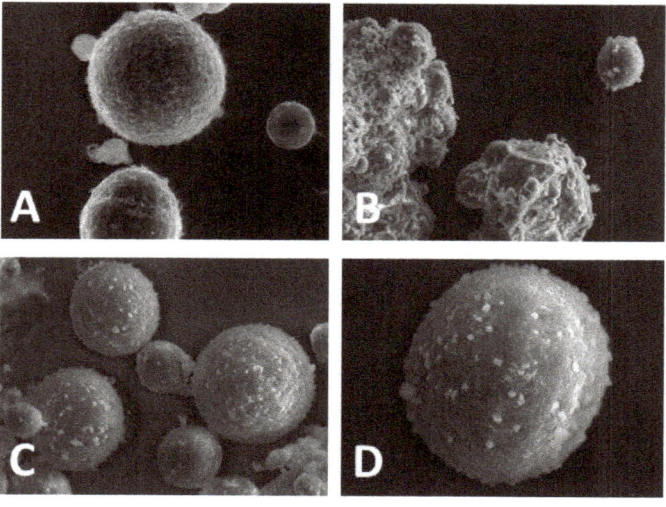

Figure 2. VPSME images of LS$_{TRIST}$-CLO (**A**), LS$_{TRIST/AL10}$-CLO (**B**), and LS$_{TRIST/AL1}$-CLO (**C,D**). Bar represents 25, 50, 60, and 15 μm in panels (**A–D**) respectively. LS acronyms are reported in Table 1.

Regarding CLO EE, the values ranged between 85% and 98%, as reported in Table 1. The highest CLO EE value was achieved in the case of LS$_{TRIST/AL10}$-CLO (98%), nevertheless, this type of LS was discharged because of aggregate formation.

3.2. Anticandidal Activity Study

LS$_{TRIST}$-CLO, LS$_{TRIST/AL1}$-CLO, and the corresponding LS produced in the absence of CLO were assayed against *Candida albicans* (Table 4).

Table 4. Minimum inhibitory concentration values (MIC, ng/mL) of clotrimazole-loaded liposheres against *Candida albicans* ATCC 10231.

Formulation	MIC (ng/mL) ± s.d. [a]
LS$_{TRIST}$-CLO	23 ± 1.6
LS$_{TRIST/AL1}$-CLO	17 ± 1.4
LS$_{TRIST}$	no activity
LS$_{TRIST/AL1}$	no activity
CLO	32 ± 2.3

[a] Standard deviation; LS acronyms are reported in Table 1.

A CLO solution in methanol was employed as a control. CLO-containing LS displayed lower MIC values with respect to the CLO solution (the MIC of LS$_{TRIST}$-CLO and LS$_{TRIST/AL1}$-CLO were, respectively, 1.4 times and 1.9 times lower than the MIC of CLO). In addition, MIC values were lower in the case of LS$_{TRIST/AL1}$-CLO with respect to LS$_{TRIST}$-CLO. The differences between MIC values were statistically significant in the case of LS$_{TRIST}$-CLO versus LS$_{TRIST/AL1}$-CLO ($p < 0.05$) and very significant when both LS were compared with CLO ($p < 0.01$). Empty LS did not display activity, as expected, suggesting that LS did not exert intrinsic antifungal activity [18,35,36].

3.3. Production and Characterization of Liposphere Gels

To obtain viscous formulations suitable for vaginal administration, LS, CLO, or AL were included in a xanthan gum gel (Table 2). Since the pH of vaginal hydrogels must be in the range 4–5 [8], we made the choice to use citrate buffer pH 4 instead of distilled water with the aim to prevent pH variation of the formulations, whose pH values were indeed 4.2–4.7. The transparency of the obtained formulations enabled to verify that the LS were homogeneously distributed within the gel.

3.3.1. Gel Viscosity

A formulation consistency is one of the most important key features for the application on mucosae or skin, thus gel viscosity plays a key role in drug permeation control [37]. The viscosities of Gel LS$_{TRIST/AL1}$-CLO and Gel$_{AL1}$-CLO were, respectively, 661 and 486 mPa/s (25 °C, shear rate 1 s^{-1}). The behavior of Gel LS$_{TRIST/AL1}$-CLO and Gel$_{AL1}$-CLO was non-Newtonian shear thinning, indeed their viscosity decreased as the shear rate increased (Figure 3A).

This behavior suggests low flow resistance when applied at high shear conditions [38]. The curves obtained for the plain and LS gels were almost superimposable, indicating that the presence of LS slightly affected the gel viscosity behavior. The symbols on the curves are the means of three experiments, and the error bars represent the standard deviations.

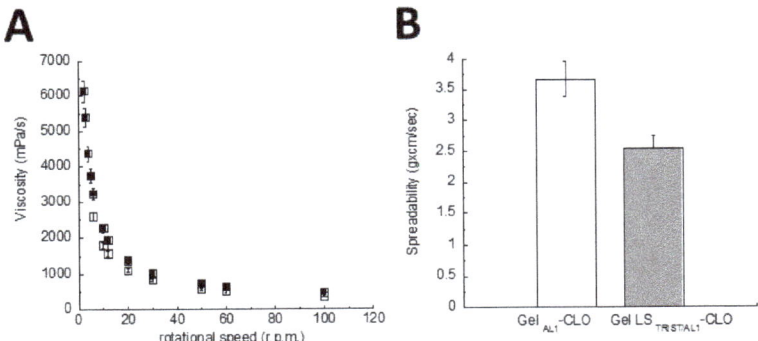

Figure 3. (**A**) Viscosity of Gel LS$_{TRIST/AL1}$-CLO (■) and Gel$_{AL1}$-CLO (□) as a function of the rotational speed; (**B**) Spreadability behavior of the indicated gels. The spreadability was calculated as reported in Section 2.2.7 (Equation (3)). Gel acronyms are reported in Table 2.

3.3.2. Gel Spreadability

Spreadability is an important parameter for topical forms since it affects patient compliance, extrudability from the package, uniform application on skin or mucosae, dosage transfer, and finally therapeutic efficacy of the active molecule [39]. As expected, LS presence in Gel LS$_{TRIST/AL1}$-CLO slightly decreased the gel spreadability with respect to Gel$_{AL1}$-CLO (Figure 3B). Namely, the spreadability ratio of Gel$_{AL1}$-CLO to Gel LS$_{TRIST/AL1}$-CLO was 1.4:1.

3.3.3. Gel Leakage

The gel leakage potential from the vagina was explored because a vaginal formulation should display a minimal leakage from the vaginal walls and, thus, a short running distance over a vertical plane, to assure a prolonged action [8]. Particularly, the running distances of Gel LS$_{TRIST/AL1}$-CLO, Gel$_{AL1}$-CLO, and LS$_{TRIST/AL1}$-CLO were compared 1 and 10 min after their application on vertical agar slides at pH 4.5, based on SVF or citrate buffer (Figure 4).

The former slides were especially designed to mimic the pH and composition of the vaginal cavity, while the latter ones simulated only the vaginal pH. In the case of the application on SVF slides, the running distance of Gel $LS_{TRIST/AL1}$-CLO was lower than that of Gel_{AL1}-CLO, whereas, in the case of the application on citrate buffer slides, the leakage trend was the opposite. Namely, the leakage distance of Gel $LS_{TRIST/AL1}$-CLO applied on cthe itrate buffer slides was almost double with respect to the leakage distance on the SVF slides. This behavior suggests an affinity of Gel $LS_{TRIST/AL1}$-CLO for the SVF slides, and thus for the vaginal fluid composition, rather than for the citrate buffer slides having only the same pH of the vagina. Dry LS remained fixed to the applied site on both type of slides even after 1 hour from placement, suggesting a high affinity for the applied pH and the SVF composition.

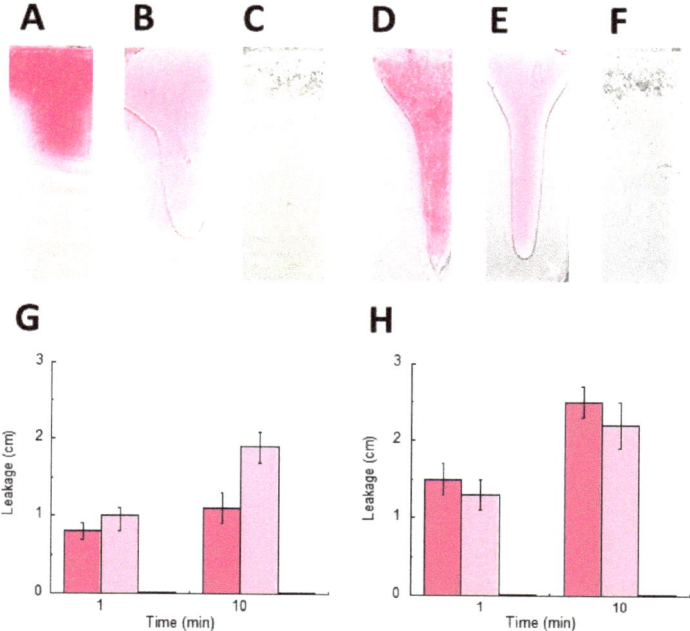

Figure 4. Comparative leakage test performed on formulations colored by rhodamine for imaging. Namely, Gel $LS_{TRIST/AL1}$-CLO (**A,D**), Gel_{AL1}-CLO (**B,E**), and $LS_{TRIST/AL1}$-CLO (**C,F**) were placed on pH 4.5 SVF (**A–C**) or citrate buffer (**D–F**) agar slides. The leakage distance was measured 1 and 10 min after the application of Gel $LS_{TRIST/AL1}$-CLO (pink), Gel_{AL1}-CLO (light pink), and $LS_{TRIST/AL1}$-CLO on pH 4.5 SVF (**G**) or citrate buffer (**H**) agar slides. (**A–F**) images were taken 1 h after placing the formulations on the slides. Gel acronyms are reported in Table 2.

3.3.4. Gel Adhesion

Adhesion can be defined as the capability of a material to adhere to a mucosal surface. A high adhesion is required to accomplish the retention of a pharmaceutical dosage form on a mucous membrane [8,9,40]. The adhesion of Gel_{AL1}-CLO, Gel $LS_{TRIST/AL1}$-CLO, or dry $LS_{TRIST/AL1}$-CLO was evaluated by comparing their residence times on slides immersed in pH 4.5 SVF or citrate buffer (Figure 5).

After 2 h, the presence of LS was clearly detectable only in the case of Gel $LS_{TRIST/AL1}$-CLO applied on SVF agar slides (Figure 5A, panel b). Indeed, only few LS were detectable in the case of citrate buffer agar slides (Figure 5B, panel b), confirming the suitability of Gel $LS_{TRIST/AL1}$-CLO for vaginal application and contact with vaginal fluids. Two hours after the placement of dry LS on SVF and citrate buffer agar slides, $LS_{TRIST/AL1}$-CLO were almost absent (panels d of Figure 5A,B), suggesting that the inclusion of LS in the gel is required to assure their adhesion. Images of Gel$_{AL1}$-CLO are not reported because the gel instantaneously dissolved after immersion in SVF or citrate buffer, indicating that the LS presence was essential to achieve gel adhesion.

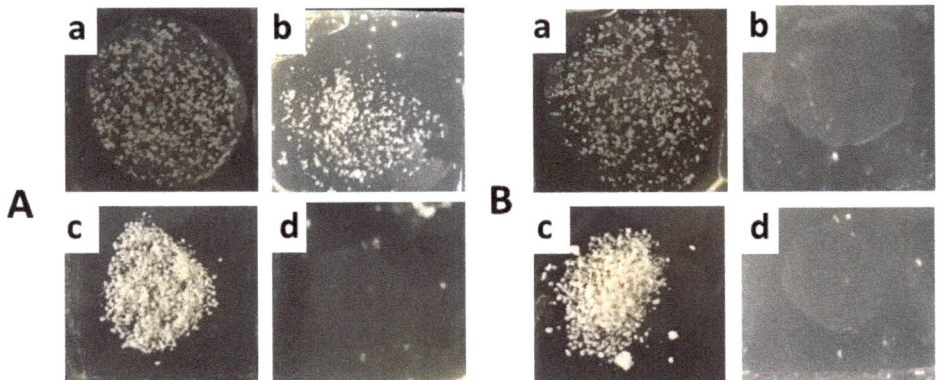

Figure 5. Comparative adhesion test performed on pH 4.5 SVF (**A**) or citrate buffer (**B**) agar plates immersed for 2 h in 10 mL of SVF or citrate buffer, respectively. The images were taken 1 (**a,c**) or 120 (**b,d**) min after the application of Gel LS$_{TRIST/AL1}$-CLO (**a,b**) and LS$_{TRIST/AL1}$-CLO (**c,d**). Gel acronyms are reported in Table 2.

3.4. In Vitro CLO Release Kinetics

To investigate and compare the performances of Gel LS$_{TRIST/AL1}$-CLO, Gel LS$_{TRIST}$-CLO, LS$_{TRIST/AL1}$-CLO, and LS$_{TRIST}$-CLO as delivery systems for CLO, the release profiles were determined in vitro by a dialysis method [11]. The release kinetics, reported in Figure 6, were in general characterized by a biphasic profile in which CLO was initially released linearly, followed by a slower phase in which the remaining drug was released.

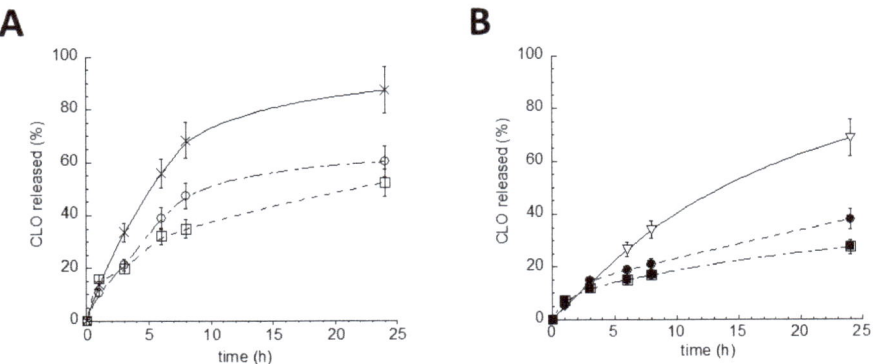

Figure 6. In vitro release kinetics of CLO from LS$_{TRIST/AL1}$-CLO (□), LS$_{TRIST}$-CLO (○) (**A**), Gel LS$_{TRIST/AL1}$-CLO (■), Gel LS$_{TRIST}$-CLO (●) (**B**). The experiments were performed by a dialysis method. For comparison, the profiles obtained using CLO in aqueous (×) (**A**) or xanthan gum (▽) (**B**) dispersions are also reported. The data are the mean of six experiments ± s.d. Gel acronyms are reported in Table 2.

The encapsulation of CLO in LS or in gel enabled to slow down the drug release with respect to the aqueous dispersion (Figure 6A) or the xanthan gum gel (Figure 6B), employed as controls. As expected, the inclusion of $LS_{TRIST/AL1}$-CLO or LS_{TRIST}-CLO in gels delayed CLO release. In addition, the presence of AL (1% w/w) in the LS matrix enabled to better control CLO release, as can be noticed in the $LS_{TRIST/AL1}$-CLO and Gel $LS_{TRIST/AL1}$-CLO kinetics, with respect to their counterparts LS_{TRIST}-CLO and Gel LS_{TRIST}-CLO (Figure 6A,B).

To determine the mechanism of CLO release from the studied formulations, a mathematical analysis of the release profile was performed. The theoretical release profiles were calculated according to the linear form of Equations (4) and (5), respectively mimicking dissolutive and diffusive model. Then, a comparison between the theoretical and the experimental release from LS_{TRIST}-CLO (Figure S2A), $LS_{TRIST/AL1}$-CLO (Figure S2B), Gel LS_{TRIST}-CLO (Figure S2C), and Gel $LS_{TRIST/AL1}$-CLO (Figure S2D) was conducted considering the first 8 h of release. Apart from LS_{TRIST}-CLO, for which the experimental curve was almost superimposable to the dissolutive theoretical curve, CLO release from the other formulations was dominated by a mixed release mechanism. Indeed, the experimental curves overlapped partly the theoretical dissolutive curve and partly the theoretical diffusive curve [32,33]. Since LS are characterized by a matrix structure, as demonstrated by VPSEM observation, it can be hypothesized that a slow LS and gel dissolution in contact with vaginal fluids and a dissolution and diffusion of CLO first through LS and then through the gel network take place.

4. Discussion

The aim of this study was to verify the anticandidal activity of CLO encapsulated in a LS-based gel and, particularly, in LS constituted of TRIST and AL. This alkyl lactate derivative was added to the LS matrix to possibly improve CLO action. Indeed, it should be considered that CLO, although effective against *Candida albicans* infection, is also destructive to components of the normal vaginal microflora, often leading to an increased risk of infection or disease [41]. Since AL is the ester of lactic acid and a mixture of monobranched C_{12}-C_{13} primary alcohols, its hydrolysis produces fatty alcohols and lactic acid [42]. The latter can inhibit bacterial proliferation, as well as the action of lipases that decompose the LS matrix after in vivo administration. Thus, the presence of AL in LS should support CLO activity by controlling bacterial proliferation, re-establishing the pH of the vaginal environment, and modulating LS metabolism.

The preformulation study enabled to select 1% w/w as the optimal AL concentration for LS production; indeed higher amounts (10–30% w/w) hindered LS formation, resulting in collapsed and aggregated LS. The aggregation phenomenon could be attributed to interchain bonds between the AL C_{12}-C_{13} alkyl chains present on the surface of this type of LS. Contrarily, TRIC (30% w/w) led to more regular and structured LS, probably because of the affinity between TRIC and TRIST, both constituted of triglycerides able to give rise to LS by crystallization. As expected, AL presence permitted to increase CLO encapsulation in LS (Table 3). Indeed, it has been demonstrated that a binary mixture of two spatially different lipid matrices, i.e., a solid lipid and a liquid lipid (or oil), results in the formation of structured lipid carriers able to solubilize and encapsulate higher amount of drug with respect to carriers containing a single component [20,21,43].

The anticandidal study indicated, on one hand, that the encapsulation of CLO in LS improved its activity and, on the other, that the combination of CLO and AL in LS further increased the anticandidal activity of CLO, supporting our hypothesis. It can be supposed that the encapsulation of CLO within LS improves its activity because of a close interaction between LS and the fungal cells. It is known that *Candida albicans* adheres to epithelial cells, endothelial cells, soluble factors, extracellular matrix, and inert materials implanted in the body of the host. Indeed, *Candida albicans* adhesion is a prerequisite for colonization and an essential step in the establishment of infection. Namely, the physical interaction between *Candida albicans* cells is mediated by adhesins, the designated cell wall constituents. Thus, it can be reasonably hypothesized that an interaction between the adhesins of the fungal cell wall and the surface of LS occurs, providing a microenvironment able to facilitate CLO release and effect. In the case of the in vitro experiments, in the culture medium, the colonized LS should slowly dissolve and release CLO from their matrix by a dissolution and diffusion mechanism, resulting in a direct close contact of the drug with the fungal cells [44,45]. Conversely, in the case of a CLO methanolic solution, it should be considered that the dilution with the aqueous medium decreases CLO solubility, since CLO is insoluble in an aqueous environment. Thus, the CLO solution would be less efficacious against fungal cells with respect to CLO encapsulated in LS.

Since LS in their dry form cannot be easily applied on mucosae, we included them in a xanthan gum gel and verified the resulting gel suitability for vaginal administration. The obtained results were very encouraging. Particularly, the shear-thinning behaviour of Gel $LS_{TRIST/AL1}$-CLO, whose viscosity decreased when applying a certain force [38], suggests that the gel can be handled and, more importantly, it can easily coat the vaginal cavity, remaining in the application site without draining [8,46], as demonstrated by the leakage experiment.

The leakage and adhesion results agree well, both demonstrating the suitability of the Gel $LS_{TRIST/AL1}$-CLO for vaginal application. In fact, the gel exhibited a minimal leakage and a long adhesion time when applied on SVF agar plates mimicking the vaginal cavity.

Noteworthily, the in vitro dialysis results confirmed that the inclusion of LS in the gel was a successful choice. Indeed, CLO release kinetics were slower in the case of Gel $LS_{TRIST/AL1}$-CLO with respect to the other formulations. The control of CLO release should be attributed to (a) LS matrix, (b) AL presence, and (c) xanthan gum network. Xanthan gum has been described by other authors as a biopolymer able to control drug release. Particularly, it has been employed as a rate-controlling polymer for the development of matrix tablets [25], as a stabilizing agent and delivery vehicle for gold, alginate or iron particles [47–50], and in combination with other polymers to produce vaginal gels [8,51].

Remarkably, Gel $LS_{TRIST/AL1}$-CLO production can be easily scaled-up for industrial production. Nonetheless, in vivo experiments are required to confirm its suitability to treat vaginal candidiasis.

Supplementary Materials: The following are available online at http://www.mdpi.com/2073-4360/10/2/160/s1, Figure S1: Variable pressure scanning electron microscopy images of LS_{TRIST}-CLO (A) and $LS_{TRIST/AL1}$-CLO (B), Figure S2: Comparison of the theoretical (x) and experimental CLO profiles from LS_{TRIST}-CLO (A), $LS_{TRIST/AL1}$-CLO, (B), Gel LS_{TRIST}-CLO (C) and Gel $LS_{TRIST/AL1}$-CLO (D), The theoretical curves were obtained using the coefficient calculated by linear regression of the linearized form of Equation (4) (□) and Equation (5) (○).

Acknowledgments: The authors are grateful to Maria Rita Bovolenta for her help in microscopic measurements.

Author Contributions: Elisabetta Esposito and Rita Cortesi conceived and designed the experiments; Maddalena Sguizzato and Christian Bories performed the experiments; Claudio Nastruzzi analyzed the data and helped full discussion; Elisabetta Esposito and Rita Cortesi wrote the paper.

Conflicts of Interest: The authors declare no conflict of interest.

Abbreviations

LS	Liposphere
AL	C_{12}-C_{13} alkyl lactate
TRIST	stearic triglyceride
TRIC	caprylic/capric trigliceride
CLO	clotrimazole
VPSEM	variable-pressure scanning electron microscopy
MIC	minimal inhibitory concentration

References

1. Mukaremera, L.; Lee, K.K.; Mora-Montes, H.M.; Gow, N.A.R. *Candida albicans* yeast, pseudohyphal, and hyphal morphogenesis differentially affects immune recognition. *Front. Immunol.* **2017**, *8*, 629. [CrossRef] [PubMed]
2. Noverr, M.C.; Huffnagle, G.B. Regulation of *Candida albicans* morphogenesis by fatty acid metabolites. *Infect. Immun.* **2004**, *72*, 6206–6210. [CrossRef] [PubMed]

3. Ferrer, J. Vaginal candidosis: Epidemiological and etiological factors. *Int. J. Gynecol. Obstet.* **2000**, *71*, S21–S27. [CrossRef]
4. Zhu, W.; Filler, S.G. Interactions of *Candida albicans* with epithelial cells. *Cell. Microbiol.* **2010**, *12*, 273–282. [CrossRef] [PubMed]
5. Ravani, L.; Esposito, E.; Bories, C.; Moal, V.L.; Loiseau, P.M.; Djabourov, M.; Cortesi, R.; Bouchemal, K. Clotrimazole-loaded nanostructured lipid carrier hydrogels: Thermal analysis and in vitro studies. *Int. J. Pharm.* **2013**, *454*, 695–702. [CrossRef] [PubMed]
6. Foxman, B.; Muraglia, R.; Dietz, J.P.; Sobel, J.D.; Wagner, J. Prevalence of recurrent vulvovaginal candidiasis in 5 European countries and the United States: Results from an internet panel survey. *J. Low. Genit. Tract Dis.* **2013**, *17*, 340–345. [CrossRef] [PubMed]
7. Kyle, A.A.; Dahl, M.V. Topical therapy for fungal infections. *Am. J. Clin. Dermatol.* **2004**, *5*, 443–451. [CrossRef] [PubMed]
8. Andrade, A.O.; Parente, M.E.; Ares, G. Brazilian Screening of mucoadhesive vaginal gel formulations. *J. Pharm. Sci.* **2014**, *50*, 931–941.
9. Aka-Any-Grah, A.; Bouchemal, K.; Koffi, A.; Agnely, F.; Zhang, M.; Djabourov, M.; Ponchel, G. Formulation of mucoadhesive vaginal hydrogels insensitive to dilution with vaginal fluids. *Eur. J. Pharm. Biopharm.* **2010**, *76*, 296–303. [CrossRef] [PubMed]
10. Santos, S.S.; Lorenzoni, A.; Ferreira, L.M.; Mattiazzi, J.; Adams, A.I.H.; Denardi, L.B.; Sydney, H.A.; Schaffazick, S.R.; Cruz, L. Clotrimazole-loaded Eudragit® RS100 nanocapsules: Preparation, characterization and in vitro evaluation of antifungal activity against Candida species. *Mater. Sci. Eng. C* **2013**, *33*, 1389–1394. [CrossRef] [PubMed]
11. Cortesi, R.; Esposito, E.; Luca, G.; Nastruzzi, C. Production of lipospheres as carriers for bioactive compounds. *Biomaterials* **2002**, *23*, 2283–2294. [CrossRef]
12. Domb, A. Lipospheres for controlled delivery of substances. In *Microencapsulation; Methods and Industrial Applications*, 2nd ed.; Benita, S., Ed.; Taylor and Francis: Boca Raton, FL, USA, 2006; pp. 297–316.
13. Maniar, M.H.; Amselem, D.; Xie, S.; Burch, X.; Domb, R.A.J. Characterization of lipospheres: Effect of carrier and phospholipid on the loading of drug into the lipospheres. *Pharm. Res.* **1991**, *8*, 175–185.
14. Elgart, A.; Cherniakov, I.; Aldouby, Y.; Domb, A.J.; Hoffman, A. Lipospheres and pro-nano lipospheres for delivery of poorly water soluble compounds. *Chem. Phys. Lipids* **2012**, *165*, 438–453. [CrossRef] [PubMed]
15. Dudala, T.B.; Yalavarthi, P.R.; Vadlamudi, H.C.; Thanniru, J.; Yaga, G.; Mudumala, N.L.; Pasupati, V.K. A perspective overview on lipospheres as lipid carrier systems. *Int. J. Pharm. Investig.* **2014**, *4*, 149–155. [PubMed]
16. Barakat, N.S.; Yassin, A.E.B. In vitro characterization of carbamazipine-loaded precifac lipospheres. *Drug Deliv.* **2006**, *13*, 95–104. [CrossRef] [PubMed]
17. Shivakumar, H.N.; Patel, P.B.; Desai, B.G.; Ashok, P.; Arulmozhi, S. Design and statistical optimization of glipizide loaded lipospheres using response surface methodology. *Acta Pharm.* **2007**, *57*, 269–285. [CrossRef] [PubMed]
18. Haller, I. Mode of action of clotrimazole: Implications for therapy. *Am. J. Obstet. Gynecol.* **1985**, *152*, 939–944. [CrossRef]
19. Esposito, E.; Ravani, L.; Contado, C.; Costenaro, A.; Drechsler, M.; Rossi, D.; Menegatti, E.; Sacchetti, G.; Cortesi, R. Clotrimazole nanoparticle gel for mucosal administration. *Mater. Sci. Eng. C Mater.* **2013**, *33*, 411–418. [CrossRef] [PubMed]
20. Esposito, E.; Cortesi, R.; Nastruzzi, C. Production of Lipospheres for Bioactive Compound Delivery. In *Lipospheres in Drug Targets and Delivery*; Nastruzzi, C., Ed.; CRC Press LLC: Boca Raton, FL, USA, 2005; pp. 23–40.
21. Jenning, V.; Thünemann, A.; Gohla, S. Characterisation of a novel solid lipid nanoparticle carrier system based on binary mixtures of liquid and solid lipids. *Int. J. Pharm.* **2000**, *199*, 167–177. [CrossRef]
22. Lind, H.; Jonsson, H.; Schnqrer, J. Antifungal effect of dairy propionibacteria—Contribution of organic acids. *Int. J. Food Microbiol.* **2005**, *98*, 157–165. [CrossRef] [PubMed]
23. Dumitriu, S. *Polysaccharides in Medicinal Applications*; Marcel Dekker: New York, NY, USA, 1996.
24. Denise, F.S.; Petri, J. Xanthan gum: A versatile biopolymer for biomedical and technological applications. *Appl. Polym. Sci.* **2015**, *132*, 42035–42048.

25. Lazzari, A.; Kleinebudde, P.; Knop, K. Xanthan gum as a rate-controlling polymer for the development of alcohol resistant matrix tablets and mini-tablets. *Int. J. Pharm.* **2018**, *536*, 440–449. [CrossRef] [PubMed]

26. Jana, S.; Gandhi, A.; Sen, K.K.; Basu, S.K. Natural polymers and their application in drug delivery and biomedical field. *J. PharmaSciTech* **2011**, *1*, 16–27.

27. Griffin, B.J. Variable pressure and environmental scanning electron microscopy: Imaging of biological samples. *Methods Mol. Biol.* **2007**, *369*, 467–495. [PubMed]

28. National Committee for Clinical Laboratory Standards. *Reference Method for Broth Dilution Antifungal Susceptibility Testing of Yeasts*, 2nd ed.; Approved Standard, NCCLS Document M27-A2, No. 15; Clinical and Laboratory Standards Institute: Villanova, PA, USA, 2002; Volume 22.

29. Jahn, B.; Martin, E.; Stueben, A.; Bhakdi, S. Susceptibility Testing of *Candida albicans* and Aspergillus Species by a Simple Microtiter Menadione-Augmented 3-(4,5-Dimethyl-2-Thiazolyl)-2,5-Diphenyl-2H-Tetrazolium Bromide Assay. *J. Clin. Microbiol.* **1995**, *33*, 661–667. [PubMed]

30. Kaur, L.P.; Garg, R.; Gupta, G.D. Development and evaluation of topical gel of minoxidil from different polymer bases in application of alopecia. *Int. J. Pharm. Pharm. Sci.* **2010**, *2*, 43–47.

31. Bachhav, Y.G.; Patravale, V.B. Microemulsion-based vaginal gel of clotrimazole: Formulation, in vitro evaluation, and stability studies. *AAPS PharmSciTech* **2009**, *10*, 476–481. [CrossRef] [PubMed]

32. Peppas, N.A. Analysis of Fickian and non-Fickian drug release from polymers. *Pharm. Acta Helv.* **1985**, *60*, 110–111. [PubMed]

33. Siepmann, J.; Siepmann, F. Mathematical modeling of drug delivery. *Int. J. Pharm.* **2008**, *364*, 328–343. [CrossRef] [PubMed]

34. Natarajan, S.B.; Lakshmanan, P. Effect of processing variables on characterization of ofloxacin loaded liposheres prepared by melt dispersion technique. *Curr. Drug Deliv.* **2013**, *10*, 517–526. [CrossRef] [PubMed]

35. Garcia-Bennett, A.E. Synthesis, toxicology and potential of ordered mesoporous materials in nanomedicine. *Nanomedicine* **2001**, *6*, 867–877. [CrossRef] [PubMed]

36. Murgia, S.; Falchi, A.M.; Mano, M.; Lampis, S.; Angius, R.; Carnerup, A.M.; Schmidt, J.; Diaz, G.; Giacca, M.; Talmon, Y.; et al. Nanoparticles from Lipid-Based Liquid Crystals: Emulsifier Influence on Morphology and Cytotoxicity. *J. Phys. Chem. B* **2010**, *114*, 3518–3525. [CrossRef] [PubMed]

37. Karadzovska, D.; Brooks, J.D.; Monteiro-Riviere, N.A.; Riviere, J.E. Predicting skin permeability from complex vehicles. *Adv. Drug Deliv. Rev.* **2013**, *65*, 265–277. [CrossRef] [PubMed]

38. Han, C.D. *Rheology and Processing of Polymeric Materials. Volume 1: Polymer Rheology*; Oxford University Press: New York, NY, USA, 2007.

39. Garg, A.; Aggarwal, D.; Garg, S.; Singla, A.K. Spreading of Semisolid Formulations. An Update. *Pharm. Technol.* **2002**, *26*, 84–105.

40. Boddupalli, B.M.; Mohammed, Z.N.K.; Nath, R.A.; Banji, D. Mucoadhesive drug delivery system: An overview. *J. Adv. Pharm. Technol. Res.* **2010**, *1*, 381–387. [CrossRef] [PubMed]

41. Ross, R.A.; Lee, M.L.; Onderdonk, A.B. Effect of *Candida albicans* infection and clotrimazole treatment on vaginal microflora in vitro. *Obstet. Gynecol.* **1995**, *86*, 925–930. [CrossRef]

42. *Cosmacol Eli Data Sheet*; Sasol Germany, GmbH: Hamburg, Germany, 2014.

43. Iqbal, M.A.; Sahni, J.K.; Baboota, S.; Dang, S.; Ali, J. Nanostructured lipid carrier system: Recent advances in drug delivery. *J. Drug Target* **2012**, *20*, 813–830. [CrossRef] [PubMed]

44. Lajean Chaffin, W.; López-Ribot, J.L.; Casanova, M.; Gozalbo, D.; Martínez, J.P. Cell Wall and Secreted Proteins of *Candida albicans*: Identification, Function, and Expression. *Microbiol. Mol. Biol. Rev.* **1998**, *62*, 130–180.

45. Pendrak, M.L.; Klotz, S.A. Adherence of *Candida albicans* to host cells *FEMS Microbiol. Lett.* **1995**, *129*, 103–113.

46. Das Neves, J.; Bahia, M.F. Gels as vaginal drug delivery systems. *Int. J. Pharm.* **2006**, *318*, 1–14. [CrossRef] [PubMed]

47. Pooja, D.; Panyaram, S.; Kulhari, H.; Rachamalla, S.S.; Sistla, R. Xanthan gum stabilized gold nanoparticles: Characterization, biocompatibility, stability and cytotoxicity. *Carbohydr. Polym.* **2014**, *110*, 1–9. [CrossRef] [PubMed]

48. Deshmukh, V.N.; Jadhav, J.K.; Masirkar, V.J.; Sakarkar, D.M. Formulation, optimization and evaluation of controlled release alginate microspheres using synergy gum blends. *Res. J. Pharm. Technol.* **2009**, *2*, 324–327.

49. Xue, D.; Sethi, R. Viscoelastic gels of guar and xanthan gum mixtures provide long-term stabilization of iron micro- and nanoparticles. *J. Nanopart. Res.* **2012**, *14*, 1239–1258. [CrossRef]
50. Dalla Vecchia, E.; Luna, M.; Sethi, R. Transport in porous media of highly concentrated iron micro- and nanoparticles in the presence of xanthan gum. *Environ. Sci. Technol.* **2009**, *43*, 8942–8947. [CrossRef] [PubMed]
51. Ahmad, F.J.; Alam, M.M.A.; Iqubal, Z.I.; Khar, R.K.; Ali, M. Development and in vitro evaluation of an acid buffering bioadhesive vaginal gel for mixed vaginal infections. *Acta Pharm.* **2008**, *58*, 407–419. [CrossRef] [PubMed]

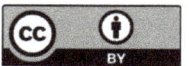

© 2018 by the authors. Licensee MDPI, Basel, Switzerland. This article is an open access article distributed under the terms and conditions of the Creative Commons Attribution (CC BY) license (http://creativecommons.org/licenses/by/4.0/).

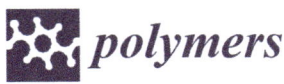

Article

Effects of Cyclodextrins (β and γ) and L-Arginine on Stability and Functional Properties of Mucoadhesive Buccal Films Loaded with Omeprazole for Pediatric Patients

Sajjad Khan and Joshua Boateng *

Department of Pharmaceutical, Chemical and Environmental Sciences, Faculty of Engineering and Science, University of Greenwich at Medway, Central Avenue, Chatham Maritime, Kent ME4 4TB, UK; sajjadkhan_1@hotmail.com
* Correspondence: j.s.boateng@gre.ac.uk or joshboat40@gmail.com; Tel.: +44-208-331-8980

Received: 13 January 2018; Accepted: 2 February 2018; Published: 7 February 2018

Abstract: Omeprazole (OME) is employed for treating ulcer in children, but is unstable and exhibits first pass metabolism via the oral route. This study aimed to stabilize OME within mucoadhesive metolose (MET) films by combining cyclodextrins (CD) and L-arginine (L-arg) as stabilizing excipients and functionally characterizing for potential delivery via the buccal mucosa of paediatric patients. Polymeric solutions at a concentration of 1% w/w were obtained by dispersing the required weight of metolose in 20% v/v ethanol as solvent at a temperature of 40 °C using polyethylene glycol (PEG 400) (0.5% w/w) as plasticizer. The films were obtained by drying the resulting polymer solutions at in an oven at 40 °C. Textural (tensile and mucoadhesion) properties, physical form (differential scanning calorimetry (DSC), X-ray diffraction (XRD) and Fourier transform infrared (FTIR) spectroscopy), residual moisture content (thermogravimetric analysis (TGA)) and surface morphology (scanning electron microscopy (SEM)) were investigated. Optimized formulations containing OME, CDs (β or γ) and L-arg (1:1:1) were selected to investigate the stabilization of the drug. The DSC, XRD, and FTIR showed possible molecular dispersion of OME in metolose film matrix. Plasticized MET films containing OME:βCD:L-arg 1:1:1 were optimum in terms of transparency and ease of handling and therefore further functionally characterized (hydration, mucoadhesion, in vitro drug dissolution and long term stability studies). The optimized formulation showed sustained drug release that was modelled by Korsmeyer–Peppas equation, while the OME showed stability under ambient temperature conditions for 28 days. The optimized OME loaded MET films stabilized with βCD and L-arg have potential for use as paediatric mucoadhesive buccal delivery system, which avoids degradation in the stomach acid as well as first pass metabolism in the liver.

Keywords: buccal mucosa drug delivery; cyclodextrins; films; L-arginine; mucoadhesive polymer; omeprazole; paediatric

1. Introduction

Gastro-oesophageal reflux involves movement of excessive acid from the stomach into the oesophagus. It affects a significant number of infants, exhibiting an array of symptoms, including physiological reflux, hematemesis, or even sudden infant death syndrome. Many of these children suffer from gastro-oesophageal reflux but with no definite causes or accompanying complications [1]. In addition, some investigations that assessed the effects of early therapeutic interventions showed that about 55% of the infants are free of any clinical symptoms by the time they are 10 months old and this increases to 81% by 18 months old [2]. That notwithstanding, it is still vital to identify which children exhibit gastro-oesophageal reflux-associated disease to allow selection of the most effective therapy for treating the manifestations of the disease [3].

Until recently, Cisapride which possesses 5HT-4 antagonist characteristics, was the drug of choice in gastro-oesophageal reflux [4]. However, due to cardiac dysrhythmias associated with its use, Cisapride is no more routinely prescribed for the condition. Although histamine receptor 2 antagonists (H$_2$RAs) can provide relief from oesophagitis, and high-dosage ranitidine (20 mg·kg^{-1}·day^{-1}) demonstrated as effective in refractory reflux oesophagitis, side effects such as nocturnal acid secretion present a limitation [5]. It has been shown that pharmacological tolerance of proton pumps inhibitors (PPIs) is good, safe for patients and an effective way of treating gastro-oesophageal reflux disease (GERD) [6]. PPIs are chemical compounds that inhibit hydrogen/potassium adenosine triphosphatase enzymes in the stomach wall, and providing relief from oesophageal, gastric and duodenal ulcers as well as from GERD [5]. They act by changing their chemical structure upon interaction with H$^+$/K$^+$ adenosine triphosphatase enzyme in the parietal cells, which leads to the formation of its active derivative through acceptance of a H$^+$ proton, thereby increasing stomach pH whilst reducing the secretion of acid from the stomach wall. Furthermore, the protonated derivative can bind with parietal cells in the stomach wall, and subsequently lowers the secretion of acid even further [7]. PPIs can be divided into: (i) competitive; and (ii) covalent, with the competitive PPIs exerting reversible inhibition of the proton pump mechanism in the wall of the stomach by binding to its extracellular surface. On the other hand, PPIs belonging to the covalent class cause inhibition, which is not reversible, and results in a longer period for the secretion of other enzymes. Initially, 2-methyl-8-(phenyl-methoxy)-imidazo-1,2-pyridin-3-acetonitrile and 3-butyryl-8-methoxy-4-(2-tolylamino) quinolone were the most common PPIs, however, more recent groups are composed mainly of benzimidazole derivatives such as omeprazole and pantoprazole [8].

Omeprazole (OME) is an effective therapy for treating ulcers of the stomach and duodenum often combined with antibacterial drugs to eliminate *Helicobacter pylori* [9]. For children suffering from GERD and demonstrating acute symptoms as well as those with erosive, ulcerative, or stricturing (narrowing) of the oesophagus caused by using endoscopy, a starting course of OME is the therapeutic regimen of choice [10]. OME is also used to prevent and treat ulcers resulting from using non-steroidal anti-inflammatory drugs (NSAID), and the dose of OME should normally be maintained in such situations even after healing of the ulcer to avoid chances of recurring [11]. Furthermore, OME is effective for treating Zollinger–Ellison syndrome and also employed to aid in reducing degradation of pancreatic enzyme supplements in children suffering from cystic fibrosis [8].

However, although OME is effectively absorbed from the gastrointestinal tract, the systemic bioavailability after oral administration is between 40% and 50% which suggests that the drug experiences significant first pass metabolism in the liver. Once it is absorbed, OME gets metabolized into three main metabolites: OME sulphone, OME sulphide and hydroxyl OME, all of which have been detected in human plasma [12]. Hydroxylation position 5 is subject to genetic polymorphism and the sulphone in plasma is accumulated in patients who metabolize S-mephenytion 4' hydroxylation poorly [13]. Another challenge with the drug is that, in aqueous solution, OME's stability is solely determined by the pH and rapidly degrades under acidic and neutral conditions, but shows better stability in alkaline environments [14]. OME is also rapidly degraded by heat, light and humidity [15]. These limitations present a formulation challenge in the design and manufacture of oral pharmaceutical delivery systems with optimum bioavailability due to its rapid gastric degradation [9]. To avoid such stomach acid breakdown, OME is formulated as enteric-coated granules in the form of capsules [2]. As a result, alternative formulations for administration via non-enteric routes such as buccal mucosa have been proposed [16,17]. These notwithstanding, the physical instability of OME remains an issue during formulation and storage and therefore requires stabilizing agents such as L-arginine and cyclodextrins.

Cyclodextrins (CDs) are oligosaccharides with cyclic configurations employed as excipients in different fields such as the preparation of inclusion complexes utilized in various dosage forms. They are able to form water-soluble complexes with poorly water soluble drugs which fit into their cavities [18]. The three main types of CDs are α, β and γ comprising 6, 7 and 8 D-glucose units respectively. The molecular structure of CDs involves glucopyranose units in 4C1-chair conformation connected through α (1 → 4) bonds. The glucose units are syn-oriented in which O-6 hydroxyls are on one side of the ring while the O-2 and O-3 hydroxyls are on the other side. The internal hydrophobic cavity of CDs facilitates their formation of inclusive complexes which allows their effective use as a drug carrier to improve drug solubility, chemical stability, dissolution and bioavailability or to decrease unfavourable side effects.

L-arginine (S-2-amino-5-guanidinopentanoic acid) is an amino acid which is basic in nature and presents naturally in human diets, especially foods such as meats and nuts. Arginine prevents the involution of thymic after surgery and helping in the increase of lymphocytes which is an essential agent for adequate wound healing. In addition, arginine is used as an auxiliary substance to increase the water molecular solubility of other compounds [19].

Metolose (MET) is a non-ionic water-soluble cellulose ether that is derived from pulp. Highly purified pulp is etherified with methyl chloride or a combination of methyl chloride and propylene oxide to form a water soluble, non-ionic cellulose ether. It can produce transparent films by casting from their gel solutions [20] and the film properties markedly depend on the moisture content [21]. MET comprises methylcellulose and three substitution types of hydroxypropylmethylcellulose (HPMC) each available in several grades (SM, SH and SE) with varying viscosities based on the type of esterification agent. The SM type is rich in methyl groups, SH type is rich in both hydroxypropyl and methyl groups while the SE type is rich in hydroxyethyl and methyl groups [22]. Some of the key properties of MET include solubility in cold water and forms transparent solutions; it forms reversible gels during heating due to its viscoelastic properties and the formed gel maintains its shape during heating [23,24].

In this study, we report on the stabilizing effects of βCD and γCD combined with L-arg for OME in polymer (MET) based mucoadhesive buccal films for potential delivery to paediatric patients. In addition, the films were functionally characterized for swelling, adhesiveness, dissolution of OME, its release kinetics and long-term stability over 28 days (four weeks). The originality of the research presented in this paper is the use of a composite stabilizing system combining CDs and L-arg within a polymer based mucoadhesive buccal formulation, which overcomes limitations of current oral gastrointestinal delivery.

2. Materials and Methods

The mucoadhesive polymer, Metolose (MET) was provided as a gift by Shin Etsu (Stevenage, Hertfordshire, UK). Polyethylene glycol (PEG 400), L-arginine (L-arg), gelatin and beta cyclodextrin (βCD) were purchased from Sigma-Aldrich (Gillingham, UK), ethanol, potassium dihydrogen phosphate and sodium hydroxide from Fisher Scientific (Leicester, UK) whilst omeprazole (OME) and gamma cyclodextrin (γCD) were purchased from TCI (Tokyo, Japan).

2.1. Formulation (Gel and Film) Development

Solvent cast films were formulated from ethanolic gels of the mucoadhesive polymer (MET) and loaded with drug (OME) as previously reported [17]. Briefly, the OME was dissolved in 20% v/v EtOH together with βCD or γCD at different ratios to form an OME solution as summarized in Table 1a. Subsequently, MET powder was slowly added to the vigorously stirred drug–CD solution at room temperature to obtain the drug loaded (DL) CD gels. The gels obtained gels were covered using parafilm, left to stand to allow the escape of air bubbles after which 20 g was poured into Petri dishes and left to dry in an oven set to a temperature of 40 °C [25]. Further, due to visually observed degradation of the drug even in the presence of either βCD or γCD alone in the ethanolic gel, L-arg was added in the CD containing gels as shown in Table 1b. During this step, L-arg (0.10% w/w) was incorporated into the gel whilst maintaining the concentration of the original OME (0.10% w/w), βCD (0.10% w/w), and γCD (0.10% w/w) constant [26].

Table 1. (a) Composition of omeprazole (OME) loaded metolose (MET) ethanolic gels containing varying concentrations of amounts of beta cyclodextrin (βCD) and gamma cyclodextrin (γCD), polyethylene glycol 400 (PEG 400) at a concentration of 0.50% w/w; and (b) optimized gels containing 0.50% w/w PEG 400, βCD and γCD as well as L-arginine (L-arg) in ratio of OME:CD:L-arg 1:1:1.

Gel Formulation Composition	Concentration (% w/w)			
	(a)			(b)
MET	1.0			1.0
OME	0.1			0.1
PEG 400	0.5			0.5
βCD	0.1	0.2	0.3	0.1
γCD	0.1	0.2	0.3	0.1
L-arg		0		0.1

2.2. Physico-Chemical Characterization

2.2.1. Tensile Properties

A texture analyser (HD plus, Stable Micro System, Surrey, UK) equipped with a 5 kg load cell and texture exponent-32 software program was employed. Thickness and width of the films were measured and entered into the software program and used to calculate the tensile parameters. The films free from any physical defects, with the average thickness of (0.07 ± 0.01 mm) were selected for testing. The films which were cut in the shape of dumb-bell strips were attached to two tensile grips which were 30 mm apart and stretched at the speed of 1.0 mm/s till they broke. The tensile strength (representing film brittleness), elastic modulus (rigidity) and percentage elongation (flexibility and elasticity) were calculated using Equations (1)–(3). Each experiment was undertaken three times (n = 3) and average values calculated.

$$Tensile\ strength = \frac{Force\ at\ failure}{cross-sectional\ area\ of\ the\ film} \quad (1)$$

$$Percent\ elongation\ at\ break = \frac{Increase\ in\ length\ at\ break}{Initial\ film\ length} \times 100 \quad (2)$$

$$Young's\ modulus = \frac{slope\ of\ stres-strain\ curve}{Film\ thickness\ \times\ Cross\ head\ speed} \quad (3)$$

2.2.2. Thermal Analysis

Hot Stage Microscopy (HSM)

These experiments were performed using a Mettler Toledo FP82HT (Greifensee, Switzerland) with a Nikon Microphot. Optimized MET DL films plasticized with 0.5% PEG 400, and containing OME:L-arg:βCD in ratio of 1:1:1 were placed on a glass slide, covered with a coverslip, and heated from ambient temperature to 200 °C at a rate of 10 °C/min. The changes in morphological behaviour with heating were collected in the form of a video recording with the help of a PixeLINK PL-A662 camera (PixeLINK, Ottawa, ON, Canada).

Differential Scanning Calorimetry (DSC)

DSC was performed for MET DL films analysed for HSM above and changes in their properties after the addition of PEG and OME within the films investigated. Small strips of each film (DL OME:L-arg:βCD 1:1:1), and starting materials (MET, OME and L-arg) weighing about 2.5 mg, were placed into hermetically sealed Tzero aluminium pans with a pin hole in the lid. The pans containing the samples were then heated in a Q2000 (TA Instruments, New Castle, DE, USA) calorimeter from a low temperature of 40 °C to 180 °C using a heating rate of 10 °C/min under constant flow of nitrogen (N_2) (100 mL/min) to evaluate the glass transition, melting point, crystallization and a possible interactions between polymer and plasticizer [27].

Thermogravimetric Analysis (TGA)

TGA analyses were performed with the help of a Q5000 (TA Instruments, New Castle, DE, USA) thermogravimetric analyser to investigate the amounts of residual moisture within the films. About 1–2.5 mg (n = 3) of the optimized DL films (films prepared from ethanolic gels plasticized with 0.5% PEG 400, and containing OME:L-arg:βCD 1:1:1) were placed into hermetically sealed Tzero aluminium pans. The films were then heated from ambient temperature (20 °C) to 200 °C at a rate of 10 °C/min under nitrogen (N_2) gas at a gas flow rate of 25 mL/min, to evaluate the residual moisture content of the starting materials (MET, OME, CD, L-arg) and DL films.

2.2.3. Scanning Electron Microscopy (SEM)

The surface morphology, general uniformity and the presence of any cracks in the optimized MET DL films were investigated with SEM. Films were mounted onto Agar Scientific G301 aluminium pin-type stubs (12 mm diameter) with Agar Scientific G3347N double-sided adhesive carbon tapes and coated with chromium (Sputter Coater S150B, 15 nm thickness). The coated films were then evaluated using a Hitachi Triple detector CFE-SEM SU8030, (Hitachi High-Technologies, Tokyo, Japan) scanning electron microscope at an accelerating voltage of 2 kV [28,29].

2.2.4. X-ray Diffraction (XRD)

XRD was used to analyse the physical form (crystalline or amorphous) of the optimized MET DL films. XRD diffractograms were obtained on a DIFFRAC plus instrument (Bruker, Coventry, UK) equipped with an XRD commander program. A Goebel mirror was used to produce a focused monochromatic CuK$\alpha_{1\&2}$ primary beam (λ = 1.54184 Å) with exit slits of 0.6 mm and a Lynx eye detector and voltage and current settings set at 40 kV and 40 mA, respectively. The samples for analysis were prepared by cutting the films into 2 cm^2 square strips to fit the square tiles of the holder. The films were subsequently mounted on the sample cell and then scanned between 2 theta of 0° to 70° with 0.1 s step size [30,31].

2.2.5. Attenuated Total Reflectance Fourier Transform Infrared (ATR-FTIR) Spectroscopy

FTIR spectra were obtained using a Perkin Elmer spectrophotometer (Spectrum Two, Perkin Elmer, San Diego, CA, USA) equipped with a crystal diamond universal ATR sampling accessory (UATR). Prior to the start of each sample measurement, the ATR crystal was cleaned thoroughly using tissue paper soaked in ethanol. During the measurement, the films made intimate contact with the universal diamond ATR top-plate, enabled by a pressure clamp to hold samples in place throughout the analysis. For each sample, the spectra representing an average of 4 scans were recorded in the range of 4000–400 cm^{-1}.

2.3. Functional Characterization

Functional characteristics were investigated for the selected optimized MET DL films (0.5% PEG 400, OME:L-arg:βCD 1:1:1).

2.3.1. Swelling Index (Capacity)

The swelling capacities of the films were determined by incubating the samples in 0.01 M PBS solution at a pH of 6.8 ± 0.1 (to simulate salivary pH) and heated to a temperature of 37 ± 0.1 °C. The films were cut into 2 × 2 cm square strips and placed into Petri-dish containing 10 mL of the hydrating solution (PBS) and initially weighed. At predetermined time intervals (5 min), the PBS solution was completely removed using a syringe and weighed again. Before the films were weighed, excess PBS solution was gently off blotted using paper towels. After weighing, 10 mL of fresh PBS solution maintained at a temperature of 37 ± 0.1 °C was placed back in the Petri dish using a syringe. The experiments were performed in triplicate (n = 3) for each set of formulated samples and the percentage swelling index (swelling capacity) was calculated using Equation (4):

$$Swelling\ Index(\%) = \frac{Ws - Wi}{Wi} \times 100 \qquad (4)$$

where Ws is the initial weight of the film before hydration and Wi is the initial weight of the film after hydration in the PBS solution.

2.3.2. In Vitro Mucoadhesion

The in vitro mucoadhesion experiments were performed using the TA HD plus Texture Analyzer (Stable Micro Systems, Surrey, UK) fitted with a 5 kg load cell. The film was attached to an adhesive rig probe having a diameter of 75 mm using double sided adhesive tape. A model mucosal substrate was prepared by first dissolving 6.67 g of gelatin in 100 mL of warm deionized water and pouring 20 g of the warm solution into Petri dishes with diameter of 88 mm diameter and allowed to set as a solid gel. To allow proper simulation of the oral buccal mucosa and the surface of the set gelatin gel was equilibrated with 0.5 mL PBS (pH 6.8) to represent the buccal mucosa [32]. The film was attached to the texture analyser probe and placed in contact with the equilibrated gelatin gel for a period of 60 s to provide optimal contact and hydration. The following settings: pre-test speed 0.5 mm/s; test speed 0.5 mm/s; post-test speed 1.0 mm/s; applied force 1 N; trigger type auto; trigger force 0.05 N and return distance of 10.0 mm, in tension mode were used during the measurements and Texture Exponent 32 software was used to record and process the data. The peak adhesive force (PAF) required to completely detach the film from the gelatin surface was determined by the maximum force, area under the curve (AUC) representing the total work of adhesion (TWA) was estimated from the force-distance plot and the cohesiveness of the sample was determined by the distance travelled by the film before complete detachment.

2.3.3. In Vitro Release of Omeprazole (OME) Using Franz-Type Diffusion Cell

Prior to investigating the drug release and dissolution profiles, drug assay and uniformity of OME within the film was determined. This was determined by first weighing the film accurately to a weight of 5 mg (n = 3) and hydrating in 8 mL of 0.01 M PBS solution at a pH of 6.8 and stirred at a temperature of 37 ± 0.5 °C until completely dissolved. The concentration of OME was analysed using HPLC (as described below).

For the in vitro drug dissolution studies, a Franz-type diffusion cell was used comprising donor compartment and receiver compartment. Five milligrams of the optimized MET DL film were placed in the donor compartment on stainless steel wire mesh (0.5 mm × 0.5 mm) which separated the donor and receiver compartments, with the mucoadhesive surface in contact with the wire mesh and facing the receiver compartment of the Franz diffusion cell [33]. The receiver chamber was filled with 8 mL of 0.01 M PBS pH 6.8, 37 °C and magnetically stirred at a speed of 250 rev/min. The chambers were held together with the help of a cell clamp and also sealed with parafilm to reduce evaporation. At predetermined time intervals, aliquots (1 mL) of the PBS medium was sampled and replaced with the same amount of fresh solution to keep the total volume constant over a 2 h period. The sampled dissolution medium was first filtered into an HPLC sample vial and analysed at 302 nm using HPLC (see Section 2.2.4). The concentration of OME released from the film was determined from the linearized calibration curve (R^2 > 0.99) and percentage cumulative drug release profiles plotted.

2.4. Drug Stability

Drug stability within the optimized films was determined by analysing the amount of drug present in the films after storing under two sets of conditions. Samples were placed in humidity controlled desiccators and placed in ovens at 40 °C representing accelerated conditions and the other at room temperature (ambient) over a period of 4 weeks. The MET DL film (OME:βCD:L-arg 1:1:1, PEG 400 (0.5% w/w) was placed in the desiccators and wrapped with aluminium foil due to its light sensitivity and to prevent moisture absorption by MET. For HPLC analysis, the stored samples were accurately weighed (5 mg) and hydrated in 0.01 M PBS solution (pH 6.8 ± 0.1 simulating salivary pH) in volumetric flasks (10 mL) and left to completely dissolve. Aliquots (1 mL) of the sample solution from each flask was removed and filtered into HPLC vials prior to analysis by HPLC.

An Agilent 1200 HPLC machine equipped with auto sampler (Agilent Technology, Cheshire, UK) with Chemstation® software program was used to analyse the samples. A Hypersil™ reversed phase ODS C18 HPLC column, with particle size of 5 µm and respective length and diameter of 250 mm × 4.6 mm (Thermo Scientific, Hampshire, UK), was used as the stationary phase. The mobile phase was prepared by mixing ammonium acetate and acetonitrile in the ratio of 60:40 v/v. The flow rate of the mobile phase was maintained at 2 mL/min and diode array UV detector wavelength for OME was set at 302 nm; with injection volume of 20 µL during each run.

3. Results and Discussion

3.1. Formulation Development and Optimization

The polymer (MET), which is a combination of hydroxypropylmethylcellulose and methyl cellulose, used in this study, was chosen because of its hydrophilic nature and well known swelling and mucoadhesive properties [34,35]. Stirring was applied during gel formulation to prevent formation of lumps which could occur through incomplete hydration, whilst heating the resulting mixture to a temperature of 40 °C reduced the viscosity of the final gels and helped air bubbles generated during stirring, to escape easily to the surface and subsequently released into the surrounding atmosphere. Furthermore, the reduced viscosity also allowed ease of pouring of the gels into the casting Petri dishes [36]. In addition, aqueous ethanolic solution (20% v/v of ethanol in water) was used as solvent because both OME and MET were more easily dissolved than water alone whilst also helping to reduce the drying time due to its volatility.

Physical Evaluation of DL Films

One of the major challenges with OME is its physical and chemical instability, and therefore a key objective of this study was to stabilize the drug within the MET films using CDs either alone or in combination with L-arg. When OME is added to water, it dissolves quickly to produce a clear solution. OME dissolves very rapidly in the presence of water to yield a clear solution, and its stability after addition of MET and PEG, plays an important role in the overall stability of the final DL gel and subsequently the film formulation [37]. However, it was observed that the drug quickly showed signs of degradation within 20 min with the colour of the gel changing to red. This is because OME is only stable in alkaline solutions above pH 6.5.

The stabilization of OME was attempted by introducing two different types of CDs (β and γ) into the DL gel in three different ratios as shown in Table 1a,b. Although the OME loaded gels remained stable over a longer period (hours) in the presence of βCD and γCD, the colour of the gel eventually changed to brownish-red suggesting that both CDs on their own could not sustain the stability of the drug during gel and film formulation. The visual observations made for the final appearance of the different films were captured with a digital camera as shown in Figure 1. On the contrary, the OME-CD complex within the gels and the final dried films was stabilized in the presence of L-arg as shown in Figure 2, clearly depicting desirable and optimum properties of homogeneity, transparency and uniform drug distribution. This is because OME is unstable at low pH but this improves at higher pH and the presence of L-arg provides a neutral to weakly alkaline environment which improved the stability.

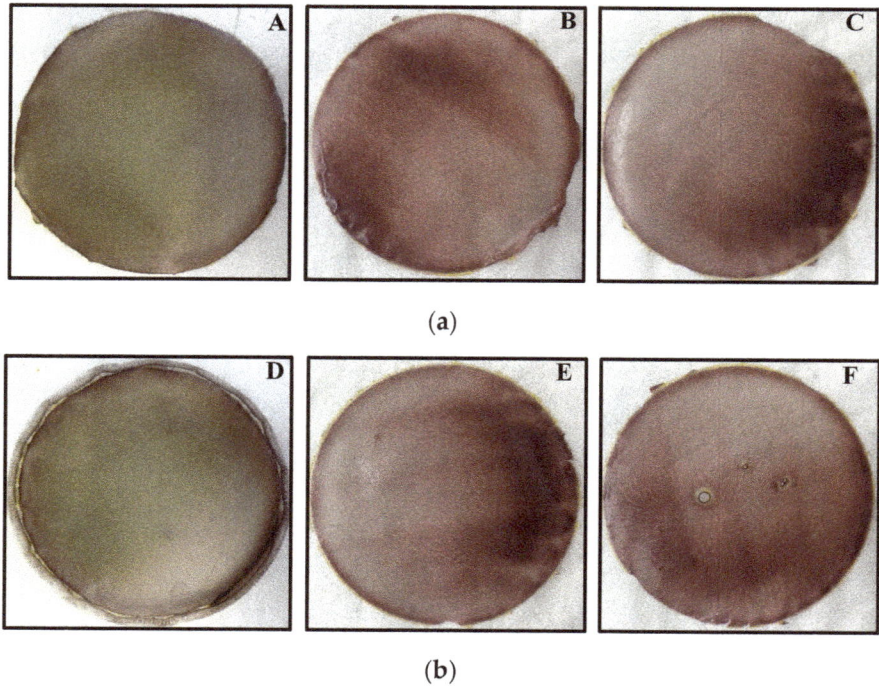

Figure 1. (a) Digital photographic images of OME and βCD loaded DL MET films in different OME:βCD ratios: (**A**) 1:1; (**B**) 1:2; and (**C**) 1:3 without L-arg, showing drug degradation indicated by brown coloration. (b) Digital photographic images of OME and γCD DL MET films in different OME:γCD ratios: (**D**) 1:1; (**E**) 1:2; and (**F**) 1:3 without L-arg showing drug degradation indicated by brown coloration.

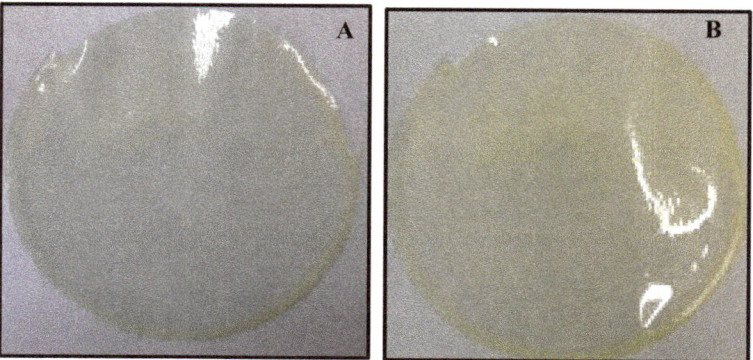

Figure 2. Photographs of OME and CD DL films: (**A**) βCD; and (**B**) γCD with L-arg ratio (1:1:1) captured using a digital camera showing stabilization of OME in the presence of L-arg combined with CD.

The molecular mechanism of how L-arg and OME interact with βCD by the formation of inclusion complexes, has been reported in the literature based on the work by Figuerias and co-workers [38]. They showed that with the presence of L-arg, the difference observed in the mean distances between the "e" and "f" atoms of OME to the centre of mass of CD's O4 atoms, which was considered as a reference to the centre of the CD inner cavity of the two complexes, was not significant [38]. They further suggested that for OME:L-arg combined in equal ratios, the H atom of the L-arg was nearer in proximity to the nitrogen atom of OME and noted that the distance between the H (L-arg) and the N (OME) was relatively small, and explained that this increased the probability of hydrogen bonds forming between the two compounds. The visual characterization for the physical appearance of the films based on the most ideal characteristics (transparency, ease of peeling and flexibility) are summarized in Table 2. In summary, based on the visual evaluation, it was determined that DL MET films combining either L-arg and βCD or L-arg and γCD in the ratio of OME:CD:L-arg 1:1:1 were most optimum and were therefore selected for further analytical and functional characterization studies.

Table 2. Ideal characteristics of optimized drug loaded (DL) films of βCD and γCD.

Polymer	Solvent	PEG (% w/w)	OME (g)	βCD (g)	L-arg (g)	Ease of Peeling	Film Characteristics
MET	20% EtOH	0.5	0.1	0.1	0.1	YES	Transparent/flexible
Polymer	Solvent	PEG (% w/w)	OME (g)	γCD (g)	L-arg (g)	Ease of Peeling	Film Characteristics
MET	20% EtOH	0.5	0.1	0.1	0.1	YES	Transparent/flexible

3.2. Physico-Chemical Characterization

3.2.1. Texture Analysis (TA)

Texture analysis was used to characterize the tensile behaviour of the films by measuring tensile strength, elastic modulus and per cent elongation at break of the DL films. The tensile properties were used to evaluate the effects of OME, βCD, γCD and L-arg on the behaviour of the plasticized MET films and the results used to further select the most appropriate formulations for further analysis. The effects of CD on the tensile strength values of the films are shown in Figure 3 and showed significant differences ($p < 0.05$) in the tensile strength (brittleness).

It has been reported that, ideally, the mean per cent elongation at break for thin films should fall somewhere between values of 30 to 60% [36] which is indicative of an appropriate balance between flexibility and elasticity. The βCD loaded film satisfied this required criterion, however, γCD loaded films gave a low per cent elongation at break as shown in Figure 3. Based on the previously identified ideal characteristics for a good film in terms of flexibility, uniformity and transparency, the formulations prepared from ethanolic gels containing 1:1:1 ratio of OME:βCD:L-arg and plasticised with 0.5% w/w PEG400 was confirmed to be the most appropriate for further investigations.

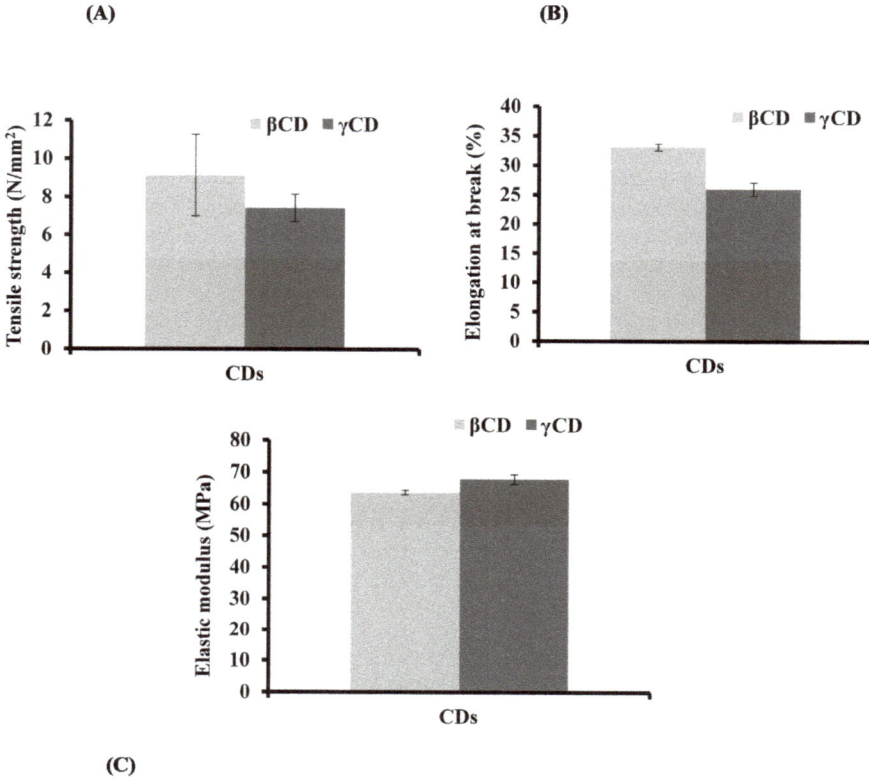

Figure 3. Tensile properties: (**A**) tensile strength; (**B**) elongation at break; and (**C**) elastic modulus of DL MET films prepared from ethanolic gels containing (0.5% w/w PEG 400), OME:βCD:L-arg (1:1:1) and OME:γCD:L-arg (1:1:1) (mean ± SD, (n = 3)).

3.2.2. Thermal Analysis

Hot Stage Microscopy (HSM)

The HSM results were used to aid the development of appropriate heating cycles during the TGA and DSC analyses and helped to determine the maximum temperature to which the samples could be heated. For the selected βCD containing films, the results showed that with increase in temperature, the surface of the film changed from rough to clear as a result of water evaporation from the film matrix as shown below in Figure 4. It has been reported in the literature [39] that βCD undergoes a melt transition between 290 °C and 300 °C. However, Figure 4 shows melting after 260 °C, followed immediately by decomposition.

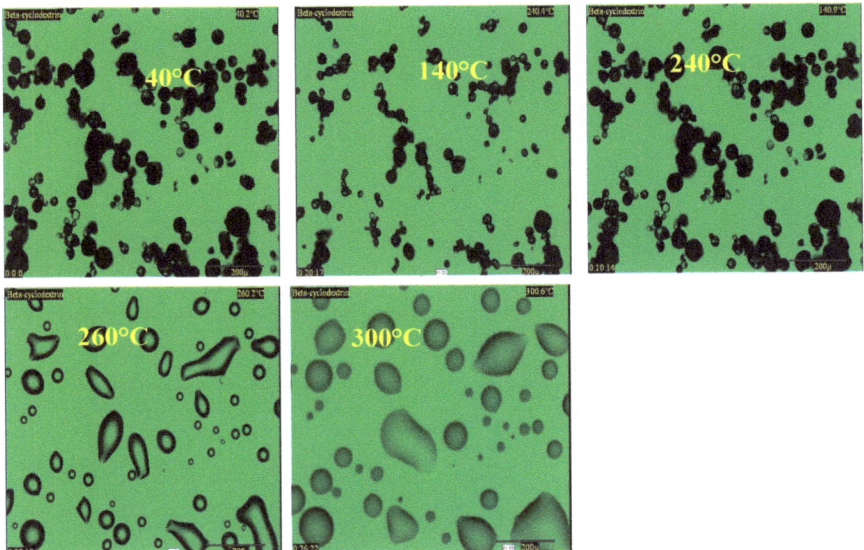

Figure 4. Hot stage microscopy (HSM) results showing selected optimized DL MET film containing βCD.

Differential Scanning Calorimetry (DSC)

DSC was employed to investigate the interactions between the components (MET, PEG 400, L-arg and model drug (OME)) of the formulation within the film matrix as shown in Figure 5a. The polymer (MET) showed a broad endothermic peak between 60–80 °C, caused by evaporation of water and no definite melt or glass transition peak, whilst pure OME showed a melting peak at 158 °C and L-arg at 100 °C, with pure βCD showing broad endothermic peak at 60.1 °C attributed to water loss with no definite melt or glass transition peaks (Figure 5b). The thermograms (Figure 5c) of plasticized MET DL films loaded with OME:βCD:L-arg in equal proportions, exhibited a broad endothermic transition with peak temperature of 62 °C and no melt peaks for OME and L-arg, suggesting films were amorphous. However, SEM and XRD analyses were further undertaken to confirm this definitively.

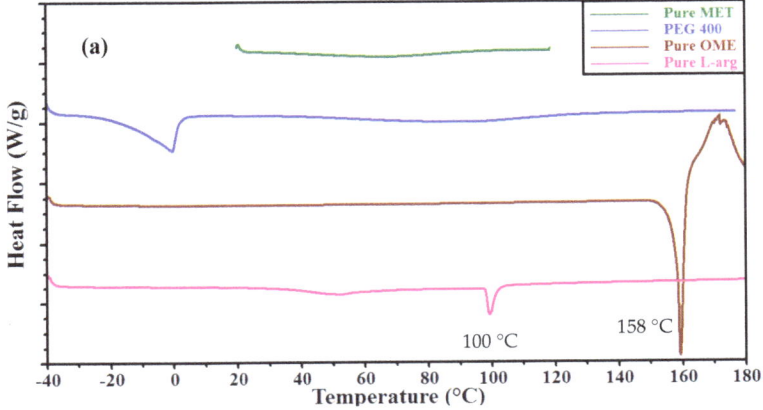

Figure 5. *Cont.*

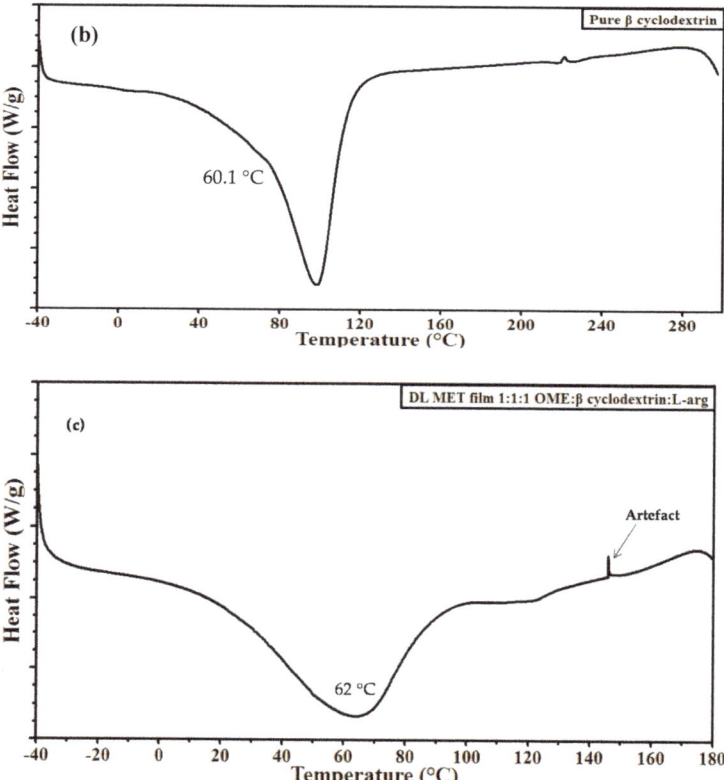

Figure 5. Differential scanning calorimetry (DSC) thermograms for: (**a**) the pure metolose (MET), pure omeprazole (OME), pure L-arginine (L-arg) and polyethylene glycol (PEG 400); (**b**) pure beta cyclodextrin (βCD); and (**c**) plasticized drug loaded (DL) MET films from gels loaded with 0.5% w/w PEG 400 and containing OME:βCD:L-arg (1:1:1).

Thermogravimetric Analysis (TGA)

TGA was employed to quantify the residual water content as a percentage of the total film weight. The water content for βCD after heating from ambient temperature (20 °C) to 100 °C was 13.09% whilst the MET DL films containing OME:βCD:L-arg (1:1:1) had a residual water content of 4.04%. The residual water was significantly lower for films compared to the pure βCD which is due to EtOH in the gels which increased the rate of water evaporation during drying to obtain the films coupled with the oven drying temperature of 40 °C. Such low residual moisture is expected to contribute towards the slower rate of OME degradation by hydrolysis, which is important given the known poor stability of OME.

3.2.3. Scanning Electron Microscopy (SEM)

The morphology and topographic appearance of DL MET films containing drug (OME) and stabilizers (L-arg and βCD) were analysed with the help of SEM, as shown in Figure 6. The results show that pure βCD appeared as irregular particles without any well-defined shapes.

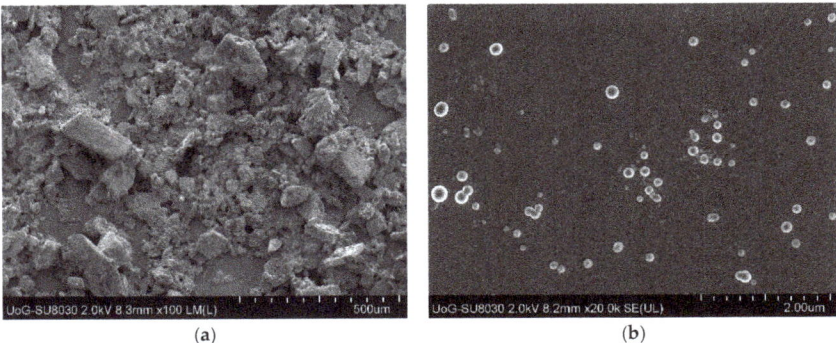

Figure 6. Scanning electron microscopy (SEM) micrograph of: (**a**) pure beta cyclodextrin (βCD); and (**b**) plasticized drug loaded (DL) metolose (MET) films cast from ethanolic (20% v/v EtOH) gels containing 0.5% w/w PEG 400 and OME:βCD:L-arg (1:1:1).

The topography of the plasticized films containing OME:βCD:L-arg (1:1:1) showed continuous sheets with relatively smooth and homogeneous surfaces and no pores observed. This suggests that all formulation constituents were uniformly mixed during gel and film formation. However, small structures with circular shapes can be seen on the film surface and could be attributed to excess OME or βCD precipitating out due to the rapid evaporation of ethanol and water during drying and film formation, but this requires further evaluation.

3.2.4. X-ray Diffraction (XRD)

XRD analysis was performed to investigate the estimated crystalline–amorphous ratio and confirm the physical form of the various components of the films. The XRD diffractograms of the pure βCD and DL MET films cast from ethanolic gels (20% v/v EtOH) gels containing OME:βCD:L-arg (1:1:1) with 0.5% w/w PEG 400 are shown in Figure 7.

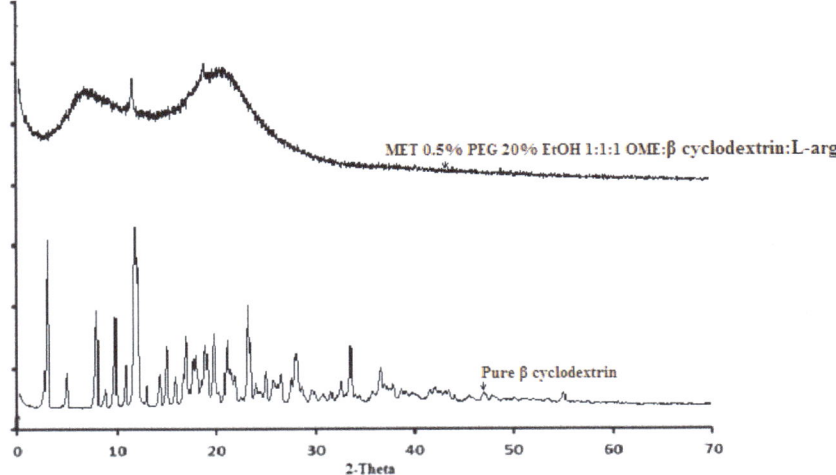

Figure 7. XRD diffractograms for pure beta cyclodextrin (βCD) and drug loaded (DL) metolose (MET) films cast from ethanolic (20% v/v EtOH) polymeric gels containing 0.5% w/w polyethylene glycol (PEG 400) and OME:βCD:L-arg (1:1:1).

The results show that pure βCD was crystalline and confirmed the DSC results. In addition, small additional peaks corresponding to pure OME and βCD were observed, which indicate small levels of crystallinity within the plasticized film, however, overall, the films were generally amorphous. The crystalline:amorphous ratio was estimated at 2% which suggests there could be small amounts of free OME and/or βCD present in these films and could be attributed to the small amounts of recrystallized structures present on the film surface according to the SEM images.

3.2.5. Fourier Transform Infrared (FTIR) Spectroscopy

FTIR analysis was employed to investigate molecular changes in the drug due to any interactions with the other additives present within the film matrix. The FTIR absorption bands of βCD are summarized in Table 3 whilst those for plasticized DL MET are shown in Figure 8. The FTIR spectra of DL MET films, showed the characteristic absorption bands of OME decreased in intensity which could be due to dilution occurring from addition of βCD. There were no new bands observed in the spectrum, which suggests that no new entities were generated from interaction between the film components, as shown in Figure 8.

Table 3. The observed characteristic FTIR bands for pure cyclodextrin (CD).

Pure Materials	Absorption Bands (cm^{-1})	Bands Assignment
βCD	998	C–H bending
	1077	–S=O stretching
	1152	C=O stretching
	1415	C–H stretching
	1644	–C=C stretching
	2925	C–H stretching
	3295	N–H stretching

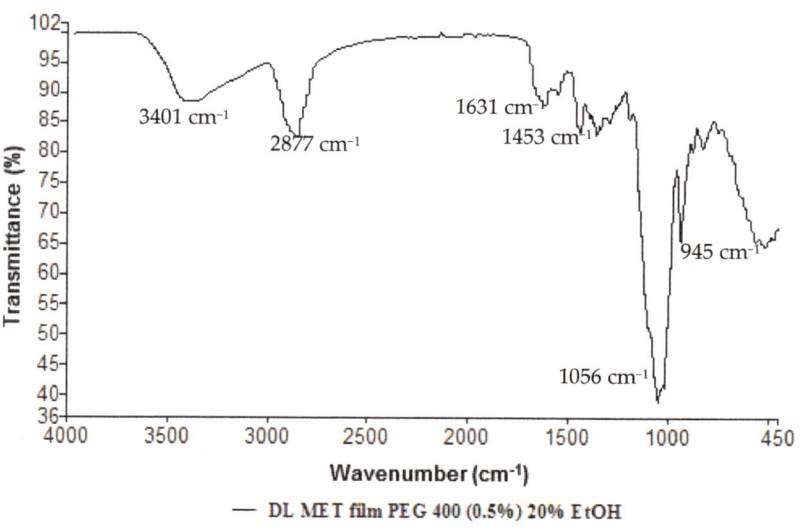

Figure 8. FTIR spectra of drug loaded (DL) metolose (MET) films obtained from ethanolic gels comprising 0.5% w/w polyethylene glycol (PEG 400) and OME:βCD:L-arg (1:1:1).

3.3. Functional Characterization

3.3.1. Hydration (Swelling) Capacities

Plasticised DL MET films containing drug (OME) and stabilizer (L-arg) (ratio: 1:1), without βCD, showed swelling index of 2630% in 20 min. After 20 min, the swelling remained constant or decreased (data not shown) due to a loss of structural integrity. On the other hand, DL film containing βCD in addition to L-arg showed swelling index value of 1197% after 20 min, which was significantly lower ($p < 0.05$) compared to the above DL film with no βCD. This can be attributed to the interaction between MET and βCD complex within the film matrix and therefore competing with water molecules for bonding interactions with the polymer chains with a consequent decrease in hydration rate and eventual swelling capacity. This is an interesting observation because it is generally known that CDs are highly hydrophilic due to a high number of available OH groups.

3.3.2. Mucoadhesion

Figure 9 shows mucoadhesion data for DL MET film with and without βCD and the results show statistically significant differences for PAF (stickiness) ($p = 0.0284$) and TWA ($p = 0.0522$) whilst differences between their cohesiveness values were not significant ($p = 0.2136$). This could be attributed to strong interaction (hydrogen bonding) between the polymer (MET) and the βCD both of which contain large numbers of OH side groups, therefore reducing interaction with the model mucosa surface.

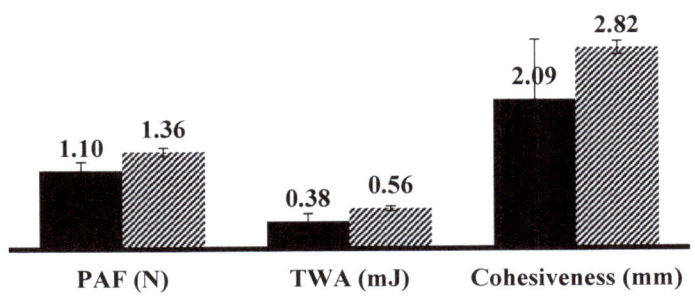

Figure 9. In vitro mucoadhesion profiles (peak adhesive force—PAF, total work of adhesion—TWA and cohesiveness) of plasticized drug loaded (DL) metolose (MET) film cast from ethanolic (20% v/v EtOH) gels containing OME:βCD:L-arg (1:1:1) using mucosal substrate equilibrated with phosphate buffered saline (PBS) (pH 6.8) of (mean ± SD, ($n = 3$)).

3.3.3. In Vitro Release of OME Using Franz-type Diffusion Cell

The release of drugs from matrix delivery systems such as films, can be controlled by diffusion from the swollen matrix, by erosion of the polymer matrix or by a combination of both drug diffusion and subsequent erosion of the matrix [40]. The dissolution profiles of the optimized OME loaded films were observed over a period of two hours because, after 60 min, the percentage of OME release remained constant. Furthermore, 2 h is the most realistic time frame for holding a formulation on the buccal mucosa surface before complete hydration or possible dislodging due to chewing or tongue movements [41]. Figure 10 shows the dissolution profile of the selected optimized DL MET film containing OME:βCD:L-arg (1:1:1) in PBS (pH 6.8). The profile shows an initial linear release phase for the first 60 min with the release reaching a maximum of 70% which did not change beyond 60 min.

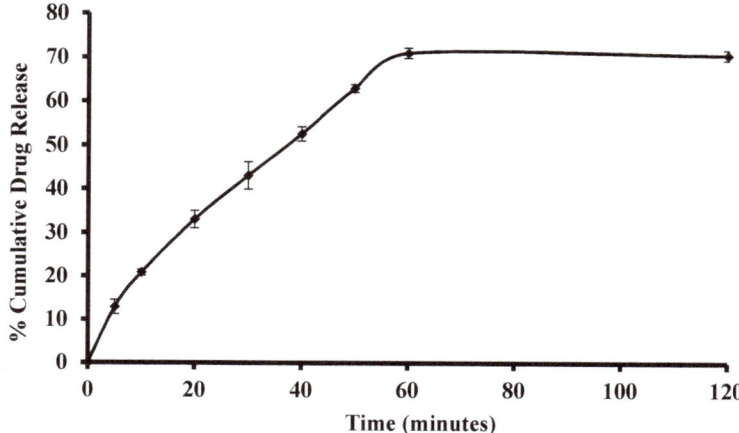

Figure 10. Drug dissolution profile of drug loaded (DL) metolose (MET) films prepared from ethanolic (20% v/v EtOH) gel containing 0.5% w/w PEG 400 and OME:βCD:L-arg 1:1:1 ratio in PBS at pH 6.8 (mean ± SD,(n = 3)).

The mechanism of OME release was investigated by fitting the drug release data to various kinetic models: zero order, first order, Higuchi and Korsmeyer–Peppas equations (coefficient, R^2 values) [42]. The release kinetics of OME in PBS (pH 6.8) showed that the drug release mechanism followed Korsmeyer–Peppas model as the R^2 value (0.9996) was the highest compared to other models. Further, evaluation of the release exponents (n) provides additional information regarding the specific molecular mechanism which controls drug release. OME release data from DL MET film containing βCD gave an n value of 0.6 which was greater than 0.45, which indicates that the drug release followed Fickian diffusion mechanism. This suggests that the OME was released through the hydrated (swollen) polymer via diffusion combined with erosion controlled drug release.

3.4. Drug Stability

The chemical stability of OME within the optimized MET DL film (OME:βCD:L-arg 1:1:1, PEG 400 (0.5% w/w), 20% v/v EtOH) was determined by way of a short-term stability study following ICH guidelines. The films were placed in desiccators and wrapped with aluminium foil due to OME's known light sensitivity. The films were also wrapped in paraffin film to prevent moisture absorption by MET and exposed to accelerated (40 ± 0.5 °C) and room temperature (ambient ± 0.5 °C) conditions (ICH guidelines) for a period of 28 days (4 weeks). The results depicted in Figure 11 show that there was a statistically significant difference ($p < 0.05$) between the per cent drug remaining within the film kept in the oven at 40 ± 0.5 °C compared to the one stored under ambient conditions with the latter remaining stable during the storage period. In the first 14 days, the drug content of OME in films kept at 40 ± 0.5 °C was 63% compared to 99% at room temperature and after 28 days the content of OME was 59% at 40 ± 0.5 °C and 99% at room temperature. These observations suggest that, when βCD and L-arg are introduced into the film, it maintains the stability of OME at room temperature (ambient ± 0.5 °C) conditions but not under accelerated conditions of 40 ± 0.5 °C. The results give an indication of the appropriate storage conditions for the formulated CD loaded films to maintain the stability of OME possibly prolonging shelf life.

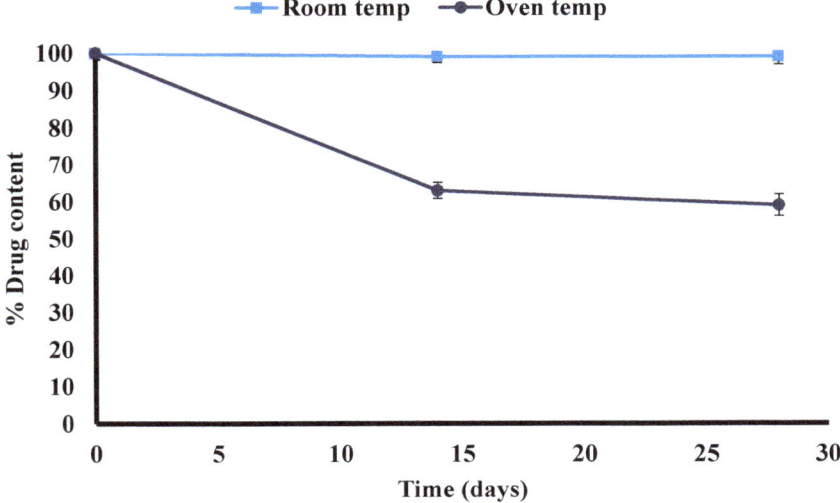

Figure 11. Plot showing the percentage of drug remaining within the film during storage at room temperature and oven temperature (40 °C) up to one month (mean ± SD, (*n* = 3)).

4. Conclusions

This study has shown the successful incorporation of both βCD and L-arg into OME loaded mucoadhesive buccal films prepared from MET for potential treatment of GERD in children. From the results obtained, it was shown that, when βCD was incorporated into the original optimized DL MET film, it did not significantly affect the DSC and FTIR profiles and drug release characteristics. However, there were changes observed in TGA, SEM, XRD, swelling and mucoadhesion properties. Furthermore, the OME present in βCD loaded mucoadhesive films remained stable at room temperature over a 28-day period. This study has also shown that, although βCD can stabilize OME, the short to long term stability of OME by βCD is also dependent on L-arg, which is known to increase pH to improve the overall stability of the drug. Finally, OME was most stable at room temperature over the 28 days compared to accelerated temperature of 40 °C, suggesting that the ideal environment to store the βCD/L-arg stabilized mucoadhesive films will be under ambient temperature and humidity conditions.

Author Contributions: Joshua Boateng conceived and designed the experiments; Sajjad Khan performed the experiments; Joshua Boateng and Sajjad Khan analysed the data; Sajjad Khan wrote the first draft of the paper; and Joshua Boateng revised a significant portion of the first draft and also interpreted the original data.

Conflicts of Interest: The authors declare no conflict of interest.

References

1. Choonara, I. Essential Drugs for Infants and Children: European Perspective. *Am. Acad. Pediatr.* **1999**, *104*, 605–607.
2. Lind, T.; Cederberg, C.; Ekenved, G.; Haglund, U.; Olbe, L. Effect of omeprazole—A gastric proton pump inhibitor—On pentagastrin stimulated acid secretion in man. *Gut* **1983**, *24*, 270–276. [CrossRef] [PubMed]
3. Melkoumov, A.; Soukrati, A.; Elkin, I.; Forest, J.M.; Hildgen, P.; Leclair, G. Quality evaluation of extemporaneous delayed-release liquid formulations of lansoprazole. *Am. J. Health Syst. Pharm.* **2011**, *68*, 2069–2074. [CrossRef] [PubMed]
4. Ameen, V.; Pobiner, B.; Giguere, G.; Carter, E. Ranitidine (Zantac) Syrup versus Ranitidine Effervescent Tablets (Zantac, EFFERdose) in children. *Pediatr. Drugs* **2016**, *8*, 265–270. [CrossRef]

5. Madanick, R. Proton pump inhibitor side effects and drug interactions: Much ado about nothing? *Clevel. Clin. J. Med.* **2011**, *781*, 39–49. [CrossRef] [PubMed]
6. Chen, L.; Chen, T.; Li, B. The efficacy and safety of proton-pump inhibitors in treating patients with non-erosive reflux disease: A network meta-analysis. *Sci. Rep.* **2016**, *6*, 32126. [CrossRef] [PubMed]
7. Chapman, B.; Rees, C.; Lippert, D.; Sataloff, R. Adverse Effects of Long-Term Proton Pump Inhibitor Use: A Review for the Otolaryngologist. *J. Voice* **2011**, *25*, 236–240. [CrossRef] [PubMed]
8. Nishioka, K.; Nagao, T.; Urushidani, T. Correlation between Acid Secretion and Proton Pump Activity during Inhibition by the Proton Pump Inhibitors Omeprazole and Pantoprazole. *Biochem. Pharmacol.* **1999**, *58*, 1349–1359. [CrossRef]
9. Stroyer, A.; McGinity, J.W.; Leopold, C.S. Solid state interactions between the proton pump inhibitor omeprazole and various enteric coating polymers. *J. Pharm. Sci.* **2006**, *95*, 1342–1353. [CrossRef] [PubMed]
10. Fass, R.; Fennerty, M.B.; Ofman, J.J.; Gralnek, I.M.; Johnson, C.; Camargo, E.; Sampliner, R.E. The Clinical and Economic Value of a Short Course of Omeprazole in Patients with Noncardiac Chest Pain. *Gastroenterol* **1998**, *115*, 42–49. [CrossRef]
11. Zimmermann, A.E.; Walters, J.K.; Katona, B.G.; Souney, P.E.; Levine, D. A Review of Omeprazole Use in the Treatment of Acid-Related Disorders in Children. *Clin. Ther.* **2001**, *23*, 660–679. [CrossRef]
12. Naseri, E.; Yenishirli, A. Proton pump inhibitors omeprazole and lansoprazole induce relaxation of isolated human arteries. *Eur. J. Pharmacol.* **2006**, *531*, 226–231. [CrossRef] [PubMed]
13. Wagner, C.; Barth, V.; Oliveira, S.; Campos, M. Effectiveness of the Proton Pump Inhibitor Omeprazole Associated with Calcium Hydroxide as Intracanal Medication: An In Vivo Study. *J. Endod.* **2011**, *37*, 1253–1257. [CrossRef] [PubMed]
14. Markovic, N.; Agotonovic-Kustrin, S.; Glass, B.; Prestidge, C.A. Physical and thermal characterization of chiral omeprazole sodium salts. *J. Pharm. Biomed. Anal.* **2006**, *42*, 25–31. [CrossRef] [PubMed]
15. Ruiz, M.; Reyes, I.; Parera, A.; Allardo, V. Determination of the stability of omeprazole by means of differential scanning calorimetry. *J. Therm. Anal.* **1998**, *51*, 29–35. [CrossRef]
16. Khan, S.; Trivedi, V.; Boateng, J.S. Functional physico-chemical, ex vivo permeation and cell viability characterization of omeprazole loaded buccal films for pediatric drug delivery. *Int. J. Pharm.* **2016**, *500*, 217–226. [CrossRef] [PubMed]
17. Khan, S.; Mitchell, J.C.; Trivedi, V.; Boateng, J.S. Conversion of sustained release omeprazole loaded buccal films into fast dissolving strips using supercritical carbon dioxide ($scCO_2$) processing. *Eur. J. Pharm. Sci.* **2016**, *93*, 45–55. [CrossRef] [PubMed]
18. Das, S.K.; Rajabalaya, R.; David, S.; Gani, N.; Khanam, J.; Nanda, A. Cyclodextrins-The Molecular Container. *Res. J. Pharm. Biol. Chem. Sci.* **2013**, *4*, 1694–1720.
19. Alvares, T.S.; Conte-Junior, C.A.; Silva, J.T.; Paschoalin, V.M. Acute L-Arginine supplementation does not increase nitric oxide production in healthy subjects. *Nutr. Metab.* **2012**, *9*, 54. [CrossRef] [PubMed]
20. Csóka, G.; Gelencsér, A.; Makó, A.; Marton, S.; Zelkó, R.; Klebovich, I.; Antal, I. Potential application of Metolose® in a thermoresponsive transdermal therapeutic system. *Int. J. Pharm.* **2007**, *338*, 15–20. [CrossRef] [PubMed]
21. Roy, S.; Pal, K.; Anis, A.; Pramanik, K.; Prabhakar, B. Polymers in Mucoadhesive Drug-Delivery Systems: A Brief Note. *Des. Monomers Polym.* **2009**, *12*, 483–495. [CrossRef]
22. Rowe, R.; Sheskey, P.; Owen, S. (Eds.) *Handbook of Pharmaceutical Excipients*, 4th ed.; Pharmaceutical Press: London, UK, 2003; pp. 386–389.
23. Pásztor, E.; Csóka, G.; Klebovich, I.; Antal, I. New formulation of in situ gelling Metolose® based liquid suppositories. *Drug Dev. Ind. Pharm.* **2011**, *37*, 1–7. [CrossRef] [PubMed]
24. Csóka, G.; Marton, S.; Gelencsér, A.; Klebovich, I. Thermoresponsive properties of different cellulose derivatives. *Eur. J. Pharm. Sci.* **2005**, *25*, S74–S75.
25. Morales, J.; McConville, J. Manufacture and characterization of mucoadhesive buccal films. *Eur. J. Pharm. Biopharm.* **2011**, *772*, 187–199. [CrossRef] [PubMed]
26. Andrews, G.; Laverty, T.; Jones, D. Mucoadhesive polymeric platforms for controlled drug delivery. *Eur. J. Pharm. Biopharm.* **2009**, *713*, 505–518. [CrossRef] [PubMed]
27. Boateng, J.; Pawar, H.; Tetteh, J. Polyox and carrageenan based composite film dressing containing anti-microbial and anti-inflammatory drugs for effective wound healing. *Int. J. Pharm.* **2013**, *441*, 181–191. [CrossRef] [PubMed]

28. Engel, A.; Colliex, C. Application of scanning transmission electron microscopy to the study of biological structure. *Curr. Opin. Biotechnol.* **1993**, *4*, 403–411. [CrossRef]
29. Frank, L.; Hovorka, M.; Konvalina, I.; Mikmekova, S.; Mullerova, I. Very low energy scanning electron microscopy. *Nucl. Instrum. Methods Phys. Res.* **2011**, *645*, 46–54. [CrossRef]
30. Brügemann, L.; Gerndt, E. Detectors for X-ray diffraction and scattering: A user's overview. *Nucl. Instrum. Methods Phys. Res.* **2004**, *531*, 292–301. [CrossRef]
31. Dittrich, H.; Bieniok, A. Measurement methods. Structural Properties: X-ray and Neutron Diffraction. In *Encyclopedia of Electrochemical Power Sources*; Garche, J., Ed.; Elsevier: Amsterdam, The Netherlands, 2009; pp. 718–737.
32. Cui, F.; He, C.; He, M.; Cui, T.; Yin, L.; Qian, F.; Yin, C. Preparation and evaluation of chitosan-ethylenediaminetetraacetic acid hydrogel films for the mucoadhesive transbuccal delivery of insulin. *J Biomed. Mater. Res. Part A* **2008**, *89*, 1064–1071. [CrossRef] [PubMed]
33. Wang, Y.; Dave, R.; Pfeffer, R. Polymer coating/encapsulation of nanoparticles using a supercritical anti-solvent process. *J. Supercrit. Fluids* **2004**, *28*, 85–99. [CrossRef]
34. Papkov, M.S.; Agashi, K.; Olaye, A.; Shakesheff, K.; Domb, A.J. Polymer carriers for drug delivery in tissue engineering. *Adv. Drug Deliv. Rev.* **2007**, *59*, 187–206. [CrossRef] [PubMed]
35. Rajabi-Siahboomi, A.R.; Bowtell, R.W.; Mansfield, P.; Davies, M.C.; Melia, C.D. NMR microscopy studies of swelling and water mobility in HPMC hydrophilic matrix systems undergoing hydration. *Proc. Int. Symp. Control Release Bioact. Mater.* **1993**, *20*, 292–293.
36. Boateng, J.; Stevens, H.N.E.; Eccleston, G.; Auffret, A.; Humphrey, J.; Matthews, K.H. Development and mechanical characterization of solvent-cast polymeric films as potential drug delivery systems to mucosal surfaces. *Drug Dev. Ind. Pharm.* **2009**, *35*, 986–996. [CrossRef] [PubMed]
37. Cui, L.; Zhang, Z.H.; Sun, E.; Jia, X.B. Effect of β-Cyclodextrin Complexation on Solubility and Enzymatic Conversion of Naringin. *Int. J. Mol. Sci.* **2012**, *13*, 14251–14261. [CrossRef] [PubMed]
38. Figueiras, A.; Sarraguça, J.; Pais, A.; Carvalho, R.; Veiga, F. The Role of L-arginine in Inclusion Complexes of Omeprazole with cyclodextrins. *AAPS PharmSciTech* **2010**, *11*, 233–240. [CrossRef] [PubMed]
39. Armspach, D. *Bioorganic Chemistry: Carbohydrates*; Hecht, S.M., Ed.; Oxford University Press: New York, NY, USA, 1999; p. 458.
40. Tuovinen, L.P.S. Drug release from starch-acetate films. *J. Control. Release* **2003**, *91*, 345–354. [CrossRef]
41. Kianfar, F.; Antonijevic, M.; Chowdhry, B.; Boateng, J.S. Lyophilized wafers comprising κ-carrageenan & pluronic acid for buccal drug delivery using model soluble and insoluble drugs. *Colloids Surf. B Biointerfaces* **2013**, *103*, 99–106. [CrossRef] [PubMed]
42. Korsmeyer, R.W.; Gurny, R.; Doelker, E.; Buri, P.; Peppas, N.A. Mechanisms of solute release from porous hydrophilic polymers. *Int. J. Pharm.* **1983**, *15*, 25–35. [CrossRef]

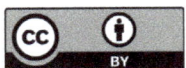

© 2018 by the authors. Licensee MDPI, Basel, Switzerland. This article is an open access article distributed under the terms and conditions of the Creative Commons Attribution (CC BY) license (http://creativecommons.org/licenses/by/4.0/).

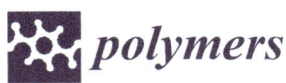

Article

Mucoadhesive Interpolyelectrolyte Complexes for the Buccal Delivery of Clobetasol

Venera R. Garipova [1], Chiara G. M. Gennari [2], Francesca Selmin [2], Francesco Cilurzo [2] and Rouslan I. Moustafine [1,*]

[1] Department of Pharmaceutical, Analytical and Toxicological Chemistry, Kazan State Medical University, 49 Butlerov Street, 420012 Kazan, Russia; venero4ka_87@mail.ru (V.R.G.)
[2] Department of Pharmaceutical Science, University of Milan, Via G. Colombo 71, 20133 Milan, Italy; chiara.gennari@unimi.it (C.G.M.G.); francesca.selmin@unimi.it (F.S.); francesco.cilurzo@unimi.it (F.C.)
* Correspondence: ruslan.mustafin@kazangmu.ru; Tel.: +7-843-252-1642

Received: 28 November 2017; Accepted: 8 January 2018; Published: 17 January 2018

Abstract: This work aimed to investigate the feasibility to design: (a) a mucoadhesive interpolyelectrolyte complex (IPEC) loaded with clobetasol propionate (CP) intended to treat oral lichen planus and (b) individuate an orodispersible dosage form suitable for its administration. IPECs were synthesized by mixing Eudragit® E PO (EPO) and different grades of cross-linked polyacrylate derivatives, in different molar ratios, namely 1:1, 1:2, and 2:1. All IPECs resulted at nanoscale independently of their composition (120–200 nm). Both zeta-potentials (ζ) and mucoadhesive performances were influenced by the ratio between polymers. On the bases of the preliminary data, IPECs made of Polycarbophil and EPO in the 1:2 ratio were loaded with CP. The encapsulation efficiency was up 88% independently of the CP-IPEC ratio. The drug encapsulation caused IPEC destabilization in water, as it was noticed by the increase of ζ values and the formation of aggregates. Oral lyophilisates were prepared by freeze-drying slurries made of placebo or CP loaded IPECs, maltodextrin with a dextrose equivalent 38 and Span®80. The optimized formulation permitted to obtain a fast disintegration upon contact with water reducing the tendency of IPECs to aggregate. Moreover, oral lyophilisates allowed improving the apparent solubility of CP throughout the in vitro release experiment.

Keywords: Carbopol; clobetasol; Eudragit® E PO; interpolyelectrolyte complex; mucoadhesion; oral lichen planus; oral lyophilisates; maltodextrin; resuspendibility

1. Introduction

Interpolyelectrolyte complexes (IPECs) are formed in aqueous dispersions by spontaneous association of oppositely charged polyelectrolytes due to strong but reversible electrostatic interactions [1]. The mild preparation procedure and responsiveness to various stimuli (i.e., pH, temperature, and osmolarity) without cross-linking agents or auxiliary molecules, e.g., catalysts, thereby reducing possible toxicity and other undesirable effects of the reagents. As the obtained polymeric networks are biocompatible and well-tolerated, they are exploited in drug delivery to administer both small drugs [2] and peptides or proteins by several routes, e.g., ocular [3], nasal [4], and oral [5].

Depending on the main features of selected polymers, IPECs exhibit peculiar physico-chemical properties due to their electrostatic interactions and flexibility. For instance, upon mixing two aqueous solutions of oppositely charged polyelectrolytes in a stoichiometric ratio, the resulting IPEC is insoluble and precipitates out [6], often as a colloid [7]. Then, the definition of a suitable drying technique, and the relative protocol, is required to improve their physical and microbiological stability. However, drying could also cause the formation of irreversible aggregates of irregular shape and size considering the IPEC dimensions.

Recently, a type of IPEC constituted by a poly(amino methacrylate) and an anionic polyacrylate derivative was proposed as mucoadhesive microparticles [8] which could be exploited in the treatment of buccal pathologies since it prolongs the residence time on a wide surface area. In contrast, the design of a suitable dosage form to administer a powder in the buccal cavity could be problematic in terms of dose accuracy and the easiness in handling. In the attempt to solve these issues, in this work we demonstrated the feasibility to prepare oral lyophilisates [9] containing mucoadhesive IPEC composed of Eudragit® E PO (EPO) and Polycarbophil®. This material was chosen among a homogenous series of cross-linked polyacrylate derivatives able to provide the original suspension with unmodified particle size and size distribution, as detailed in Scheme 1. IPECs were loaded with Clobetasol proprionate (CP) selected as a model drug since it is mainstay of topical treatment for oral lichen planus (OLP) [10]. It should be noted that despite many international guidelines refer that its topical application allows good management of this condition reducing systemic side-effects [11], dosage forms intended for buccal route are still not available.

The experimental work was organized in three steps, as detailed in Scheme 1, which summarizesthe the selection criteria and the most important variables to be considered. Firstly, placebo IPECs made of EPO and four different types of carbomers were produced to elucidate the effect of the polycomplex composition on mucoadhesive properties and physico-chemical features. IPECs with satisfactory mucoadhesive properties were loaded with different amounts of CP to investigate the maximum loading ability of IPECs. Secondly, placebo and CP loaded IPECs were formulated as oral lyophisates using maltodextrin as main matrix forming materials due to its excellent water solubility [12]. Finally, considering the low aqueous solubility of CP (~4 mg/mL) [13], the possibility to improve the drug apparent solubility was also investigated.

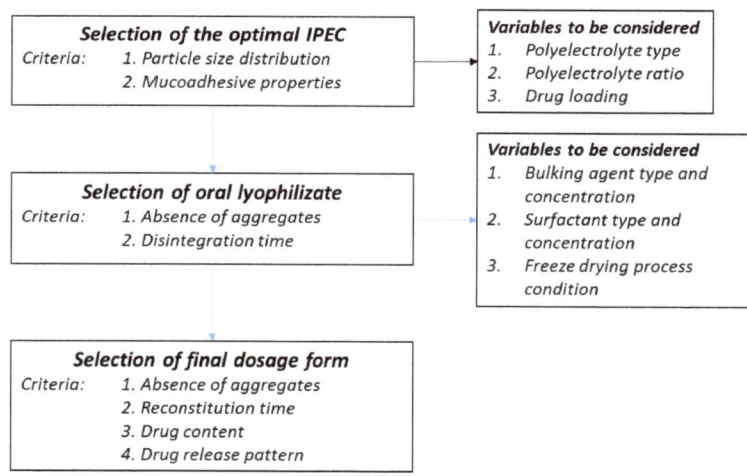

Scheme 1. Technological steps of preparing oral lyophilisates containing IPECs.

2. Materials and Methods

2.1. Materials

Eudragit® E PO (EPO)—a terpolymer of N,N-dimethylaminoethyl methacrylate (DMAEMA) with methylmethacrylate (MMA) and butylmethacrylate (BuMA), (PDMAEMA–co–MMA–co–BuMA) (mole ratio 2:1:1, MW 150 kDa) was used in this study as a cationic copolymer. Different grades of carbomer derivatives (Carbopol® 71G NF polymer (C71G), Carbopol® ETD 2020 NF polymer (C2020), Carbopol® Ultrez 10 NF polymer (C10) and Noveon® AA-1 Polycarbophil USP (NAA-1)) were used as polyanions. EPO and different types of Carbopol® (C71G, C2020, C10) as well as Noveon® AA-1 (NAA-1) were generously donated by Evonik Röhm GmbH (Darmstadt, Germany) and Lubrizol Advanced Materials (Wickliffe, OH, USA), respectively. Their main relevant physicochemical characteristics as specified by manufacturers are summarized in Table 1. The polymers were used after drying at 40 °C under vacuum over a 2 day-period. Maltodextrin with a dextrose equivalent 38 (Glucidex IT38, DS) was kindly gifted by Roquette (Lestrem, France). Span®80 and Tween®80 were provided by Croda Lubricants (Snaith, UK) and Carlo Erba Reagenti, (Milan, Italy), respectively. Clobetasol 17-propionate (CP) was purchased from SICOR (Pero, Italy). All solvents were of analytical grade, unless specified.

Table 1. Physicochemical characteristics as specified by Evonik (healthcare.evonik.com) for Eudragit® E PO (EPO) and Lubrizol Advanced Materials (lubrizol.com) for polycarbophil and different grades of carbomer used to prepare interpolyelectrolyte complex (IPEC). (Abbreviation: Monomers: AA—acrylic acid; EG—ethylene glycol; PAA—polyacrylic acid; crosslinking agents: AEPE—allyl ester of pentaerythritol; DVG—divinyl glycol).

Grade (Code)	Type of Polymer	Viscosity (0.5%, pH 7.5), cP	MW (kDa)	Mesh Size—Distance between Crosslinks (kDa)	ζ (mV)
C2020	Carbomer interpolymer. Type B (copolymer of AA and EG crosslinked with AEPE)	47,000–77,000	4500	11.4	-36.2 ± 2.7
C71G	Carbomer homopolymer. Type A (PAA, crosslinked with AEPE)	4000–11,000	3000	237.6	-51.0 ± 2.0
C10 *	Carbomer interpolymer. Type A (block copolymer of EG and a long chain alkyl acid ester)	45,000–65,000	3000	- *	-33.3 ± 2.1
NAA-1 *	Polycarbophil (PAA, crosslinked with DVG)	2000–12,000	3000	- *	-40.1 ± 2.1
EPO	Butylated methacrylate copolymer	-	150	-	45.7 ± 2.1

* No data available.

2.2. Synthesis of Placebo and CP Loaded IPECs

The conditions to optimize the interaction between chemically complementary grades of a polycationic (EPO) and a polyanionic (C71G, C2020, C10, NAA-1) polymer in the presence of CP were evaluated in an aqueous medium. EPO solution was obtained dissolving EPO in 1 M CH_3COOH. Then, it was diluted with deionized water to the required volume and the pH was adjusted to 7.0 with 1 M NaOH. Carbomer dispersions were prepared by dispersing and swelling the polymer in 1 M NaOH. This dispersion was diluted with demineralized water to the desired volume and the pH was adjusted to 7.0 with 1 M CH_3COOH. The EPO solutions were slowly poured into carbomer-CP dispersions [10]. The solutions and dispersions of copolymers and CP were mixed in different IPEC-CP weight ratios (e.g., 90:10, 80:20, 70:30, 60:40, 50:50 w/w), using three Carbomer/EPO ratios in synthesized IPECs (in equal quantities and with an excess of EPO or Carbopol®).

The optimal composition of IPEC (placebo) and IPEC-CP systems were obtained in a reactor system LR 1000 control equipped with pH- and temperature controlling units (IKA®, Staufen, Germany) under continuous agitation using overhead stirrer Eurostar 60 control (IKA®, Staufen, Germany) at 500 rpm. The feeding rate of EPO solution was about 2 mL/min and mixtures were stirred over a 7 day period. After the isolation, IPEC-CP particles were washed with ultrapure water (Smart2Pure UV/UF, Thermo Fisher Scientific, Waltham, MA, USA) and subsequently dried under vacuum at 40 °C (vacuum oven VD 23, Binder, Germany) over a 2 day period until constant weight. The samples were stored in tightly sealed containers at room temperature until use. The elementary analysis on placebo

IPEC samples was carried out by a Thermo Flash 2000 CHNS/O elemental analyzer (Thermo Fisher Scientific, Paisley, UK).

2.3. IPEC Characterization

2.3.1. Dynamic Light Scattering

To determine the hydrodynamic diameter (D_h) of IPECs, laser diffraction analysis was carried out using a Zetasizer Nano ZS (Malvern Instruments, Worcestershire, UK). This technology determines particle sizes in the range from 0.5 nm to 5 µm allowing the detection of particle aggregates in a suspension. Since the particle stability was not sufficient in pure water during a single measurement, Span®80 at the concentration of 0.25% was used as a steric stabilizer. The analysis was conducted at a scattering angle of 173° and a temperature of 25 °C.

2.3.2. Zeta-Potential Measurements

Charge was determined as the zeta potential (ζ) by using folded capillary cell at 25 °C using a Zetasizer Nano ZS (Malvern Instruments, Worcestershire, UK). The results are reported as mean ± standard deviation (n = 3).

2.3.3. Modulated DSC Analysis

Thermal analysis on IPEC, CP, IPEC-CP were carried out using a modulated differential scanning calorimetry (MDSC; Discovery DSC™, TA Instruments, Newcaste, DE, USA), equipped with a refrigerated cooling system (RCS90, TA Instruments, Newcastle, DE, USA). Samples of about 5 mg exactly weighted were sealed in Tzero aluminium pans (TA Instruments, Newcastle, DE, USA) and empty pan was used as a reference. The mass of the reference and sample pans were considered to normalize the data. Dry nitrogen at a flow rate of 50 mL/min was used to purge the DSC cell. Indium and *n*-octadecane standards were used to calibrate the DSC temperature scale; enthalpic response and heat capacity were calibrated with indium and sapphire, respectively. The modulation parameters were set as follows: 2 °C/min heating rate, 40 s period and 1 °C amplitude. Samples were analyzed from 25 to 250 °C. Glass transition temperature was determined in the reversing heat flow signals by using TRIOS™ software (version 3.1.5.3696, TA Instruments, Newcastle, DE, USA).

2.3.4. FTIR-Spectroscopy

ATR-FTIR-spectra were recorded using a Nicolet iS5 FTIR-spectrometer (Thermo Fisher Scientific, Waltham, MA, USA) equipped with a DTGS detector (Thermo Fisher Scientific, Waltham, MA, USA). IPECs, raw polymers (i.e., C71G, C2020, C10, NAA-1) and vacuum-dried IPEC-CP were directly placed on the iD5 smart single bounce ZnSe ATR crystal. The spectra were analysed using OMNIC spectra software (Thermo Fisher Scientific, Waltham, MA, USA).

2.4. In Vitro Mucoadhesive Properties of Placebo IPECs

The texture analysis was performed as previously described [14] using mucin as the adherent substrate [15]. Mucoadhesive properties were determined by using a software-controlled texture analyzer (Instron 5965, Instron, Pianezza, Italy) equipped with a 50 N force cell in adhesion mode. A flat faced compact of testing materials (weight: 170 mg, diameter: 11.28 mm) was obtained by applying a compression force of 10 tons for 30 s by means of a hydraulic press (Glenrothes, UK). Compacts were glued to the mobile steel punch. A mucin compact (weight: 130 mg, diameter: 11.28 mm) obtained applying a compression force of 10 tons for 60 s, was glued to a steel plate fixed at the bottom of the tensile apparatus. Both compacts were hydrated with 50 µL deionized water for 5 min to obtain a jelly layer. Upon making contact between the two hydrated compacts, a constant force of 1.3 N was applied over 360 s. The mucoadhesive properties were expressed as maximum detachment force (MDF), namely the force required to separate the IPEC compact from mucin upon

2.5. Preparation of Oral Lyophilisates

To set-up the freeze-drying parameters, the glass transition temperature of the maximally freeze-concentrated phase (T_g') of the aqueous solution of DS in the presence of different components was determined by a DSC 1 STARe System (Mettler Toledo, Greifensee, Switzerland). In brief, aliquots of about 30–40 mg were cooled below the expected T_g' at 1 K/min and kept at the temperature for 5 min. Thereafter, samples were re-heated at 5 K/min to room temperature. To optimize the tablet formulation, the effect of DS concentration and the presence of a surfactant (Span®80 or Tween®80) in different concentrations on the tablet disaggregation time and IPEC size were evaluated. The composition of tablets loaded with placebo IPECs is reported in Table 2.

Table 2. Tablet composition and its influence on hydrodynamic diameter (D_h) and zeta potential (ζ) of placebo IPECs after disintegration.

Tablet Code	Tablet Composition (%, w/w)					Disintegration Time (s)	D_h (nm)	ζ (mV)
	IPEC 1	IPEC 8	DS	S80	T80			
1	10%	-	40.9	-	-	6	149 ± 42 (54.9%)	n.d.
2	10%	-	81.8	-	-	n.d. *	-	-
3	-	10%	40.9	-	-	11	136 ± 16 (95.6%)	−26.6 ± 0.7
4	-	10%	81.8	-	-	n.d. *	-	-
5	10%	-	40.9	0.01	-	20	141 ± 0 (97.8%)	−26.6 ± 0.6
6	10%	-	40.9	0.1	-	6	132 ± 8 (90.0%)	−25.8 ± 0.1
7	10%	-	40.9	0.5	-	26	145 ± 8 (98.4%)	−26.0 ± 1.3
8	10%	-	40.9	-	0.01	n.d. **	-	-
9	10%	-	40.9	-	0.1	n.d. **	-	-
10	10%	-	40.9	-	0.5	n.d. **	-	-
11	-	10%	40.9	0.01	-	33	125 ± 10 (100%)	−26.3 ± 1.9
12	-	10%	40.9	0.1	-	12	111 ± 9 (100%)	−25.1 ± 3.0
13	-	10%	40.9	0.5	-	15	114 ± 12 (98.2%)	−19.0 ± 2.1
14	-	10%	40.9	-	0.01	n.d. **	-	-
15	-	10%	40.9	-	0.1	n.d. **	-	-
16	-	10%	40.9	-	0.5	n.d. **	-	-
17	20%	-	40.9	0.5	-	26	165 ± 1 (100%)	−46.9 ± 1.2

* Tablets presented an irregular surface due to the presence of bubbles. ** Tablets were sticky and, therefore, difficult to handle.

Aliquots of 200 μL were poured into the cavity of PVC/OPA/Al/OPA/PVC laminate blister (Catalent Pharma Solutions, Somerset, NJ, USA) and loaded into an Epsilon 2–6 laboratory scale freeze-dryer (Martin Christ Freeze Dryers, Osterode, Germany). The samples were frozen at the rate of 1 K/min to a minimum shelf temperature of −25 °C including two equilibration steps at 5 and −5 °C for 15 min to achieve similar nucleation temperatures. After holding samples at −25 °C for 1 h, the chamber pressure was decreased to 0.120 mbar and the shelf temperature was increased to −10 °C at 1 K/min to initiate the main drying. After 6 h of sublimation, the shelf temperature was further increased to 40 °C at the rate of 1 K/min to initiate the secondary drying. The sublimation phase was carried out over a 5 h period. Then, samples sealed under vacuum in glass vials were stored at room temperature.

Tablets containing CP loaded IPECs were similarly prepared by weighing the exact amounts of IPEC containing 120 μg drug per single unit.

The oral lyophilisates were characterized in terms of uniformity of mass and disintegration time according to the Ph. Eur. 9th edition. After disintegrating one or two tablets in 10 mL of filtered deionized water (Milli-Q™ Water system, Millipore Corporation, Vimodrone, Italy), particle size and zeta potential of placebo and loaded IPECs were also measured.

2.6. In Vitro Drug Release Test

The in vitro drug release test was performed according to a "sample-and-separate" method [10]. Considering the limited volumes of fluids in the buccal cavity, the in vitro release test was carried out in oversaturation condition in order to better discriminate the different features of CP loaded IPECs. Oral lyophilisates were placed in closed glass vials containing 20 mL deionized water and shaken in a horizontal incubator at 50 strokes/min and 37 ± 0.5 °C. At each time point, a volume of 4 mL medium was diluted with 1 mL acetonitrile, and the amount of CP released was quantified by the high-performance liquid chromatography (HPLC) method reported in Section 2.7. The withdrawn medium was replaced with equal volumes of deionized water.

2.7. HPLC Method

The CP content loaded into IPECs and released in the in vitro release test was assayed by an HPLC method using HP1100 Chemstation (Agilent Technologies, Cernusco sul Naviglio, Italy). Chromatographic conditions: column: Spherisorb ODS2, 4.6 mm × 150 mm, 3 µm (Waters, Vimodrone, Italy); mobile phase: 50:50 (%v/v) acetonitrile:water; flow rate: 1.0 mL/min; wavelength: 240 nm; injection volume: 20 µL. The drug concentrations were determined from standard curves ranging from 0.1 to 50 µg/mL [9].

3. Results

3.1. Characterization of Placebo IPECs

All IPECs obtained by mixing EPO and four types of carbomers differing in chemical composition, molecular weight, or cross-linking were insoluble in water. To evaluate the possible interactions between components, a physicochemical study was carried out by MDSC and FTIR spectroscopy. According to the FTIR spectra, a new absorption band at 1560 cm^{-1} appeared in the IPEC with respect to the raw materials, suggesting the formation of a new chemically individual compound (Figure 1).

This absorption band is diagnostic of the formation of ionic bonds between carboxyl groups of Carbopol® and dimethylamino groups of EPO [16–19] and responsible for complex insolubilization. MDSC data supported the formation of such interaction at a molecular level. EPO and carbomer are both amorphous polymers with a characteristic T_g value (Table 3). After IPEC formation, a single value of T_g was detected independently of the nature of anionic polyelectrolytes suggesting the absence of microdomains of free copolymer. Moreover, the shift of T_g towards higher values with respect to the starting polymers, suggests the formation of a stiffer material. The elementary analysis of IPEC after washing revealed the presence of an excess of carbomer polymers in all samples (Table 3).

Regarding the particle size and particle size distribution, C10 and C2020, which provide substantially more viscous solutions than the low molecular weight counterpart, allowed the formation of nanoparticles (Table 4) and aggregates sizing about 5 µm. The percentage of this population of large particles considerably increased decreasing the EPO content (Table 4). In contrast, the mixing of NAA-1 and EPO led to the formation of nanoparticles of about 160 nm with a monomodal distribution (Table 4).

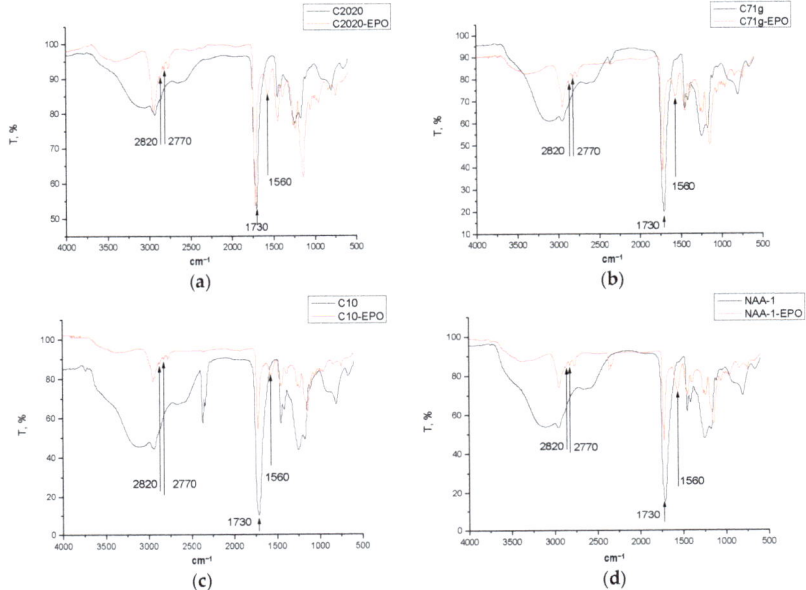

Figure 1. ATR-FTIR-spectra of C2020 and IPEC C2020/EPO (**a**); C71G and IPEC C71G/EPO (**b**); C10 and IPEC C10/EPO (**c**); and NAA-1 and IPEC NAA-1/EPO (**d**).

Table 3. MDSC data on raw materials and placebo IPECs.

Samples Name	T_g (°C)	Composition (mol/mol)
EPO	52.1 ± 1.2	-
C71G	129.5 ± 1.2	-
C2020	125.2 ± 1.2	-
C10	126.5 ± 1.2	-
NAA-1	131.3 ± 1.5	-
C71G/EPO	132.8 ± 1.2	2.12:1 *
C2020/EPO	133.5 ± 1.2	1.73:1 *
C10/EPO	134.8 ± 1.1	2.11:1 *
NAA-1/EPO	138.5 ± 1.3	1.66:1 *

* The composition of carbomer/EPO (mol/mol) IPECs is referred to the elementary analysis.

Table 4. Main physical features, namely hydrodynamic diameter (D_h), zeta potential (ζ), and mucoadhesive properties of placebo IPECs. The value in the brackets refers to the percentage of the main population.

IPEC Code	Composition (%, w/w)					ζ (mV)	D_h (nm)	MDF (kPa)	WA (mJ)
	EPO	NAA1	C10	C71G	C2020				
1	67	33	-	-	-	14.7 ± 0.5	154 ± 9 (98.0%)	111 ± 10	2611 ± 413
2	50	50	-	-	-	−5.5 ± 2.5	154 ± 0 (97.6%)	100 ± 13	1848 ± 335
3	33	67	-	-	-	−16.0 ± 0.4	168 ± 4 (96.1%)	49 ± 6	741 ± 33
4	67	-	33	-	-	7.7 ± 1.0	222 ± 9 (94.1%)	85 ± 20	1462 ± 210
5	50	-	50	-	-	−5.1 ± 0.9	158 ± 4 (96.2%)	103 ± 1	2154 ± 66
6	33	-	67	-	-	−13.7 ± 0.5	149 ± 13 (52.7%)	45 ± 6	643 ± 57
7	67	-	-	33	-	4.3 ± 1.6	195 ± 12 (63.7%)	94 ± 17	1902 ± 322
8	50	-	-	50	-	−47.8 ± 2.7	175 ± 17 (97.2%)	67 ± 31	1272 ± 448
9	33	-	-	67	-	−28.8 ± 1.7	188 ± 9 (96.4%)	55 ± 9	1010 ± 95
10	67	-	-	-	33	−28.2 ± 4.0	166 ± 9 (90.0%)	89 ± 25	656 ± 51
11	50	-	-	-	50	−28.2 ± 3.5	192 ± 11 (83.3%)	43 ± 2	678 ± 25
12	33	-	-	-	67	−20.6 ± 1.8	225 ± 9 (71.9%)	57 ± 5	802 ± 109

Chitosan (positive control): MDF = 62 ± 10 kPa; WA = 1682 ± 162 mJ. Polyethylene (negative control): MDF = 13 ± 1 kPa; WA = 407 ± 175 mJ.

The evolution of zeta potential as a function of IPEC composition, which can be considered as an indication of the degree of inter-particle interaction, is summarized in Table 4. As the carbomer concentration increased from 33% to 67%, the zeta potential values shifted from 15 mV to a negative value according to the extent and the type of anionic copolymer used for the preparation of IPEC. This feature can be attributed to the presence of negatively charged carboxyl groups of Carbopol®, which do not participate to the formation of ionic bonds with the positively charged dimethylamino groups of EPO. Moreover, increasing the concentration of polyacrylate within the complex, the number of such carboxylic groups also increases, which give a negative charge to the IPEC particles.

The mucoadhesive properties (in terms of both WA and MDF) of the complexes made with EPO and different types of polyacrylate are reported in Table 4. All the IPEC compositions showed good mucoadhesive properties, since both MDF and WA were statistically higher than those measured using the negative control. As expected, the mucoadhesive performances of IPECs were influenced by the ratio between the polymers. The higher the EPO amount in each IPEC series, the higher the mucoadhesive properties. Indeed, when EPO concentration was 67%, the change of the IPEC charge from negative to positive values, as estimated by the zeta potential, allows the dimethylamino groups of EPO to interact by ionic bonds with the negatively charged ionized groups of sialic acid at the terminus of mucin subunits. The lower values of MDF, associated to a more negative of zeta potential, might be the result of greater repulsion between negative charges of mucin and IPECs.

These results indicate that mucoadhesion of IPECs made of C10, C71G, and NAA-1 are mainly attributed to the formation of electrostatic interactions. On the other hand, such mechanism of interaction cannot help to explain the behaviour of IPEC made with C2020, for which a less negative zeta potential in comparison with the raw polymer (C2020) was related to weaker mucoadhesion. Indeed, beyond the zeta potential values, other features of polymers (e.g., chemical composition and structure) can influence their ability to adhere to mucosa [20]. In the case of raw polymers, the more negative zeta potential may establish a better uncoiling to interpenetrate with oligosaccharide mucin chains. The mucoadhesion of C2020/EPO IPEC can be attributed by the formation of hydrogen bonds between carboxyl groups of Carbopol® and mucin, since mucoadhesion of polymers containing weak anionic carboxyl, such as polyacrylic acid (Carbopol®), is often related to the formation of hydrogen bonds with mucin [21].

3.2. Oral Lyophilisates Containing Placebo IPEC

The physico-chemical characterization of placebo IPECs permitted to consider two materials worth of further characterization. In particular, C71G/EPO (50:50) and NAA-1/EPO (33:67) were chosen based on the zeta potential value (Table 4) to evaluate how the superficial properties can affect the formulation of oral lyophilisates and resuspendibility. In addition, IPEC made of NAA-1/EPO (33:67) is characterized by the highest rates of mucoadhesion (Table 4), which can also influence the properties of the final dosage form. To obtain oral lyophilisates with suitable characteristics, it is necessary to tune up both the formulation and the lyophilization parameters. Of fundamental importance to preserve IPEC nano-size during the lyophilization process is the selection of the type and concentration of lyoprotectants and steric stabilizers. The "vitrification hypothesis" suggests the possible role of lyoprotectants during freezing: saccharides form a glassy system, known also as cryo-concentrated phase, where nanoparticles are immobilized and preserved from the ice crystals [22]. Besides lyoprotectants, steric stabilizers can improve the nanoparticles stability during the lyophilization according to the "water replacement theory". This theory suggests that the hydrogen bonds between water and nanoparticles are replaced by interactions occurring onto nanoparticles surface with the adsorbed steric stabilizer, thus avoiding particle aggregation or fusion [23]. Steric stabilizers are generally polymers and surfactants, such as polysorbates and poly(vinyl alcohol).

Once both lyoprotectants and steric stabilizers are defined, an adequate lyophilization cycle is designed based on the T_g' and the T_c. Indeed, the formulation is required to be cooled below its T_g'

to assure the complete solidification [24] and Tc, which is the maximum allowable temperature of product during primary drying, to avoid the collapse [25]. Thermal analysis indicated that the T_g' of a DS solution at 40% was -21.81 ± 0.3 °C without being significantly affected by the presence of the surfactant ($T_g' = -20.56 \pm 0.25$ °C); meanwhile the dispersion of 10% IPEC caused a slight increase in T_g' value to -19.10 ± 0.04 °C, as exemplified in Figure 2. Hence, the samples were frozen at the temperature of -25 °C, considering a safety product margin of about 2 °C [21].

The final concentrations of the additives (i.e., lyoprotectants and steric stabilizers) in the formulations containing IPEC are reported in Table 2. All freeze-dried tablets loaded with IPEC presented as a white spongy texture. The tablets occupied the same volume of the original frozen mass and no shrinkage or cake collapse was observed, demonstrating that the process parameters yielded good lyophilisates.

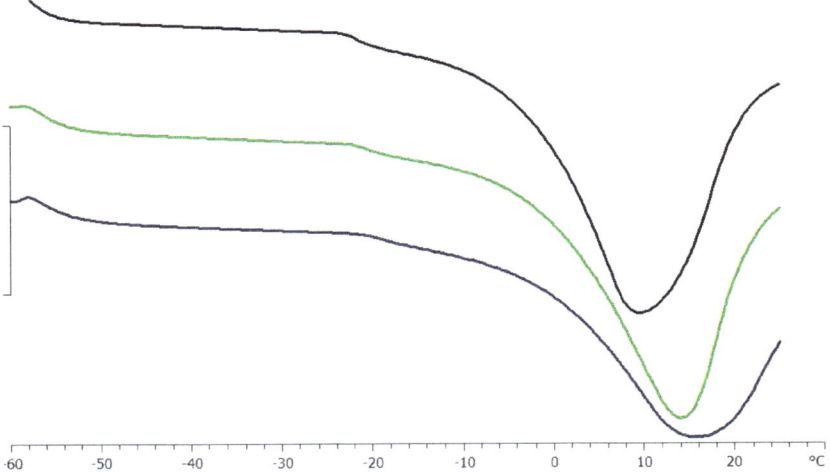

Figure 2. DSC analysis of 40% solution of DS 38 (black line) in the presence of 0.5% Span®80 (green line) and 10% IPEC No.1 (blue line).

Tablets obtained by the DS solution at the highest concentration presented a very irregular surface due to the presence of bubble after filling the blisters. Decreasing the DS concentration to about 40%, visually acceptable tablets were obtained and, therefore, they were disintegrated in water in order to characterize IPECs in terms of particle size and PDI. The presence of a steric stabilizer was essential during lyophilization since DS as such was not able to avoid the formation of large and irreversible aggregates (Table 2). However, sticky tablets, difficult to handle, were obtained by using Tween®80 independently of its concentration and, therefore, discarded from further evaluation. Span®80 was effective as a steric stabilizer as a function of its concentration since only the formulation containing DS in combination with 0.5% of Span®80 preserved the IPEC size upon lyophilization (Table 2). Additionally, the ratio between the cryoprotectant and IPEC influenced the freeze-drying process, since at 20% IPEC loading the resuspended particles exhibited a monomodal distribution with a low size heterogeneity (PDI ~0.15). This evidence agreed with the results on the lyopresevation effect of threalose on diblock and triblock poly(lactic acid)-poly(ethylene oxide) copolymer nanoparticles—the lyoprotective efficiency increased at higher nanoparticles concentration [26].

After lyophilization and redispersion, IPECs shifted their characteristic surface charge from about 15 to -25 mV (Table 2). This variation can be the result of a "masking-effect" due to the adsorption of maltodextrin on the positive surface of IPEC. This result is in line with literature data since the entrapment of nanoparticles in some polymers usually modifies the zeta potential because the coating layers shield the surface charge and move the shear plane out wards from the particle surface [27–29].

According to the obtained results, the optimal composition was 20%, IPEC NAA-1/EPO (33:67), 40.9% DS, and 0.5% Span®80 since the resulting oral lyophilisates have the required disintegration time (<30 s) and after disintegration test IPEC particles had a monomodal distribution without aggregates. Thus, this composition was selected to produce oral lyophilisates loaded with CP.

3.3. CP Loaded IPECs

The effect of different CP loading on the main features of IPEC made of NAA-1 and EPO in the ratio 33:67 was evaluated. The loading procedure gave a high encapsulation efficiency in all considered ratios (Table 5).

Table 5. Characterization of clobetasol propionate (CP) loaded into IPEC formed by NAA-1 and EPO in the ratio 33:67 %.

Composition	CP Content (%)		D_h (nm)	ζ (mV)	MDF (kPa)	WA (mJ)
	Theoretic	Actual				
CP-IPEC 50:50	50	53.2 ± 0.3	401 ± 295	−11.3 ± 2.1	30 ± 6	2530 ± 58
CP-IPEC 60:40	60	56.1 ± 1.4	435 ± 197	−9.0 ± 1.2	22 ± 5	2988 ± 110
CP-IPEC 70:30	70	62.1 ± 5.3	431 ± 119	−10.8 ± 1.2	18 ± 2	2550 ± 27
CP-IPEC 80:20	80	79.4 ± 0.2	560 ± 116	6.8 ± 2.8	16 ± 2	1400 ± 26
CP-IPEC 90:10	90	88.5 ± 12.6	416 ± 6	3.8 ± 2.2	15 ± 1	820 ± 19

The FTIR spectra of CP loaded IPECs revealed that no interactions occurred independently on their ratio (Figure 3).

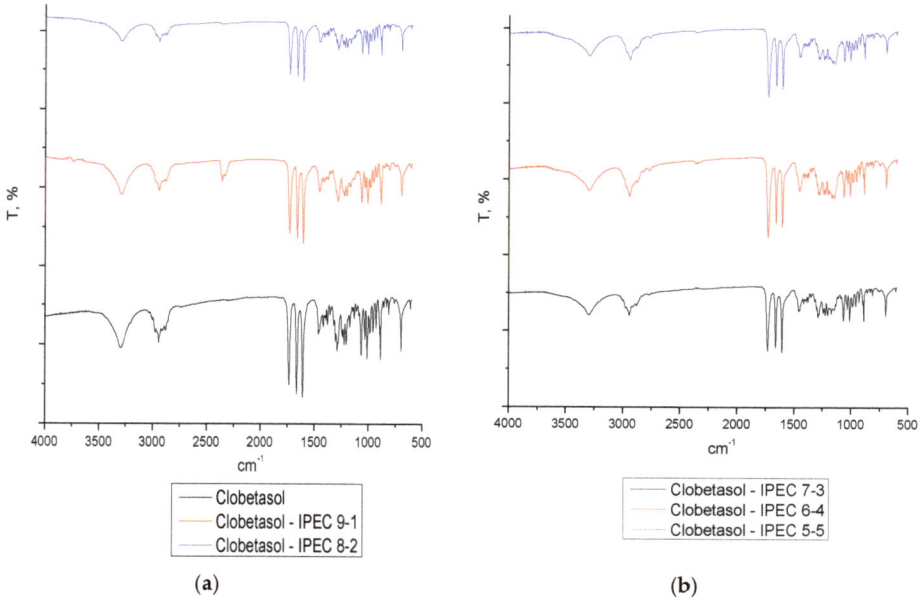

Figure 3. ATR-FTIR-spectra of raw material CP (panel (**a**)) and CP loaded IPECs in the following ratio: (panel (**a**)) 9:1, 8:2; (panel (**b**)) 7:3, 6:4, 5:5.

This result is consistent with the MDSC data as the endothermic event attributed to CP melting was observed in all samples and it increased the drug content accordingly (Figure 4). Independently of the drug content, IPEC dimension increased from around 160 to 450 nm (Table 5). This behavior can be due to the presence of aggregates since the drug loading caused a shift of zeta potential value in the range of instability (Table 5).

As far as the mucoadhesion is concerned, the drug loading led to a decrease in the MDF values of IPECs (Table 5), at a higher extent with increasing CP content. As a matter of fact, the values obtained for CP content higher than 70% (i.e., formulations CP-IPEC 80:20 and 90:10) resulted not significantly different from the negative control. On the other hand, for all the tested formulations, WA was higher than the negative control and, for those with low CP content (i.e., formulations CP-IPEC 50:50, 60:40, and 70:30), it was of the same order of magnitude of the corresponding placebo IPECs.

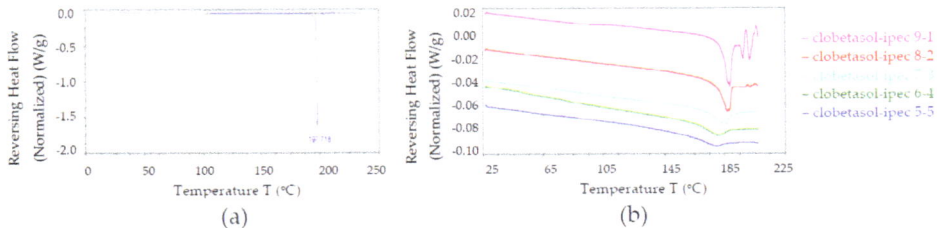

Figure 4. MDSC thermograms of (**a**) CP raw material and (**b**) CP loaded CP—in different ratios, namely 90:10, 80:20, 70:30, 60:40, and 50:50.

In the case of drug loaded IPECs, the decrease in MDF, not concurrent with a decrease in WA, could be due to an increase of the viscous modulus of the hydrated interpolymeric complex/mucin mixture. As a matter of fact, the last phase during the separation of the drug loaded IPECs showed a resistance to the detachment in terms of elongation and time, higher than the placebo. Indeed, the mucin compact was not totally detached from IPEC compact due to the formation of visually observed fibrils. Oral lyophilisates were obtained by dispersing an appropriate amount of CP loaded IPECs in the DS solution in order to have a drug content of 120 µg/unit. The final composition is reported in Table 6. After freeze-drying all tablets appeared as elegant solids without defects or sign of collapse, easy to remove from blister and to handle. The disintegration time of all oral lyophilisates was less than 30 s and no aggregates were detected confirming suitability of components to stabilize IPECs during the lyophilization process (Table 6). The zeta potential values of all resuspended IPECs shifted towards the neutrality probably because the excipients remained adsorbed on the IPEC surface.

Table 6. Composition of oral lyophilisates containing CP loaded IPECs formed by NAA-1 and EPO in the ratio 33:67 %. The amount of IPEC was defined in order to have 120 µg drug per unit. The main features of CP loaded IPECs after disintegration were evaluated in terms of particle size (D_h) and zeta-potential (ζ).

Formulation	Tablet Composition (%w/w)				D_h	Disintegration		
	Composition	IPEC	Span®80	DS		Time (s)	D_h (nm)	ζ (mV)
1	CP-IPEC 50:50	0.29	1.20	98.50	299 ± 122 (95.6%)	<30	323 ± 69	1.08 ± 0.16
2	CP-IPEC 60:40	0.24	1.21	98.55	419 ± 81	<30	363 ± 122	−0.99 ± 1.25
3	CP-IPEC 70:30	0.21	1.21	98.59	306 ± 198	<30	350 ± 87	−4.42 ± 0.46
4	CP-IPEC 80:20	0.18	1.21	98.61	369 ± 178	<30	448 ± 122	−2.90 ± 1.64
5	CP-IPEC 90:10	0.16	1.21	98.63	518 ± 88	<30	356 ± 70	3.27 ± 0.60

The dissolution profiles showed that the CP encapsulation into IPEC improved its apparent solubility as a function of the loaded drug amount (Figure 5). Indeed, the CP-IPEC ratio of 50:50 exhibited the highest supersaturation degree, which was conversely unstable, since after 120 min the concentration of CP in the dissolution medium was superimposable to that of CP solubility. On the other hand, at the CP-IPEC ratio of 90:10 (Formulation 5) the steady state was reached in about 2 h. Based on these observations, it can be assumed that IPEC not only controlled the drug release rate, but also favored the stabilization of the supersaturated system. Indeed, when the CP amount ranged from 80% to 60% (Formulations 2–4, Table 6), a stable supersatured solution was obtained over the entire considered period of time.

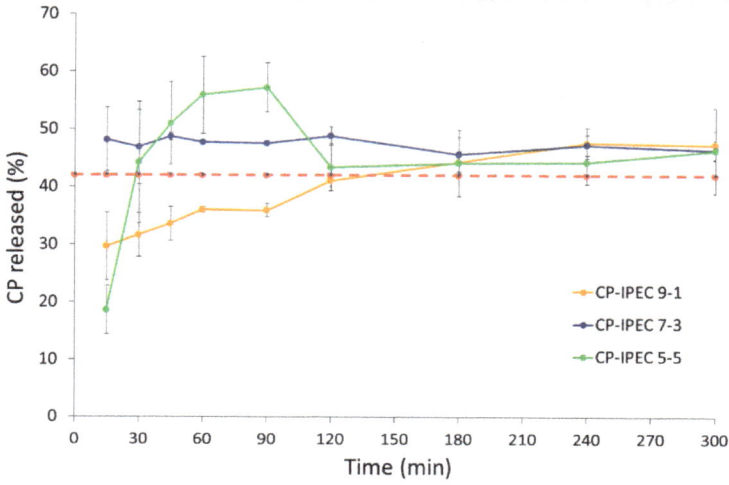

Figure 5. In vitro dissolution profile of CP from oral lyophilisates containing CP-IPEC w/w: 9:1 (90:10), 7:3 (70:30), and 5:5 (50:50) under oversaturation conditions. The dotted line corresponds to the CP solubility at the saturation.

4. Conclusions

A new drug delivery system obtained combining the colloidal and mucoadhesive properties of IPEC formed by Carbopol® and EPO, was proposed to treat buccal pathologies. In particular, the ability to interact with mucin was attributed to the IPEC structural features, namely the presence of free dimethylamino groups of EPO or carboxylate groups of Carbopol®. Indeed, the higher the mucoadhesion, the higher the excess of unbalanced charge in IPEC. Regarding oral lyophilisates, the use of maltodextrin DE 38 and Span®80 preserved the IPEC size during the thermal stress so that it was possible to reconstitute the original nanosuspension upon contact with water in few seconds. Moreover, this approach allowed to improve the CP apparent solubility thanks to the formation of a stable supersaturated system.

Hence, the overall data suggest that this dosage form could be advantageously exploited in drug delivery systems as demonstrated in the case of clobetasol propionate.

The performed work also permitted us to withdraw general information on the design of oral lyophilisates loaded with nanosized particles. Scheme 1 detained the general approach, underling the selection criteria of each phase and the most important variables to be considered.

Acknowledgments: This work was carried out in the framework of the activities of the Cooperation Agreement stipulated between the Kazan State Medical University and the University of Milan, 2014–2019. It is partially supported by the Russian Foundation for Basic Research via grant 16-04-01692 (to Venera R. Garipova and Rouslan I. Moustafine).

Author Contributions: Rouslan I. Moustafine and Francesco Cilurzo conceived and designed the experiments; Venera R. Garipova, Chiara G. M. Gennari, and Francesca Selmin carried out the experiments; all authors analyzed the data and wrote the paper.

Conflicts of Interest: The authors declare no conflict of interest.

References

1. Bourganis, V.; Karamanidou, T.; Kammona, O.; Kiparissides, C. Polyelectrolyte complexes as prospective carriers for the oral delivery of protein therapeutics. *Eur. J. Pharm. Biopharm.* **2017**, *111*, 44–60. [CrossRef] [PubMed]
2. Alfurhood, J.A.; Sun, H.; Kabb, C.P.; Tucker, B.S.; Matthews, J.H.; Luesch, H.; Sumerlin, B.S. Poly(*N*-(2-hydroxypropyl)methacrylamide)–valproic acid conjugates as block copolymer nanocarriers. *Polym. Chem.* **2017**, *8*, 4983–4987. [CrossRef] [PubMed]
3. Dillen, K.; Vandervoort, J.; Van den Mooter, G.; Ludwig, A. Evaluation of ciprofloxacin-loaded Eudragit® RS100 or RL100/PLGA nanoparticles. *Int. J. Pharm.* **2006**, *314*, 72–82. [CrossRef] [PubMed]
4. Luppi, B.; Bigucci, F.; Mercolini, L.; Musenga, A.; Sorrenti, M.; Catenacci, L.; Zecchi, V. Novel mucoadhesive nasal inserts based on chitosan/hyaluronate polyelectrolyte complexes for peptide and protein delivery. *J. Pharm. Pharmacol.* **2009**, *61*, 151–157. [CrossRef] [PubMed]
5. Mustafin, R.I. Interpolymer combinations of chemically complementary grades of Eudragit copolymers: A new direction in the design of peroral solid dosage forms of drug delivery systems with controlled release. *Pharm. Chem. J.* **2011**, *45*, 285–295. [CrossRef]
6. Kramarenko, E.Y.; Khokhlov, A.R.; Reineker, P. Stoichiometric polyelectrolyte complexes of ionic block copolymers and oppositely charged polyions. *J. Chem. Phys.* **2006**, *125*, 194902. [CrossRef] [PubMed]
7. Hartig, M.S.; Greene, R.R.; Dikov, M.M.; Prokop, A.; Davidson, J.M. Multifunctional nanoparticulate polyelectrolyte complexes. *Pharm. Res.* **2007**, *24*, 2353–2369. [CrossRef] [PubMed]
8. Mustafin (Moustafine), R.I.; Semina, I.I.; Garipova, V.A.; Bukhovets, A.V.; Sitenkov, Y.A.; Salakhova, A.R.; Gennari, C.G.M.; Cilurzo, F. Comparative study of polycomplexes based on Carbopol® and oppositely charged polyelectrolytes as a new oral drug delivery system. *Pharm. Chem. J.* **2015**, *49*, 1–6. [CrossRef]
9. Cilurzo, F.; Musazzi, U.M.; Franzè, S.; Selmin, F.; Minghetti, P. Orodispersible dosage forms: Biopharmaceutical improvements and regulatory requirements. *Drug Discov. Today* **2017**. [CrossRef] [PubMed]
10. Cilurzo, F.; Gennari, C.G.M.; Selmin, F.; Epstein, J.B.; Gaeta, G.M.; Colella, G.; Minghetti, P. A new mucoadhesive dosage form for the management of oral lichen planus: Formulation and clinical study. *Eur. J. Pharm. Biopharm.* **2010**, *76*, 437–442. [CrossRef] [PubMed]
11. Guidelines for the Management of Oral Lichen Planus in Secondary Care—October 2010. Available online: www.bsom.org.uk/LP_guidelines_-_BSOM.pdf (accessed on 14 January 2018).
12. Selmin, F.; Franceschini, I.; Cupone, I.E.; Minghetti, P.; Cilurzo, F. Aminoacids as non-traditional plasticizers of maltodextrins fast-dissolving films. *Carbohyd. Pol.* **2015**, *115*, 613–616. [CrossRef] [PubMed]
13. Herbig, M.E.; Evers, D.H. Correlation of hydrotropic solubilization by urea with log D of drug molecules and utilization of this effect for topical formulations. *Eur. J. Pharm. Biopharm.* **2013**, *85*, 158–160. [CrossRef] [PubMed]
14. Cilurzo, F.; Minghetti, P.; Selmin, F.; Casiraghi, A.; Montanari, L. Polymethacrylate salts as new low-swellable mucoadhesive materials. *J. Control. Release* **2003**, *88*, 43–53. [CrossRef]
15. Jabbari, E.; Wisniewski, N.; Peppas, N.A. Evidence of mucoadhesion by chain interpenetration at a poly(acrylic acid)/mucin interface using ATR–FTIR spectroscopy. *J. Control. Release* **1993**, *26*, 99–108. [CrossRef]
16. Mustafin, R.I.; Kabanova, T.V.; Zhdanova, E.R.; Bukhovets, A.V.; Garipova, V.A.; Nasibullin, S.F.; Kemenova, V.A. Synthesis and physicochemical evaluation of new carrier based on interpolyelecrtolyte complex formed by Eudragit® EPO and Carbomer 940. *Pharm. Chem. J.* **2010**, *44*, 271–273. [CrossRef]
17. Mustafin, R.I.; Kabanova, T.V.; Semina, I.I.; Bukhovets, A.V.; Garipova, V.A.; Shilovskaya, E.V.; Nasibullin, S.F.; Sitenkov, A.Y.; Kazakova, R.R.; Kemenova, V.A. Biopharmaceutical assessment of a polycomplex matrix system based on Carbomer 940 and Eudragit® EPO for colon-specific drug delivery. *Pharm. Chem. J.* **2011**, *45*, 491–494. [CrossRef]
18. Mustafin, R.I.; Kabanova, T.V.; Zhdanova, E.R.; Bukhovets, A.V.; Garipova, V.A.; Nasibullin, S.F.; Kemenova, V.A. Diffusion-transport properties of a polycomplex matrix system based on Eudragit® EPO and Carbomer 940. *Pharm. Chem. J.* **2010**, *44*, 147–150. [CrossRef]

19. Moustafine, R.I.; Kabanova, T.V.; Kemenova, V.A.; Van den Mooter, G. Characteristics of interpolyelectrolyte complexes of Eudragit E 100 with Eudragit L 100. *J. Control. Release* **2005**, *103*, 191–198. [CrossRef] [PubMed]
20. Russo, E.; Selmin, F.; Baldassari, S.; Gennari, C.G.M.; Caviglioli, G.; Cilurzo, F.; Minghetti, P.; Parodi, B. A focus on mucoadhesive polymers and their application in buccal dosage forms. *J. Drug Deliv. Sci. Technol.* **2016**, *32*, 113–125. [CrossRef]
21. Albarkah, Y.; Green, R.J.; Khutoryanskiy, V.V. Probing the mucoadhesive interactions between porcine gastric mucin and some water-soluble polymers. *Macromol. Biosci.* **2015**, *15*, 1546–1553. [CrossRef] [PubMed]
22. Levine, H.; Slade, L. Another view of trehalose for drying and stabilizing biological materials. *Eur. J. Pharm. Biopharm.* **1992**, *5*, 36–40.
23. Crowe, J.H.; Crowe, L.M.; Carpenter, J.F. Preserving dry biomaterials: The water replacement hypothesis. *Eur. J. Pharm. Biopharm.* **1993**, *6*, 28–37.
24. Tang, X.; Pikal, M. Design of freeze-drying processes for pharmaceuticals: Practical advice. *Pharm Res.* **2004**, *21*, 191–200. [CrossRef] [PubMed]
25. Pikal, M.J.; Shah, S.; Roy, M.L.; Putman, R. The secondary drying stage of freeze drying: Drying kinetics as a function of temperature and chamber pressure. *Int. J. Pharm.* **1990**, *60*, 203–207. [CrossRef]
26. De Jaeghere, F.; Allémann, E.; Feijen, J.; Kissel, T.; Doelker, E.; Gurny, R. Freeze-drying and lyopreservation of diblock and triblock poly (lactic acid)-poly (ethylene oxide)(PLA-PEO) copolymer nanoparticles. *Pharm. Dev. Technol.* **2000**, *5*, 473–483. [CrossRef] [PubMed]
27. Hawley, A.E.; Illum, L.; Davis, S.S. Preparation of biodegradable, surface engineered PLGA nanospheres with enhanced lymphatic drainage and lymph node uptake. *Pharm. Res.* **1997**, *14*, 657–661. [CrossRef] [PubMed]
28. Tobio, M.; Gref, R.; Sanchez, A.; Langer, R.; Alonso, M.J. Stealth PLA–PEG nanoparticles as protein carriers for nasal administration. *Pharm. Res.* **1998**, *15*, 270–275. [CrossRef] [PubMed]
29. Redhead, H.M.; Davis, S.S.; Illum, L. Drug delivery in poly (lactide-*co*-glycolide) nanoparticles surface modified with poloxamer 407 and poloxamine 908: In Vitro characterization and in vivo evaluation. *J. Control. Release* **2001**, *70*, 353–363. [CrossRef]

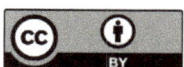

© 2018 by the authors. Licensee MDPI, Basel, Switzerland. This article is an open access article distributed under the terms and conditions of the Creative Commons Attribution (CC BY) license (http://creativecommons.org/licenses/by/4.0/).

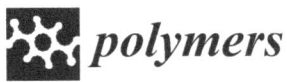

Article

Gellan Gum/Pectin Beads Are Safe and Efficient for the Targeted Colonic Delivery of Resveratrol

Fabíola Garavello Prezotti [1], Fernanda Isadora Boni [1], Natália Noronha Ferreira [1], Daniella de Souza e Silva [2], Sérgio Paulo Campana-Filho [2], Andreia Almeida [3,4,5], Teófilo Vasconcelos [3,4], Maria Palmira Daflon Gremião [1], Beatriz Stringhetti Ferreira Cury [1] and Bruno Sarmento [3,4,5,6,*]

1. Faculdade de Ciências Farmacêuticas, Universidade Estadual Paulista (UNESP), Araraquara, Rodovia Araraquara–Jaú, Km 1, Araraquara 14801-902, Brazil; fabiolagp@gmail.com (F.G.P.); boni.fernanda@gmail.com (F.I.B.); noronhanat@fcfar.unesp.br (N.N.F.); pgremiao@fcfar.unesp.br (M.P.D.G.); curybsf@fcfar.unesp.br (B.S.F.C.)
2. Instituto de Química de São Carlos, Universidade de São Paulo (USP), Avenida Trabalhador São-Carlense, 400, São Carlos 13560-970, Brazil; danyss1986@gmail.com (D.d.S.e.S.); scampana@iqsc.usp.br (S.P.C.-F.)
3. I3S-Instituto de Investigação e Inovação em Saúde, Universidade do Porto, Rua Alfredo Allen, 208, 4200-135 Porto, Portugal; andreia.almeida@ineb.up.pt (A.A.); teofilo.vasconcelos@bial.com (T.V.)
4. INEB-Instituto de Engenharia Biomédica, Universidade do Porto, Rua Alfredo Allen, 208, 4200-135 Porto, Portugal
5. CESPU-Instituto de Investigação e Formação Avançada em Ciências e Tecnologias da Saúde, Rua Central de Gandra 1317, 4585-116 Gandra, Portugal
6. School of Pharmacy, Queen's University Belfast, Medical Biology Centre, 97 Lisburn Road, Belfast BT9 7BL, UK
* Correspondence: bruno.sarmento@ineb.up.pt; Tel.: +351-226-074-949

Received: 6 November 2017; Accepted: 3 January 2018; Published: 8 January 2018

Abstract: This work addresses the establishment and characterization of gellan gum:pectin (GG:P) biodegradable mucoadhesive beads intended for the colon-targeted delivery of resveratrol (RES). The impact of the polymer carrier system on the cytotoxicity and permeability of RES was evaluated. Beads of circular shape (circularity index of 0.81) with an average diameter of 914 µm, Span index of 0.29, and RES entrapment efficiency of 76% were developed. In vitro drug release demonstrated that beads were able to reduce release rates in gastric media and control release for up to 48 h at an intestinal pH of 6.8. Weibull's model correlated better with release data and *b* parameter (0.79) indicated that the release process was driven by a combination of Fickian diffusion and Case II transport, indicating that both diffusion and swelling/polymer chains relaxation are processes that contribute equally to control drug release rates. Beads and isolated polymers were observed to be safe for Caco-2 and HT29-MTX intestinal cell lines. RES encapsulation into the beads allowed for an expressive reduction of drug permeation in an in vitro triple intestinal model. This feature, associated with low RES release rates in acidic media, can favor targeted drug delivery from the beads in the colon, a promising behavior to improve the local activity of RES.

Keywords: gellan gum; pectin; resveratrol; mucoadhesive microspheres; cytotoxicity; in vitro permeability; Caco-2 cells; triple co-culture model

1. Introduction

Gellan gum (GG) and pectin (P) are widespread available, low-cost, nontoxic, stable, biocompatible polysaccharides which exhibit gelling properties and have several structures able to be chemically and/or physically modified, providing promising characteristics for the design of drug delivery systems in the pharmaceutical field [1,2]. They have been also investigated as technological platforms due to their mucoadhesive properties—their ability to establish supramolecular interactions with mucosal components, such as mucin chains—which contribute to drug immobilization and retention in a target organ through more intimate contact over an extended period of time, favoring a local concentration gradient [3]. Additionally, while GG is degraded specifically in the colon by galactomannanas enzymes [4], P exhibits resistance to gastric and intestinal bacteria, being specifically fermented by *Bifidobacteria* and *Bacteroides* in the colon environment [5]. Since both polymers are degraded specifically by the colonic microbiota, it is noteworthy that they represent promising materials in the development of carrier systems to target drugs to the colon [1,5–8].

Mucoadhesion is a complex phenomenon and mucoadhesive ability can be related to the presence of reactive functional groups in the polymer chain capable of interacting with mucin present in the mucus [9]. Both GG and P are anionic polysaccharides with well-known mucoadhesiveness, related mainly to their numerous carboxyl groups that can interact through hydrogen bonds with mucin oligosaccharide chains [1,10–16].

Considering the ability of GG and P to form mucoadhesive microcapsules in the presence of cations such as Ca^{2+} and Al^{3+}, ionically crosslinked beads based on GG or GG:P blends were previously designed by our research group, since mucoadhesiveness is an important property for multiparticulate systems intended for the colon-targeted delivery of drugs by the oral route [1,8]. The colon has a low mucus turnover rate and slow motility, which facilitates contact between polymeric systems and mucin glycoproteins and is responsible for the initial adhesive interaction that might involve chain interpenetration, prolonging residence time at the action site [1,8,17].

Blending P with GG was proposed in order to form a material with suitable properties in relation to the isolated polymers—improved mucoadhesiveness and mechanical properties—to allow for the effective control of drug release at different sites in the gastrointestinal tract (GIT) [8]. The control of drug release rates is based on a swellable polymer matrix that resists premature dissolution and/or degradation in the upper portions of the GIT at an acidic pH. The crosslinking process is a rational strategy to modulate such properties, and the correlation between the degree crosslinking of a polymer with the control of release rates of the entrapped drug has been demonstrated [1,8,18–20]. Additionally, effective drug targeting to the colon should be achieved since specific enzymatic degradation of the matrix should happen at this site by specific enzymes produced by the colonic microbiota [6,21].

The GG:P beads previously developed by Prezotti and co-authors (2014) were prepared by ionotropic gelation using $AlCl_3$ as a crosslinking agent, and their high mucoadhesive ability was evidenced by in vitro and ex vivo experiments. In addition, the beads were able to reduce release rates of the loaded drug (ketoprofen) in acidic media (pH 1.2) and prolong drug release in phosphate buffer (pH 7.4) for up to 6 h. The advantageous features of these beads reveal that they are a promising carrier for protecting drugs and targeting them to specific sites in the GIT in order to treat local diseases or modulate drug permeability [8].

RES has attracted great attention due to its wide range of beneficial effects in humans and several drug delivery systems have been proposed to carry this drug. It has been recognized as a promising compound for the treatment of several illnesses, such as metabolic and cardiovascular diseases, neurodegeneration, and ischemic injuries, and for both the prevention and treatment of several types of cancer [22–25].

Resveratrol (RES), a class II in the Biopharmaceutical Classification System, is a natural polyphenol with recognized antioxidant properties found in grapes, red wine, peanuts, mulberries, and some medicinal plants [26], and is potentially useful as a dietary supplement or for use in natural medicine [22,23]. However, the labile properties, low solubility, and rapid and extensive metabolism of RES impose great challenges for its applications in therapeutics, mainly, by the oral route [25,27].

Such features make the amount of RES that reaches the colon following oral administration insufficient to promote the desired beneficial effects at the target site, making a carrier system necessary for the effective delivery of RES to the colon. Additionally, the high permeability of RES opposes the accumulation of the drug in the colon [28].

The in vitro intestinal permeability of RES was evaluated using an innovative triple co-culture model consisting of Caco-2 cells, to reproduce the characteristics of the enterocytes; HT29-MTX cells, capable of secreting mucus; and Raji-B cells, which induce differentiation of Caco-2 cells into M cells [29–31]. Co-culture models that use multiple cell lines together enable accurate reproduction of an organ of interest, as is the case in this triple co-culture which consists of three different cell lines, exactly mimicking the human intestinal epithelium [30], being more physiological, functional, and reproducible for the study of drug permeability [29].

In this study, we showed that crosslinked mucoadhesive GG:P beads are a rational strategy to protect RES from the harsh environment of the stomach and modulate its release rates and biological interactions, and is an efficient and safe system for the targeted colonic delivery of this promising drug by the oral route.

2. Materials and Methods

2.1. Chemicals

Pectin (type LM-5206 CS) and gellan gum (Kelcogel® CG-LA) were kindly provided by CP Kelco (Limeira, Brazil). Resveratrol was purchased from Sigma-Aldrich (São Paulo, Brazil). Transwell® cell culture inserts were from Corning (Madrid, Spain). Dulbecco's Modified Eagle's Medium (DMEM) was from Lonza (Basel, Switzerland). Non-essential amino acids and fetal bovine serum were purchased from Biochrom GmbH (Berlin, Germany). Hank's Balanced Salt Solution (HBSS) was from Gibco (Invitrogen Corporation, Life Technologies, Paisley, UK). Phosphate Buffered Saline and 3-(4,5-dimethyl-2-thiazolyl)-2,5-diphenyl-2H-tetrazolium bromide (MTT reagent) were from Sigma-Aldrich (Sintra, Portugal). Triton® X-100 was from Merck (Oeiras, Portugal). All other materials used were of analytical grade and obtained from commercial suppliers.

2.2. Bead Preparation

Beads were prepared as previously described [8]. Briefly, aqueous dispersions of GG:P (4:1) at a concentration of 2% (w/v) were prepared under magnetic stirring at 80 °C until complete homogenization. RES was added to the dispersion at 0.5% (w/v) at 40 °C and kept under magnetic stirring for an additional 15 min. The dispersions were dropped through flat-tipped needles (23 G, 25 × 0.6 mm) into a cooled solution (8 °C) of $AlCl_3$ (3%, w/v) under magnetic stirring (60 rpm). The crosslinking reaction was kept for an additional 45 min in an ice bath for strengthening of the beads. After, beads were separated by filtration, washed with distilled water to remove unreacted crosslinking agent, and dried at room temperature. Beads were prepared in duplicate and were stored in a desiccator containing silica gel.

2.3. Bead Characterization

2.3.1. Particle Size, Size Distribution, and Morphology

Images of RES-loaded beads were taken on a Leica MZ APO® stereoscope (Leica Microsystems, Wetzlar, Germany) coupled to the Motic Images Advance 2.0® program. Fifty beads, previously dried until constant weight, were used to determine the average particle size, size distribution (Span index), and average circularity [1,8]. Span index was determined using the following Equation (1):

$$\text{Span} = (D_{90} - D_{10})/D_{50} \tag{1}$$

where D_{90}, D_{10}, and D_{50} are the diameters (μm) determined for the 90th, 10th, and 50th percentiles, respectively.

2.3.2. Attenuated Total Reflectance-Fourier Transform Infrared (ATR-FTIR) Spectroscopy

Infrared spectroscopy of GG, P, RES, empty beads, and RES-loaded beads was performed using a Vertex 70 Fourier Transform Infrared (FTIR) spectrometer (Bruker Optics Inc., Billerica, MA, USA) equipped with a Golden Gate single reflection ATR accessory and DLaTGS detector to investigate polymer–drug interactions [32,33]. Powdered samples were scanned over a wave region of 400–4000 cm^{-1}.

2.3.3. Entrapment Efficiency (%EE)

Immediately after being prepared, eight beads were grounded with 20 mL of phosphate buffer (pH 7.4) in a centrifuge tube using a high-shear homogenizer (Ultra-turrax IKA®, Campinas, Brazil) at 11,000 rpm for 2 min in order to extract the encapsulated drug. Sodium lauryl sulphate (1%, w/v) was added to ensure total drug solubilization. After 1 h, the dispersions were centrifuged to remove polymeric debris (2500 rpm; 5 min) and the amount of RES in the supernatant was quantified using a Cary 60 UV-Vis spectrophotometer (Agilent Technologies, Santa Clara, CA, USA) at 320 nm, in five replicates. The measured drug loaded (%DL$_m$), theoretical drug loaded (%DL$_t$), and entrapment efficiency (%EE) were calculated according to Equations (2)–(4), respectively [34]:

$$\%DL_m = (weight_{drug\ in\ beads}/weight_{beads}) \times 100 \quad (2)$$

$$\%DL_t = (weight_{added\ drug}/weight_{polymers+drug}) \times 100 \quad (3)$$

$$\%EE = (\%DL_m/\%DL_t) \times 100 \quad (4)$$

where weight$_{drug\ in\ beads}$ (µg) is the amount of RES in eight beads and weight$_{beads}$ is the average mass (µg) of eight dried beads determined after drying the batches until constant weight. The %DL$_t$ was determined based on bead composition, where weight$_{added\ drug}$ is the mass (µg) of RES added during bead preparation, and weight$_{polymers+drug}$ is the sum of the masses (µg) of GG, P, and RES added during bead preparation.

2.4. Drug Release Studies

In vitro drug release was performed using an SR8-Plus Hanson Dissolution Test Station (Chastworth, CA, USA) equipped with USP apparatus 1 (basket) at 50 rpm and 37 ± 0.5 °C. Solutions with different pH values were used to simulate the variations in pH along the GIT according to previously published methodology with minor modifications [1,8]. Initially, dissolution was carried out in acid media (0.1N HCl pH 1.2) containing sodium lauryl sulfate (1%, w/v) as surfactant over 2 h. Posteriorly, 0.2 M of tribasic sodium phosphate was added to achieve a pH of 6.8 (enteric media). Aliquots of 2 mL were withdrawn at pre-established intervals and immediately replaced with the same volume of fresh dissolution media at 37 ± 0.5 °C. The amount of RES released was quantified on a Cary 60 UV-Vis spectrophotometer (Agilent Technologies, Santa Clara, CA, USA) at 320 nm. Tests were performed in triplicate, using a mass of beads corresponding to 5 mg of RES and the same amount of free RES.

Kinetics of Drug Release

RES release data were fitted to different mathematical models (Korsmeyer-Peppas, Higuchi, First-order, Weibull, Hixson-Crowell, and Baker-Lonsdale) to evaluate the mechanism of drug release from the beads.

2.5. Cell Lines

The Caco-2 (C2BBe1) cell line (passages 64–66) was obtained from the American Type Culture Collection (ATCC, Manassas, VA, USA). Mucus-secreting HT29-MTX (passages 38–40) and Raji-B cell lines were kindly provided by Dr. T. Lesuffleur (INSERM U178, Villejuif, France) and Dr. Alexandre Carmo (Cellular and Molecular Biology Institute (IBMC), Porto, Portugal), respectively. Cells were cultured in plastic cell culture flasks (75 cm^3) using Dulbecco's Modified Eagle's Medium (DMEM) supplemented with 10% fetal bovine serum (FBS), 100 U/mL penicillin, 100 mg/mL streptomycin, and 1% non-essential amino acids, and incubated in a humidified atmosphere with 5% CO_2 at 37 °C using a conventional incubator (Binder®, Tuttlingen, Germany). Adherent cells (Caco-2 and HT29-MTX) were harvested at a confluence of 70–80%, using trypsin to detach them, and seeded in new flasks. The medium was changed every third day. Raji-B cells were grown in suspension cultures and had their medium changed when necessary.

2.6. Cell Viability

Cell viability was assessed by methyl-thiazolyl-tetrazolium (MTT) assay which allows for measurement of the percentage of viable cells due to living cells having to metabolize the MTT reagent into a colored, reduced product: purple formazan crystals [35]. The cytotoxicity of polymers, free RES, RES-loaded beads, and empty beads was studied in Caco-2 and HT29-MTX cell lines.

Cells were seeded at a density of 0.12×10^6 cells/well in 24-well plates using supplemented DMEM. After 24 h incubation in a Binder® incubator at 37 °C with a humidified atmosphere and 5% CO_2, the medium was removed, the wells were washed with phosphate buffered saline solution (PBS) at 37 °C, and cells were incubated in the presence of isolated polymers (GG or P; 500–2500 µg/mL), empty and RES-loaded beads (suspended in HBSS—6, 8 and 10 beads/well) and free RES (diluted in HBSS) in concentrations corresponding to the amount of RES loaded in the beads (350, 450 and 600 µg/mL). The positive control (100% cell viability) was obtained by incubating them in the presence of HBSS or HBSS containing 0.5% DMSO (as found in free-RES stock solution). The negative control (cell death) was obtained by incubating cells in the presence of Triton® X-100 (1% w/v in PBS). Cells were incubated under the same conditions described above for 24 h in the presence of the polymers and 4 h in the presence of beads and free RES. After this period, the wells were washed twice with PBS at 37 °C to remove the drug and the beads, and 1 mL of the MTT reagent (0.5 mg/mL in PBS) was added to each well. Plates were incubated for an additional 4 h at 37 °C. Subsequently, the content of the wells was carefully removed and 1 mL of dimethyl sulfoxide (DMSO) was added to each well in order to solubilize the formazan crystals originated by living cells. Plates were allowed a period of 10 min of continuous stirring inside a Synergy 2® microplate reader (Biotek Instruments Inc., Winooski, VT, USA) before reading the absorbance at 590 nm (test wavelength) and 630 nm (background wavelength). Tests were performed in at least two independent experiments, each performed in quadruplicate.

2.7. In Vitro Intestinal Permeability

Permeability experiments were performed on a triple co-culture cell model. Co-cultures of Caco-2 and HT29-MTX at a 90:10 ratio were seeded in Transwell® inserts of 24 mm diameter, with a translucent permeable membrane of polycarbonate, pore size of 3 µm, and a growth area of 4.67 cm^2, at a density of 1.0×10^5 cells/cm^2 to a final volume of 1.5 mL (the apical compartment) in each insert. The inserts were placed in 6-well plates and 2.5 mL of supplemented DMEM was added to the basolateral compartment. The plates were maintained inside a Binder® incubator at 37 °C with a humidified atmosphere and 5% CO_2 [29,30]. Then, after 14 days, 1.0×10^6 Raji-B cells was added to the basolateral chamber. After the addition of these cells, the media in this compartment was kept without changes until the permeability tests on the 21st day.

To perform the in vitro permeability experiments, media was carefully removed from the apical and the basolateral compartments; the inserts and wells were gently washed twice with PBS (pH 7.4) at 37 °C to remove all supplemented DMEM, filled with HBSS (1.5 and 2.5 mL, respectively), and allowed to equilibrate for 30 min. Afterwards, the media from the apical compartment was removed and 1.5 mL of free RES at 50 µg/mL in HBSS was added. The beads were placed directly in the apical compartment without removing the media. Plates were placed inside an orbital shaking incubator (IKA® KS 4000 IC,

IKA, Staufen, Germany) at 100 rpm and 37 °C. Aliquots (200 µL) were withdrawn from the basolateral chamber at predetermined times (5, 15, 30, 45, 60, 90, 120, and 180 min) and immediately replaced with HBSS. At the end, an aliquot from the apical compartment was collected [36]. Tests were performed in triplicate and an insert without the addition of sample was used as a control.

Before, during, and at the end of the permeability experiments, the Transepithelial Electrical Resistance (TEER) was measured using an EVOM2® epithelial voltohmmeter with chopstick electrodes (World Precision Instruments, Sarasota, FL, USA) in order to monitor the formation, confluence, and integrity of the cell monolayers. Experiments were performed in triplicate.

The concentration of RES in the samples was determined by high-performance liquid chromatography (HPLC) analysis using a Waters HPLC system and data was processed with Empower 3® Software (Waters Corporation, Milford, MA, USA). The stationary phase consisted of a C18 reversed-phase column Waters Symmetry Shield RP18 (3.5 µm, 100 × 4.6 mm) at 30 °C. The mobile phase consisted of (A) water and (B) acetonitrile (65:35, v/v) in isocratic mode and a flow rate of 1 mL/min. The run time was set at 10 min, the injection volume used was 50 µL, and the detection by UV was fixed at 307 nm.

The drug apparent permeability (P_{app}) was calculated from the following Equation (5):

$$P_{app} = [(dQ/dt) \times V]/(A \times C_0) \tag{5}$$

where P_{app} is the apparent permeability (cm/s); dQ/dt (µM/s) is the flux across the monolayer obtained from the angular coefficient of the curve of the amount of drug transported versus time; V (cm^3) is the acceptor chamber volume, which in this case corresponds to 2.5 cm^3 (basolateral chamber); A (cm^2) is the insert membrane growth area (equal to 4.67 cm^2 for a 6 well plate); and C_0 (µM) is the initial concentration in the apical compartment [37,38].

2.8. Statistical Analysis

Experiments were performed in triplicate and represented as mean ± standard deviation (SD). Statistical significance between different treatments was determined using analysis of variance (ANOVA) and post hoc Tukey's test. Cytotoxicity results were analyzed by two-way analysis of variance (ANOVA) with Bonferroni Multiple/Post Hoc Group Comparisons (GraphPadPrism Software Inc., La Jolla, CA, USA). A 5% level of significance was adopted.

3. Results and Discussion

3.1. Bead Characterization

Beads were prepared by an ionotropic gelation technique, by dripping the negatively-charged polymer dispersion containing RES into a crosslinking solution containing the positively-charged aluminum ions. Beads are formed as the droplets enter the crosslinking solution, and are strengthened due to the crosslinking reaction between the polyanions (GG and P) and the trivalent ions (Al^{3+}) [8]. Beads presented an average diameter of 913.70 ± 102.73 µm and a unimodal size distribution with a Span index of 0.29, indicating low polydispersity. The high circularity index values (0.81 ± 0.12) demonstrated the circular shape of the beads. Photomicrographs of GG:P beads evidencing their spherical morfology can be seen in the previous work from our research group [8].

The chemical interactions between bead components and RES were investigated by analyzing peak variation of GG, P, RES, empty bead, and RES-loaded bead spectra using ATR-FTIR (Figure 1).

GG spectra exhibited a broad band between 3400–3100 cm^{-1} due to O–H stretch vibrations of hydroxyl groups; C–H stretch vibrations of –CH$_2$ groups were recorded at around 2925 cm^{-1}, asymmetric and symmetric carboxylate anions were recorded stretching at 1600 and 1400 cm^{-1}, respectively, while C–O stretching occurred at 1033 cm^{-1} [8,39]. Pectin showed a broad band related to O–H stretching vibrations between 3400–3100 cm^{-1}. Characteristic C=O stretching of COOH groups close to 1700 cm^{-1} and asymmetric and symmetric carboxylate anion stretching resulted in a profile similar to that presented by GG [40]. The fingerprint region of pectin spectra comprises the pyranose cycle vibrations region with five characteristic bands around 1000 cm^{-1} [41]. Characteristic peaks of RES can be observed at around 990 cm^{-1} related to the trans-olefinic band, at 1380 cm^{-1} related to C–O stretching, and at 1580 cm^{-1} related to C–C olefinic stretching. A striking sign at 1600 cm^{-1} refers to the aromatic double band stretching [33]. Empty beads exhibited a profile similar to GG and P spectra, while RES-loaded beads presented characteristics peaks of RES. These data highlight the chemical stability of the drug inside the beads and the absence of chemical interactions between polymers and RES, suggesting that it might be physically entrapped within the polymer chains.

Beads presented a %EE of 75.7% ± 0.8%. The high drug loading may be related to the low solubility of RES in aqueous solutions that hindered drug diffusion to the crosslinking media during beads preparation. Similar results were achieved with other systems based on GG and blends of GG:P using AlCl$_3$ as a crosslinking agent and containing ketoprofen [1,8].

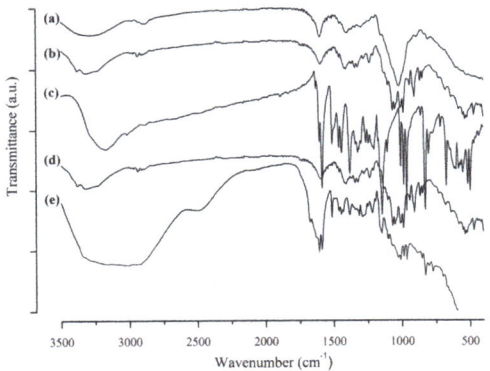

Figure 1. ATR-FTIR spectra of (**a**) gellan gum, (**b**) pectin, (**c**) resveratrol, (**d**) empty beads, and (**e**) RES-loaded beads.

3.2. Drug Release Studies

The main challenge in targeting drugs to lower segments of the GIT relates to the great variations in pH and enzymatic content that the system will face in its transit along different organs until reaching the colon. Subsequently, a successful colon-specific drug delivery system should protect the encapsulated drug against the low pH and enzymes of the stomach, preventing premature drug release in this organ, and should release it when reaching a higher pH, such as that of the colonic environment [42].

Beads were able to significantly reduce release rates in acid media compared to the free drug. From the in vitro release profile of free RES and RES-loaded beads (Figure 2) it is possible to observe that only 17.6% ± 0.3% of the drug was released from the beads in acidic media (pH 1.2) after 120 min of experiment, while 83.5% ± 2.5% of free RES was already dissolved at the same time. Free RES completed its dissolution in only 150 min, right after changing the pH to 6.8. However, GG:P beads were able to control drug release for up to 48 h without any burst effect.

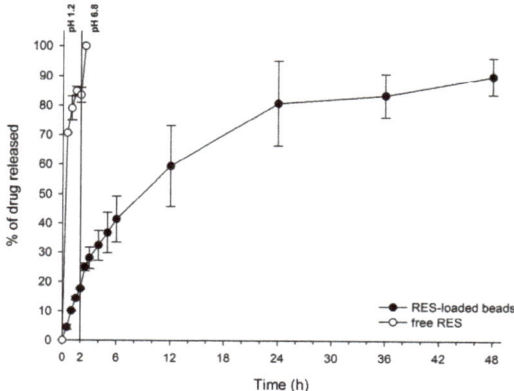

Figure 2. Dissolution profile of RES (free and loaded in GG:P beads) in media that mimic gastric (1.2) and enteric pH (6.8) (n = 3; mean ± SD).

Weibull's mathematical model fitted better with drug release data (r^2 = 0.998). For this model, the b parameter can be used to indicate the mechanism of drug transport throughout the polymer matrix. Values of $b \leq 0.75$ are related to release by Fickian diffusion, while values of $0.75 < b < 1$ correspond to a combination of Fickian diffusion and Case II transport. When $b > 1$, drug transport follows a complex release mechanism. The value of the b parameter obtained was 0.79, indicating that the release mechanism of RES from the bead matrix was governed by both Fickian diffusion, in which drug release occurs due to a concentration gradient between the polymeric matrix and the dissolution media, and Case II transport, which is related to matrix swelling [19,43,44]. Thus, it can be concluded that both diffusion and swelling/polymer chains relaxation are processes that contribute equally to the control of drug release rates, i.e., the rates of chains relaxation and drug diffusion through the swelled matrix must be similar and are limiting to the release process [19,45].

3.3. Cell Viability

The in vitro cytotoxicity and cell permeability of crosslinked mucoadhesive GG:P beads were analyzed in order to assure safety of oral administration and evaluate the potential for modulating interactions with the cells; a feature favoring the local treatment of colonic disorders such as ulcerative colitis and colonic cancer. Cytotoxicity was evaluated using cell lines from the human intestine (Caco-2 and HT29-MTX).

In vitro cell viability assays are extremely important in the development phase of new drug delivery systems once they can predict the biocompatibility and the cytotoxicity. The colorimetric MTT assay is one of the most used methods for screening of cytotoxicity. Cells with intact metabolic activity are able to reduce the MTT reagent (3-(4,5-dimethylthiazol-2-yl)-2,5-diphenyl tetrazolium bromide), originating a purple formazan product that precipitates and it is then solubilized with an organic solvent—usually DMSO. This assay can, therefore, by the amount of purple product formed, determine cell viability and infer the harmful intracellular effects of the systems on cell metabolic activity [35,46], indicating drug carrier toxicity. A threshold of 70% cell viability was considered as the toxic level according to the ISO 10993-5 guideline [47].

Analyzing Figure 3, it is possible to observe that both polymers used to prepare the beads did not decrease cell viability after 24 h of incubation for both cell lines. After incubation with GG, HT29-MTX and Caco-2 cell viabilities were found to be higher than 89.4% and 90.2%, respectively, for all concentrations. Similar behavior was found for P, in which the percentage of viable cells for the HT29-MTX cell line was higher than 98.5%, and higher than 96.0% for Caco-2 cells. The increase in GG concentration did not significantly affect HT29-MTX or Caco-2 cell viability ($p > 0.05$). The same was observed for P, since no significant differences were observed in cell viability among the different polymer concentrations ($p > 0.05$). These results show that, within the evaluated concentrations, GG and P are nontoxic polymers to Caco-2 and HT29-MTX cell lines.

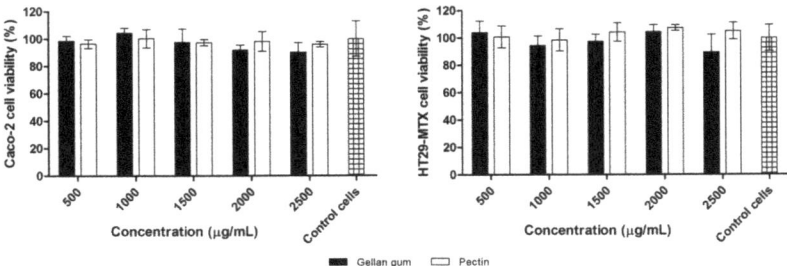

Figure 3. Cell viability (%) of Caco-2 and HT29-MTX cell lines after 24 h of incubation with increasing concentrations (500–2500 μg/mL) of GG and P (mean ± SD).

Beads biocompatibility, and therefore their safety to act as drug carriers for the delivery of RES to the colon, was evaluated by cell viability experiments. The percentage of viable cells from the different cell lines treated with empty beads, RES-loaded beads, and free RES, after 4 h of incubation with increasing concentrations of samples, is shown in Figure 4.

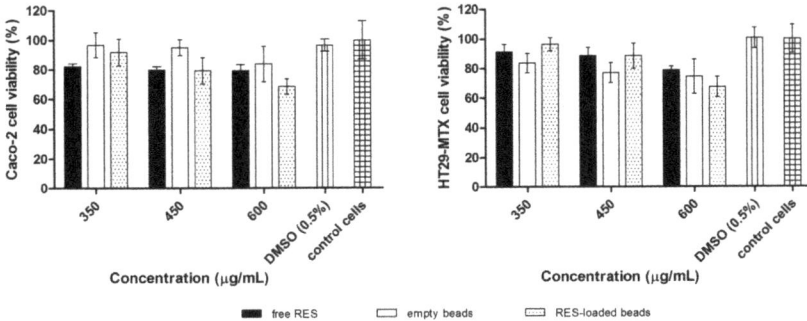

Figure 4. Cell viability (%) of Caco-2 and HT29-MTX cell lines after 4 h of incubation with increasing concentrations of free RES, and empty and RES-loaded beads (mean ± SD).

No significant cytotoxicity was observed when Caco-2 or HT29-MTX cell lines were incubated with HBSS containing 0.5% DMSO, indicating that DMSO up to 0.5% (v/v) can be used to prepare RES solutions for cytotoxicity studies. It was also observed that free RES and empty beads did not present a cytotoxic effect within the evaluated concentrations for both cell lines.

RES-loaded beads in concentrations of 6 and 8 beads/well did not reduce cell viability, however, at the highest concentration (10 beads/well) a discrete cytotoxic effect was observed, with 67.40% and 68.44% of cell viability for HT29-MTX and Caco-2 cell lines, respectively.

Comparing empty with RES-loaded beads reveals that the encapsulated RES did not influence the cell viability of both cell lines after 4 h of incubation ($p > 0.05$).

The cells were incubated in the presence of increasing concentrations of free RES (350–600 μg/mL), equivalent to the total amount of drug encapsulated in the beads (6 to 10 beads/well). The cell viability of HT29-MTX and Caco-2 cell lines after 4 h in the presence of RES-loaded beads was equal to that of free RES in all tested concentrations ($p > 0.05$).

Moreover, it is noteworthy that this assay was performed to evaluate the oral safety of the materials and to select non-toxic concentrations for the in vitro permeability experiments using the same cell lines, once the concentration of drug or drug carrier cannot present toxicity towards the cells that form the monolayer in the insert. Altogether, from the cell viability experiments, it can be concluded that GG:P beads are safe towards HT29-MTX and Caco-2 cells.

3.4. In Vitro Intestinal Permeability

The use of cell-based in vitro models allows the evaluation of drug permeability in conditions close to in vivo. These studies are of fundamental importance in the early stages of new drug delivery system development to ensure both success and reproducibility. Additionally, in vitro techniques avoid the use of laboratory animals and are less laborious and more economic than in vivo experiments [29].

The triple co-culture model used in this work has been recently established and optimized, gaining attraction as a more reliable model that more closely resembles intestinal mucosal architecture and, thus, the in vivo conditions found in humans to study drug permeability. It also allows evaluation of the effects of mucus on drug transport, and, therefore, it is a useful tool in studies with mucoadhesive systems [29,30].

In order to perform the in vitro permeability experiments, non-toxic concentrations of free RES and RES-loaded beads were selected based on cell viability results (Section 3.3). Tests were carried out uni-directionally from the apical to the basolateral compartment. The drug permeability profile is shown in Figure 5.

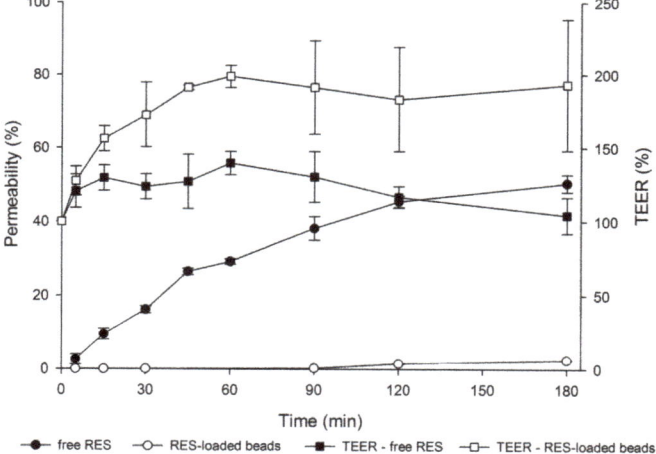

Figure 5. Permeability profile of free RES and RES-loaded beads across a triple co-culture model and TEER (%) of the cell monolayer as a function of time during the experiment ($n = 3$; mean ± SD).

Regarding RES permeability data (Figure 5), it is evident that there is a significant reduction in the permeability of RES carried in mucoadhesive beads compared to that of RES solution, which reached 50.4% permeation versus 2.49% for the encapsulated drug ($p < 0.05$).

The high P_{app} value of free RES (14.2×10^{-6} cm/s), 16 times higher than that of the encapsulated drug (0.87×10^{-6} cm/s), evidences the ability of GG:P beads to modulate the permeation of the drug. In fact, the high permeability of free RES is in agreement with previous studies on RES permeability through Caco-2 cells [48].

The significant impact of the bead carrier on the permeability of RES is a relevant and promising feature that may favor the accumulation of the RES in the colon. Regarding this behavior, important concerns must be considered. Firstly, the high permeability of free RES through this cell model indicates that the mucus layer that covers the cell in the triple co-culture model did not impose great resistance against the diffusion of RES molecules.

From this appointment, it may be possible to suppose that the retention of beads on the outer side of the mucus layer and the low drug release rates even at pH 6.8 (Section 3.2), near to 7.4 of this test, may be imperative for the low permeability of RES. Additionally, the mucoadhesiveness of the GG:P beads [8] may improve the interaction of RES with cells, prolonging the contact with the colonic cells, which might improve local activity at this site.

In addition, it was observed that for free RES, a decrease in TEER percentage occurred during the permeability test (Figure 5). It has been described in the literature that the opening of the tight junctions leads to a reduction in TEER. However, a minor damage in the monolayer is also able to drastically reduce the values of TEER. According to Odijk and co-authors, a change of around 0.4% in the area of cell coverage inside the insert could reduce TEER by 80% [49]. According to these authors, TEER values can be lower due to damage or small gaps, but the monolayer can still show good barrier function with strong tight junctions as demonstrated by fluorescent staining [49].

In contrast, for the encapsulated drug, increased TEER values (%) were observed during the experiment (from ~150% to 250%). This behavior may be related to the deposition of polymeric debris due to bead erosion on the cell layer, since significant erosion of these beads (~25%) after 2 h at a pH of 7.4 was previously reported [8].

Hence, observing the final TEER percentages of the triple co-culture model after contact with free RES and the encapsulated drug, it can be concluded that the monolayers remained relatively intact at the end of the experiments and that the variations in TEER values might not be related to cell death. In this way, the permeability results really reflect the drug transport across the cell monolayers.

4. Conclusions

In this work, RES was successfully encapsulated in mucoadhesive beads of GG:P ionically crosslinked with Al^{3+} ions, achieving a high %EE (around 75%). The system was characterized and evaluated regarding cytotoxicity and in vitro intestinal permeability using a triple co-culture cell model. Beads were circular, with an average diameter of 913 μm. FTIR analysis showed that RES must be physically entrapped within the polymer network. The system was able to reduce drug release in acidic media compared to free RES, releasing only 17.6% in a pH of 1.2, and control drug release for up to 48 h in a pH of 6.8. Release data of RES from the beads correlated better with Weibull's model and drug transport followed Fickian diffusion and Case II transport mechanisms. Cell viability studies showed that beads did not show toxicity towards a triple co-culture cell model, and even when a discrete cytotoxic effect was observed at the highest concentration evaluated in this work, the viability results were very close to the threshold value of 70%. The encapsulation of RES allowed for a significant reduction in its permeability across a triple co-culture cell model: a favorable feature for the targeted action of RES on colonic cells. In this way, the ionically-crosslinked GG:P beads represent a promising carrier system for the control of drug release throughout the GIT and the targeting of RES to the colon for the treatment of local diseases with the potential to improve the local action of the drug for the treatment of several pathologies in this organ.

Acknowledgments: Financial support from Capes. Andreia Almeida would like to thank Fundação para a Ciência e a Tecnologia (FCT), Portugal, for financial support (Grant SFRH/BD/118721/2016). This article is a result of the NORTE-01-0145-FEDER-000012 project, supported by the Norte Portugal Regional Operational Programme (NORTE 2020), under the PORTUGAL 2020 Partnership Agreement, through the European Regional Development Fund (ERDF). This work was also financed by Fundo Europeu de Desenvolvimento Regional (FEDER) funds through the COMPETE 2020 Operacional Programme for Competitiveness and Internationalisation (POCI), Portugal 2020, and by Portuguese funds through Fundação para a Ciência e a Tecnologia (FCT)/Ministério da Ciência, Tecnologia e Ensino Superior in the framework of the project "Institute for Research and Innovation in Health Sciences" (POCI-01-0145-FEDER-007274) and NETDIAMOND (POCI-01-0145-FEDER-016385).

Author Contributions: Fabíola Garavello Prezotti, Fernanda Isadora Boni, Natália Noronha Ferreira, Daniella de Souza e Silva, and Andreia Almeida conceived, designed, and performed the experiments; Teófilo Vasconcelos performed HPLC analyses; Maria Palmira Daflon Gremião, Beatriz Stringhetti Ferreira Cury, Teófilo Vasconcelos, and Bruno Sarmento contributed reagents/materials/analysis tools. The manuscript was jointly written by all authors. The manuscript has been reviewed by Sérgio Paulo Campana-Filho, Maria Palmira Daflon Gremião, Beatriz Stringhetti Ferreira Cury, and Bruno Sarmento.

Conflicts of Interest: The authors declare no conflict of interest.

References

1. Boni, F.I.; Prezotti, F.G.; Cury, B.S.F. Gellan gum microspheres crosslinked with trivalent ion: Effect of polymer and crosslinker concentrations on drug release and mucoadhesive properties. *Drug Dev. Ind. Pharm.* **2016**, *42*, 1283–1290. [CrossRef] [PubMed]
2. Prezotti, F.G.; Meneguin, A.B.; Evangelista, R.C.; Cury, B.S.F. Preparation and characterization of free films of high amylose/pectin mixtures cross-linked with sodium trimetaphosphate. *Drug Dev. Ind. Pharm.* **2012**, *38*, 1354–1359. [CrossRef] [PubMed]
3. Meneguin, A.B.; Beyssac, E.; Garrait, G.; Hsein, H.; Cury, B.S.F. Retrograded starch/pectin coated gellan gum-microparticles for oral administration of insulin: A technological platform for protection against enzymatic degradation and improvement of intestinal permeability. *Eur. J. Pharm. Biopharm.* **2018**, *123*, 84–94. [CrossRef] [PubMed]
4. Singh, B.N.; Trombetta, L.D.; Kim, K.H. Biodegradation behavior of gellan gum in simulated colonic media. *Pharm. Dev. Technol.* **2005**, *9*, 399–407. [CrossRef]
5. Vandamme, T.F.; Lenourry, A.; Charrueau, C.; Chaumeil, J.C. The use of polysaccharides to target drugs to the colon. *Carbohydr. Polym.* **2002**, *48*, 219–231. [CrossRef]
6. Sinha, V.R.; Kumria, R. Microbially triggered drug delivery to the colon. *Eur. J. Pharm. Sci.* **2003**, *18*, 3–18. [CrossRef]
7. Osmałek, T.; Froelich, A.; Tasarek, S. Application of gellan gum in pharmacy and medicine. *Int. J. Pharm.* **2014**, *466*, 328–340. [CrossRef] [PubMed]
8. Prezotti, F.G.; Cury, B.S.F.; Evangelista, R.C. Mucoadhesive beads of gellan gum/pectin intended to controlled delivery of drugs. *Carbohydr. Polym.* **2014**, *113*, 286–295. [CrossRef] [PubMed]
9. Crcarevska, M.S.; Dodov, M.G.; Goracinova, K. Chitosan coated Ca–alginate microparticles loaded with budesonide for delivery to the inflamed colonic mucosa. *Eur. J. Pharm. Biopharm.* **2008**, *68*, 565–578. [CrossRef]
10. Thirawong, N.; Nunthanid, J.; Puttipipatkhachorn, S.; Sriamornsak, P. Mucoadhesive properties of various pectins on gastrointestinal mucosa: An in vitro evaluation using texture analyzer. *Eur. J. Pharm. Biopharm.* **2007**, *67*, 132–140. [CrossRef] [PubMed]
11. Thirawong, N.; Kennedy, R.A.; Sriamornsak, P. Viscometric study of pectin–mucin interaction and its mucoadhesive bond strength. *Carbohydr. Polym.* **2008**, *71*, 170–179. [CrossRef]
12. Carvalho, F.C.; Bruschi, M.L.; Evangelista, R.C.; Gremião, M.P.D. Mucoadhesive drug delivery systems. *Braz. J. Pharm. Sci.* **2010**, *46*, 1–17. [CrossRef]
13. Sriamornsak, P.; Wattanakorn, N.; Nunthanid, J.; Puttipipatkhachorn, S. Mucoadhesion of pectin as evidence by wettability and chain interpenetration. *Carbohydr. Polym.* **2008**, *74*, 458–467. [CrossRef]
14. Liu, L.; Fishman, M.L.; Hicks, K.B.; Kende, M. Interaction of various pectin formulations with porcine colonic tissues. *Biomaterials* **2005**, *26*, 5907–5916. [CrossRef] [PubMed]
15. Mahdi, M.H.; Conway, B.R.; Smith, A.M. Development of mucoadhesive sprayable gellan gum fluid gels. *Int. J. Pharm.* **2015**, *488*, 12–19. [CrossRef] [PubMed]
16. Sosnik, A.; Das Neves, J.; Sarmento, B. Mucoadhesive polymers in the design of nano-drug delivery systems for administration by non-parenteral routes: A review. *Prog. Polym. Sci.* **2014**, *39*, 2030–2075. [CrossRef]
17. Varum, F.J.O.; Veiga, F.; Sousa, J.S.; Basit, A.W. An investigation into the role of mucus thickness on mucoadhesion in the gastrointestinal tract of pig. *Eur. J. Pharm. Sci.* **2010**, *40*, 335–341. [CrossRef] [PubMed]
18. Cury, B.S.F.; De Castro, A.D.; Klein, S.I.; Evangelista, R.C. Influence of phosphated cross-linked high amylose on in vitro release of different drugs. *Carbohydr. Polym.* **2009**, *78*, 789–793. [CrossRef]

19. Cury, B.S.F.; Castro, A.D.; Klein, S.I.; Evangelista, R.C. Modeling a system of phosphated cross-linked high amylose for controlled drug release. Part 2: Physical parameters, cross-linking degrees and drug delivery relationships. *Int. J. Pharm.* **2009**, *371*, 8–15. [CrossRef] [PubMed]
20. Cardoso, V.M.D.O.; Cury, B.S.F.; Evangelista, R.C.; Gremião, M.P.D. Development and characterization of cross-linked gellan gum and retrograded starch blend hydrogels for drug delivery applications. *J. Mech. Behav. Biomed. Mater.* **2017**, *65*, 317–333. [CrossRef] [PubMed]
21. Leopold, C.S. Coated dosage forms for colon-specific drug delivery. *Pharm. Sci. Technol. Today* **1999**, *2*, 197–204. [CrossRef]
22. Kulkarni, S.S.; Cantó, C. The molecular targets of resveratrol. *Biochim. Biophys. Acta Mol. Basis Dis.* **2015**, *1852*, 1114–1123. [CrossRef] [PubMed]
23. Walle, T.; Hsieh, F.; Delegge, M.H.; Oatis, J.E.; Walle, U.K. High absorption but very low bioavailability of oral resveratrol in humans. *Drug Metab. Dispos.* **2004**, *32*, 1377–1382. [CrossRef] [PubMed]
24. Delmas, D.; Lancon, A.; Colin, D.; Jannin, B.; Latruffe, N. Resveratrol as a chemopreventive agent: A promising molecule for fighting cancer. *Curr. Drug Targets* **2006**, *7*, 423–442. [CrossRef] [PubMed]
25. Baur, J.A.; Sinclair, D.A. Therapeutic potential of resveratrol: The in vivo evidence. *Nat. Rev. Drug Discov.* **2006**, *5*, 493–506. [CrossRef] [PubMed]
26. Camins, A.; Junyent, F.; Verdaguer, E.; Beas-Zarate, C.; Rojas-Mayorquín, A.; Ortuño-Sahagún, D.; Pallàs, M. Resveratrol: An antiaging drug with potential therapeutic applications in treating diseases. *Pharmaceuticals* **2009**, *2*, 194–205. [CrossRef] [PubMed]
27. Wenzel, E.; Somoza, V. Metabolism and bioavailability of trans-resveratrol. *Mol. Nutr. Food Res.* **2005**, *49*, 472–481. [CrossRef] [PubMed]
28. Das, S.; Lin, H.-S.; Ho, P.; Ng, K.-Y. The Impact of Aqueous Solubility and Dose on the Pharmacokinetic Profiles of Resveratrol. *Pharm. Res.* **2008**, *25*, 2593–2600. [CrossRef] [PubMed]
29. Antunes, F.; Andrade, F.; Araújo, F.; Ferreira, D.; Sarmento, B. Establishment of a triple co-culture in vitro cell models to study intestinal absorption of peptide drugs. *Eur. J. Pharm. Biopharm.* **2013**, *83*, 427–435. [CrossRef] [PubMed]
30. Araújo, F.; Sarmento, B. Towards the characterization of an in vitro triple co-culture intestine cell model for permeability studies. *Int. J. Pharm.* **2013**, *458*, 128–134. [CrossRef] [PubMed]
31. Pereira, C.; Araújo, F.; Barrias, C.C.; Granja, P.L.; Sarmento, B. Dissecting stromal-epithelial interactions in a 3D in vitro cellularized intestinal model for permeability studies. *Biomaterials* **2015**, *56*, 36–45. [CrossRef] [PubMed]
32. Munarin, F.; Petrini, P.; Farè, S.; Tanzi, M.C. Structural properties of polysaccharide-based microcapsules for soft tissue regeneration. *J. Mater. Sci. Mater. Med.* **2010**, *21*, 365–375. [CrossRef] [PubMed]
33. Das, S.; Ng, K.-Y.; Ho, P.C. Design of a pectin-based microparticle formulation using zinc ions as the cross-linking agent and glutaraldehyde as the hardening agent for colonic-specific delivery of resveratrol: In vitro and in vivo evaluations. *J. Drug Target.* **2011**, *19*, 446–457. [CrossRef] [PubMed]
34. Angadi, S.C.; Manjeshwar, L.S.; Aminabhavi, T.M. Coated interpenetrating blend microparticles of chitosan and guar gum for controlled release of isoniazid. *Ind. Eng. Chem. Res.* **2013**, *52*, 6399–6409. [CrossRef]
35. Sangsen, Y.; Wiwattanawongsa, K.; Likhitwitayawuid, K.; Sritularak, B.; Graidist, P.; Wiwattanapatapee, R. Influence of surfactants in self-microemulsifying formulations on enhancing oral bioavailability of oxyresveratrol: Studies in Caco-2 cells and in vivo. *Int. J. Pharm.* **2016**, *498*, 294–303. [CrossRef] [PubMed]
36. Silva, D.S.; Almeida, A.; Prezotti, F.; Cury, B.; Campana-Filho, S.P.; Sarmento, B. Synthesis and characterization of 3,6-O,O'-dimyristoyl chitosan micelles for oral delivery of paclitaxel. *Colloids Surf. B. Biointerfaces* **2017**, *152*, 220–228. [CrossRef] [PubMed]
37. Hilgendorf, C.; Spahn-Langguth, H.; Regårdh, C.G.; Lipka, E.; Amidon, G.L.; Langguth, P. Caco-2 versus Caco-2/HT29-MTX co-cultured cell lines: Permeabilities via diffusion, inside- and outside-directed carrier-mediated transport. *J. Pharm. Sci.* **2000**, *89*, 63–75. [CrossRef]
38. Behrens, I.; Stenberg, P.; Artursson, P.; Kissel, T. Transport of lipophilic drug molecules in a new mucus-secreting cell culture model based on HT29-MTX cells. *Pharm. Res.* **2001**, *18*, 1138–1145. [CrossRef] [PubMed]
39. Yang, F.; Xia, S.; Tan, C.; Zhang, X. Preparation and evaluation of chitosan-calcium-gellan gum beads for controlled release of protein. *Eur. Food Res. Technol.* **2013**, *237*, 467–479. [CrossRef]

40. Ramasamy, T.; Ruttala, H.B.; Shanmugam, S.; Umadevi, S.K. Eudragit-coated aceclofenac-loaded pectin microspheres in chronopharmacological treatment of rheumatoid arthritis. *Drug Deliv.* **2013**, *20*, 65–77. [CrossRef] [PubMed]
41. Kamnev, A.A.; Colina, M.; Rodriguez, J.; Ptitchkina, N.M.; Ignatov, V.V. Comparative spectroscopic characterization of different pectins and their sources. *Food Hydrocoll.* **1998**, *12*, 263–271. [CrossRef]
42. Wang, Q.-S.; Wang, G.-F.; Zhou, J.; Gao, L.-N.; Cui, Y.-L. Colon targeted oral drug delivery system based on alginate-chitosan microspheres loaded with icariin in the treatment of ulcerative colitis. *Int. J. Pharm.* **2016**, *515*, 176–185. [CrossRef] [PubMed]
43. Carbinatto, F.M.; De Castro, A.D.; Evangelista, R.C.; Cury, B.S.F. Insights into the swelling process and drug release mechanisms from cross-linked pectin/high amylose starch matrices. *Asian J. Pharm. Sci.* **2014**, *9*, 27–34. [CrossRef]
44. Papadopoulou, V.; Kosmidis, K.; Vlachou, M.; Macheras, P. On the use of the Weibull function for the discernment of drug release mechanisms. *Int. J. Pharm.* **2006**, *309*, 44–50. [CrossRef] [PubMed]
45. Masaro, L.; Zhu, X.X. Physical models of diffusion for polymer solutions, gels and solids. *Prog. Polym. Sci.* **1999**, *24*, 731–775. [CrossRef]
46. Fischer, D.; Li, Y.; Ahlemeyer, B.; Krieglstein, J.; Kissel, T. In vitro cytotoxicity testing of polycations: Influence of polymer structure on cell viability and hemolysis. *Biomaterials* **2003**, *24*, 1121–1131. [CrossRef]
47. International Organization for Standardization. *ISO 10993-5. Biological Evaluation of Medical Devices—Part 5: Tests for In Vitro Cytotoxicity*; International Organization for Standardization: Geneva, Switzerland, 2009.
48. Seljak, K.B.; Berginc, K.; Trontelj, J.; Zvonar, A.; Kristl, A.; Gašperlin, M. A self-microemulsifying drug delivery system to overcome intestinal resveratrol toxicity and presystemic metabolism. *J. Pharm. Sci.* **2014**, *103*, 3491–3500. [CrossRef] [PubMed]
49. Odijk, M.; Meer, A.D.V.D.; Levner, D.; Kim, H.J.; Helm, M.W.V.D.; Segerink, L.I.; Frimat, J.-P.; Hamilton, G.A.; Ingber, D.E.; Berga, A.V.D. Measuring direct current trans-epithelial electrical resistance in organ-on-a-chip microsystems. *Lab Chip* **2015**, *15*, 745–752. [CrossRef] [PubMed]

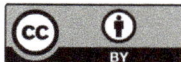

© 2018 by the authors. Licensee MDPI, Basel, Switzerland. This article is an open access article distributed under the terms and conditions of the Creative Commons Attribution (CC BY) license (http://creativecommons.org/licenses/by/4.0/).

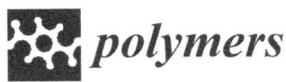

Article

Preformulation Studies of Furosemide-Loaded Electrospun Nanofibrous Systems for Buccal Administration

Andrea Kovács [1,3], Balázs Démuth [2], Andrea Meskó [3] and Romána Zelkó [3,*]

1. Gedeon Richter Plc., Formulation R&D, Gyömrői Street 19-21, H-1103 Budapest, Hungary; kovacs.andrea@pharma.semmelweis-univ.hu
2. Department of Organic Chemistry and Technology, Budapest University of Technology and Economics, Budafoki út 8. 3, H-1103 Budapest, Hungary; demuth@oct.bme.hu
3. University Pharmacy Department of Pharmacy Administration, Semmelweis University, Hőgyes Endre Street 7-9, H-1092 Budapest, Hungary; mesko.attilane@pharma.semmelweis-univ.hu
* Correspondence: zelko.romana@pharma.semmelweis-univ.hu; Tel.: +36-217-0927

Received: 18 October 2017; Accepted: 22 November 2017; Published: 25 November 2017

Abstract: Furosemide loaded electrospun fibers were prepared for buccal administration, with the aim of improving the oral bioavailability of the poorly soluble and permeable crystalline drug, which can be achieved by the increased solubility and by the circumvention of the intensive first pass metabolism. The water soluble hydroxypropyl cellulose (HPC) was chosen as a mucoadhesive polymer. In order to improve the electrospinnability of HPC, poly (vinylpyrrolidone) (PVP) was used. During the experiments, the total polymer concentration was kept constant at 15% (w/w), and only the ratio of the two polymers (HPC-PVP = 5:5, 6:4, 7:3, 8:2, 9:1) was changed. A combination of rheological measurements with scanning electron microscopic morphological images of electrospun samples was applied for the determination of the optimum composition of the gels for fiber formation. The crystalline–amorphous transition of furosemide was tracked by Fourier transform infrared spectroscopy. A correlation was found between the rheological properties of the polymer solutions and their electrospinnability, and the consequent morphology of the resultant samples. With decreasing HPC ratio of the system, a transition from the spray-dried droplets to the randomly oriented fibrous structures was observed. The results enable the determination of the polymer ratio for the formation of applicable quality of electrospun fibers.

Keywords: furosemide; electrospinning; hydroxypropyl cellulose; poly (vinylpyrrolidone); storage and loss moduli; scanning electron microscopic images

1. Introduction

Electrospinning is an emerging technology by which mats of micro- and nanofibers can be produced using an electrostatically driven jet of polymer solution or melt. A wide variety of micro- and nanofibers have been formulated by this process using several natural and synthetic polymers. The use of electrospinning for the fabrication of drug-loaded nanofibrous scaffolds is a promising alternative for developing delivery systems of high efficiency. Many types of drugs can be easily incorporated into electrospun materials. Along with the changes of the morphology, the porosity and the composition of the nanofibers, and the release profile of the incorporated drug can be fine-tuned [1].

Furosemide is used as a loop diuretic in treatment of hypertension, and in renal, cardiac, and hepatic oedematous status. It belongs to the BCS (Biopharmaceutical Classification System) IV class, due to its poor water soluble properties (5–20 µg/mL at pH = 7) and low membrane permeability, and thus, poor bioavailability [2–7]. The low and variable absorption from the stomach and upper part of the duodenum in the gastrointestinal tract, and presence of intestinal efflux proteins, make its therapeutic use difficult. The reason of the slight absorption is partly the presence of the intestinal efflux proteins, mentioned previously, and in part the ionization (the ionization is 94.06% at pH = 5 and 99.97% at pH = 7.4). In the ileum, the expression of the MDR1 (multidrug resistance P-glycoprotein; PgP) efflux protein is much more than in the jejunum. Therefore, the absorption in the ileum is 2.5 times slower than in the jejunum [8].

Furosemide is commonly applied in oral and intravenous therapies, but many systemic side effects occur during the traditional administrations, like polyuria, mouth drying, dizziness, and gastric problems [9]. Because of the low oral bioavailability and the slow onset of action (even 60 min) the administration of the conventional tablets is not appropriate in emergency situations [10].

The registered furosemide containing medicines are mostly tablets (40, 80, 500 mg) and injections in Hungary [11]. However, several research groups deal with developing new formulations, owing to the enhancement of the water solubility of the furosemide and its consequent bioavailability. Some of these formulations are fast dissolving tablets [10], supramolecular complexes [4,7], melt extrusion methods [12], micro/nanoparticles for drug delivery [13], mucoadhesive microspheres [3], and halloysites [14]. The primary focus of the recent studies was to improve the solubility and permeability of the BCS IV drugs by the use of special formulation strategies.

An alternative formulation of active ingredients with poor water solubility and low bioavailability, is to make a mucoadhesive buccal drug delivery system. It is also a good opportunity to use the drugs in emergency situations without invasive administration. The transmucosal formulations could be an option in the case of enhancing the bioavailability of the furosemide. Using buccal administration, it can be possible to circumvent the first pass metabolism. As consequence of the rich vascularization of the buccal mucosa, the drug can be easily taken to the systemic circulation. On the other hand, the buccal epithelium has a barrier function, which makes penetration difficult, therefore, it is necessary the use of permeation enhancers during the formulation [15–17].

Electrospun nanofibrous drug delivery systems could be promising alternative forms with their advantages, like high porosity, high surface to volume ratio, and the transition of crystalline to amorphous form, thus enhancing solubility [18–20].

The aim of the present study was to prepare amorphous furosemide-loaded mucoadhesive fibrous formulations containing solubilizer, which could also act as a penetration enhancer for buccal application. Aqueous solution was used for the electrospinning to generate nanofibers of environmentally friendly conditions, and consequently, there was no need to define the residual solvent content. In order to select the optimum composition, the authors provide detail and adequate characterization of the fibers with rheology, size, morphology, and solid-state characterization. The correlation between the fiber forming ability and the rheological properties of the initial drug-containing HPC-PVP solutions and their electrospinnability, and the consequent morphology of the resultant samples, was also determined.

2. Materials and Methods

2.1. Materials

Hydroxypropyl cellulose (Klucel EXF Pharm, Ashland, Covington, KY, USA; Mw ~80,000, the moles of substitution = 3.8), poly(vinylpyrrolidone) (Kollidon 90 F, BASF, Ludwigshafen, Germany; Mw ~1,000,000–1,500,000) as polymers (Figure 1b,c), trolamine (Ph. Eur., Molar Chemicals, Budapest, Hungary) as surfactant, and purified water was used as solvent for the polymers. Furosemide (Ph. Eur., Figure 1a) was used as model drug from the BCS IV class.

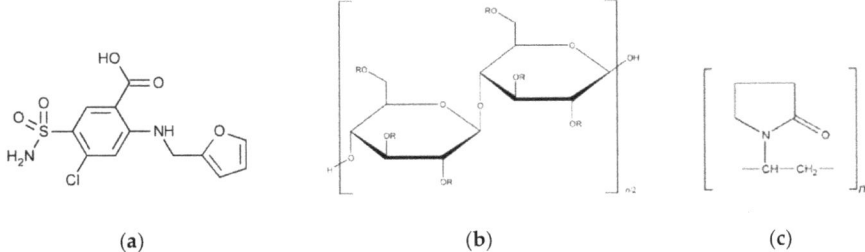

Figure 1. Chemical structure of furosemide (**a**) and the structural units of fiber forming polymers ((**b**) HPC, (**c**) PVP).

2.2. Preparation of Furosemide Containing HPC-PVP Gels

The stock solution of furosemide was prepared by adding 0.2 furosemide into a dark beaker, and it was dissolved with 17.2 g purified water in a few minutes under magnetic stirring by adding 0.3 g trolamine as solubilizer. The gels were prepared by using the furosemide solution in each case, and a different added amount of PVP. These compositions were being mixed at room temperature ($T = 25\ ^\circ C$), until they had reached a totally homogenous condition. The necessary amount of HPC was added in small portions to the prepared drug loading PVP gels during stirring, also at room temperature ($T = 25\ ^\circ C$) to achieve the homogeneity. The total polymer concentration of the gels was 15 wt %, but the w/w ratio of the applied two polymers was different. The different HPC-PVP ratios were 5:5, 6:4, 7:3, 8:2, 9:1.

2.3. Preparation of the Physical Mixtures

For the fourier transform infrared (FT-IR) measurements the powder physical mixtures of the gel components (containing furosemide, polymers, and surfactant) were prepared and homogenized by stirring for 5 min in a porcelain mortar.

2.4. Rheological Properties of the Gels

Kinexus Pro Rheometer (Malvern Instruments Ltd., Malvern, UK) was used for measuring the rheological properties of the prepared gels at room temperature ($T = 25 \pm 0.1\ ^\circ C$). During the measurement, data were registered with software of rSpace for Kinexus Pro 1.3 (Malvern Instruments Ltd., Malvern, UK). Parallel plates geometry (diameter: 50 mm) was applied during the tests; the gap between the plates was 0.0300 mm. Elastic (G') and viscous moduli (G'') were determined by oscillatory rheological tests. The oscillatory shear measurements were performed at amplitude within the linear region, which was chosen to 30% within the viscoelastic region, and the frequency was in the range of 0.1–$10\ s^{-1}$. Three parallel measurements were done with each gel in both tests.

2.5. Electrospinning

The nanofibers were prepared by electrospinning at room temperature ($25\ ^\circ C$). The gels were put into syringes, after that, silicon tubes with needles (internal diameter: 1.2) on their ends were connected to the syringes. High voltage was applied (25 kV) at 15 cm collector-needle distance. The flow rate was 0.3 mL/h during the spinning process. The prepared fibers and droplets were dried at room temperature during the electrospinning process.

2.6. ATR-FTIR (Attenuated Total Reflectance-Fourier Transform Infrared) Spectroscopy Measurements

The ATR-FTIR spectra of the fibers, physical mixtures and raw substances were measured by using Jasco FT/IR-4200 spectrophotometer (Jasco Inc., Easton, MD, USA), which was equipped with Jasco ATR PRO470-H single reflection accessory. The spectra were collected over a wavenumber range of 4000 and 1800 cm^{-1}. After 100 scans, the measurements were evaluated with Spectra Manager-II, Jasco software.

2.7. Scanning Electron Microscopy (SEM) Measurements

The morphology was examined by JEOL 6380LVa (JEOL, Tokyo, Japan) scanning electron microscope using secondary electron imaging detection method. The collected samples on aluminum foil were fixed with conductive double-sided carbon adhesive tape, and their surface was covered by sputtered gold before the measurement. Accelerating voltage (15 kV) was applied, and the working distance was 10 mm during the examination.

2.8. Statistical Analysis of the Fiber Diameters

Statistical comparisons of samples were conducted using SPSS 20.0 software package (SPSS Inc., Chicago, IL, USA). The SEM images were used for the measurement, and the mean diameters were calculated by using Image J program (https://imagej.nih.gov/nih-image/). Fifty measurements from the fibrous elements were carried out in each SEM image. Only the fibers were examined, and the droplets were not considered for the determination of the average diameter size.

3. Results and Discussion

3.1. Rheological Properties

Figure 2 represents the loss (G'')/storage (G') moduli as a function of HPC-PVP ratio. The results indicate, as a function of the SEM images, that there is an optimum viscoelastic behavior of the composite gels, which results in the best fiber forming ability, and thus, more homogeneous randomly-oriented fibrous mats. Similarly to the previous experiences [21], the scanning electron microscopic images of the samples revealed that revealed that there exists a viscoelastic range, which provides an advantageous macrostructural arrangement of the macromolecules for the fiber formation. The latter can be explained by phenomenon that the prevalent viscoelasticity of the sample could be disadvantageous from the point of the formation of homogeneous nanostructured fiber elements, since the electrical forces cannot be effectively transferred to the viscoelastic elongation of the polymer jets in the course of the fiber formation. The most elastic sample (HPC-PVP = 6:4) resulted the most homogenous nanofibrous system.

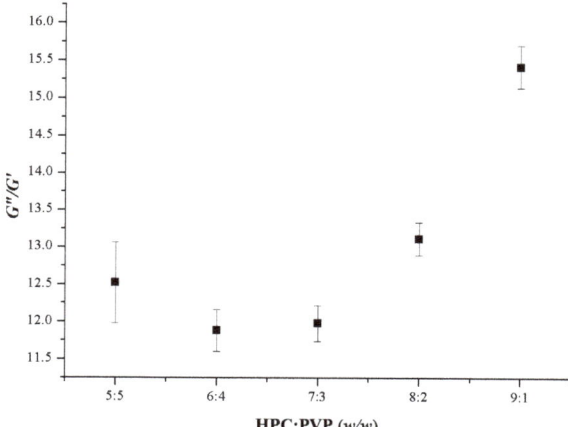

Figure 2. Ratio of loss (G'') and storage (G') moduli of furosemide-loaded gels as a function of HPC-PVP mass ratio (oscillatory shear measurements at a frequency 1.995 Hz).

3.2. ATR-FTIR Analysis

The FT-IR spectra of the raw materials, the physical mixtures and the prepared formulations are presented in the Figure 3. Furosemide has three characteristic peaks in the range of 3400–3200 cm^{-1}. The peaks are sulphonamide NH stretching at 3397 cm^{-1} and 3281 cm^{-1}, and there is a peak of secondary amine NH stretching at 3349 cm^{-1}, which are in good agreement with previous studies [7]. The Figure 3 clearly indicates similar peaks belonging to the sulphonamide NH stretching, and a peak of the secondary amine NH stretching, which are missing in the fibrous sample, meanwhile, these peaks can be distinguished in the physical mixture of the components. In the 1600–500 cm^{-1} "fingerprint region" of the fibers, the characteristic peaks of the fiber-forming polymers (PVP at 1653 cm^{-1} NH bending, HPC at 1100 cm^{-1} C–O stretching) can be identified (indicated in the Figure 3). The solubilized furosemide complexes are situated in the polymeric chains, thus forming an amorphous solid dispersion.

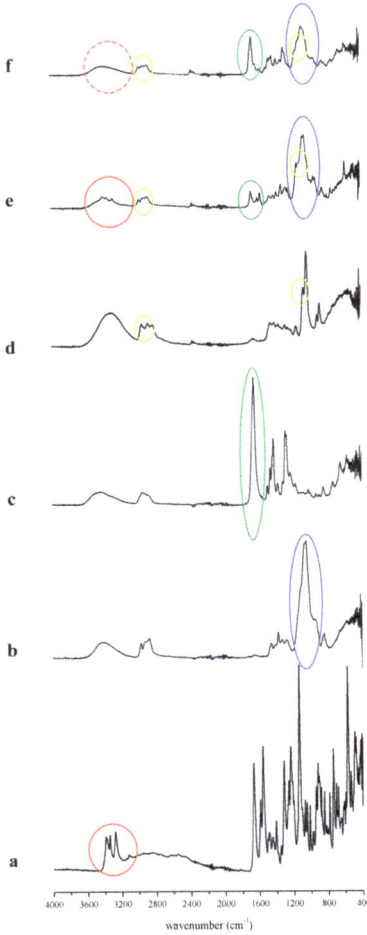

Figure 3. FT-IR spectra of the raw materials, physical mixture and the furosemide containing fibers. (**a**) furosemide; (**b**) HPC EXF; (**c**) PVP 90F; (**d**) trolamine; (**e**) physical mixture (HPC-PVP = 6:4 molar ratio); (**f**) furosemide containing fiber of HPC-PVP = 6:4 molar ratio.

3.3. Morphological Analysis

Along with the changes of the polymer ratio, the corresponding morphology of the electrospun samples also varied. On the scanning electron microscopic images (Figure 4), nanofibers and spray-dried droplets were distinguished. In case of images A and B, the fibrous structural elements are the most dominant, while on images C–E, droplets and randomly oriented fibers can be found, as well. Along with the increase of the HPC ratio in the composites, more droplets formed in the fibrous mats. Based on the SEM images, sample B (HPC-PVP = 6:4) can be considered the most homogeneous fibrous system.

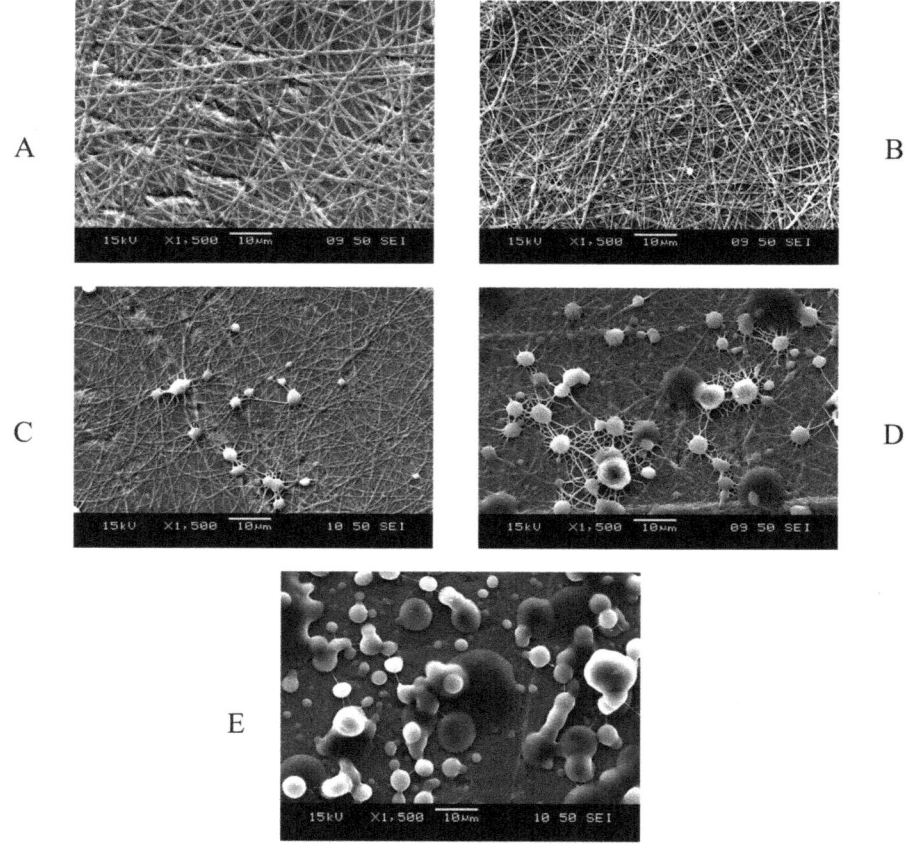

Figure 4. SEM images of the fibers consisting of different HPC-PVP molar ratios. (**A**) HPC-PVP = 5:5 molar ratio; (**B**) HPC-PVP = 6:4 molar ratio; (**C**) HPC-PVP = 7:3 molar ratio; (**D**) HPC-PVP = 8:2 molar ratio; (**E**) HPC-PVP = 9:1 molar ratio.

3.4. Statistical Analysis of the Fiber Diameters

For the statistical analysis of the fiber diameters, only the fibrous samples of HPC-PVP = 5:5; 6:4; 7:3; 8:2 molar ratios were investigated. In the case of HPC-PVP = 9:1 ratio, the diameter distribution cannot be determined, since almost totally electrosprayed structure was formed. The distributions of the four samples were tested using the Kolmogorov–Smirnov test. In all four cases, normality was confirmed (the corresponding p values are 0.964; 0.992; 0.641; 0.410). The difference of the sample distributions was analyzed by variance, and significant differences found ($p < 0.001$). Further, pairwise comparisons using the Bonferroni and Scheffe post hoc tests were conducted. The first sample (HPC-PVP = 5:5) shows significant difference from the other three ($p < 0.001$); the other samples are all normally distributed compared to each other. The results of the statistical analysis are illustrated in the Figure 5. The statistical evaluation confirmed that a sample of HPC-PVP = 6:4 ratio is the principally suitable concentration for electrospinning under given preparation conditions, which suggests that in case of the optimum concentration, the characteristics of the fibers are more predictable than in other concentrations.

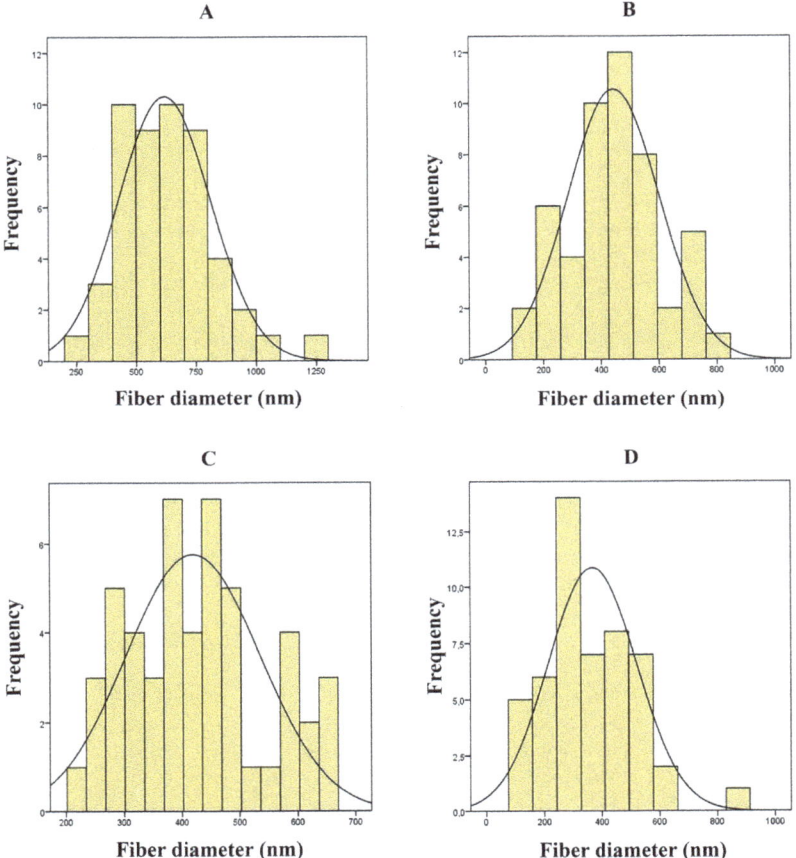

Figure 5. Distribution of fiber diameters. (**A**) HPC-PVP = 5:5 molar ratio; average diameter: 618.76 ± 193.617 nm; (**B**) HPC-PVP = 6:4 molar ratio; average diameter: 443.89 ± 158.376 nm; (**C**) HPC-PVP = 7:3 molar ratio; average diameter: 419.43 ± 116.048 nm; (**D**) HPC-PVP = 8:2 molar ratio; average diameter: 367.50 ± 153.908 nm.

4. Conclusions

Furosemide loaded HPC-PVP composite nanofibrous systems were prepared successfully by electrospinning process. The optimum composition of HPC-PVP fibers was determined based on the rheological examination of polymeric solutions and the scanning electron microscopic morphological characterization of the corresponding electrospun samples. This formulation could enable the transmucosal amorphous drug delivery of the poorly soluble and permeable drug (BCS IV), thus improving the oral bioavailability of furosemide, meanwhile, avoiding its first pass metabolism.

Acknowledgments: The authors are grateful to Péter Szabó for the valuable discussions and advices.

Author Contributions: Andrea Kovács designed and accomplished the experiments, like preparation of the gels and electrospun fibrous mats, rheological and ATR-FTIR measurements of the samples. Balázs Demuth performed the SEM measurements. Andrea Meskó statistically analyzed the results. Romána Zelkó and Andrea Kovács evaluated the results.

Conflicts of Interest: The authors declare no conflict of interest.

References

1. Andrady, A.L. Biomedical applications of nanofibers. In *Science and Technology of Polymer Nanofibers*; John W. Sons, Inc.: Hoboken, NJ, USA, 2008; pp. 183–223. ISBN 978-0-471-79059-4.
2. De Zordi, N.; Moneghini, M.; Kikic, I.; Grassi, M.; Del Rio Castillo, A.E.; Solinas, D.; Bolger, M.B. Applications of supercritical fluids to enhance the dissolution behaviors of furosemide by generation of microparticles and solid dispersions. *Eur. J. Pharm. Biopharm.* **2012**, *81*, 131–141. [CrossRef] [PubMed]
3. Lemieux, M.; Gosselin, P.; Mateescu, M.A. Carboxymethyl starch mucoadhesive microspheres as gastroretentive dosage form. *Int. J. Pharm.* **2015**, *496*, 497–508. [CrossRef] [PubMed]
4. Garnero, C.; Chattah, A.K.; Longhi, M. Improving furosemide polymorphs properties through supramolecular complexes of beta-cyclodextrin. *J. Pharm. Biomed. Anal.* **2014**, *95*, 139–145. [CrossRef] [PubMed]
5. Sahu, B.P.; Das, M.K. Nanoprecipitation with sonication for enhancement of oral bioavailability of furosemide. *Acta Pol. Pharm.* **2014**, *71*, 129–137. [PubMed]
6. Nielsen, L.H.; Gordon, S.; Holm, R.; Selen, A.; Rades, T.; Müllertz, A. Preparation of an amorphous sodium furosemide salt improves solubility and dissolution rate and leads to a faster T_{max} after oral dosing to rats. *Eur. J. Pharm. Biopharm.* **2013**, *85*, 942–951. [CrossRef] [PubMed]
7. Garnero, C.; Chattah, A.K.; Longhi, M. Supramolecular complexes of maltodextrin and furosemide polymorphs: A new approach for delivery systems. *Carbohydr. Polym.* **2013**, *94*, 292–300. [CrossRef] [PubMed]
8. Kortejarvi, H.; Malkki, J.; Shawahna, R.; Scherrmann, J.M.; Urtti, A.; Yliperttula, M. Pharmacokinetic simulations to explore dissolution criteria of BCS I and III biowaivers with and without MDR-1 efflux transporter. *Eur. J. Pharm. Sci.* **2014**, *61*, 18–26. [CrossRef] [PubMed]
9. Cho, C.W.; Choi, J.S.; Shin, S.C. Controlled release of furosemide from the ethylene-vinyl acetate matrix. *Int. J. Pharm.* **2005**, *299*, 127–133. [CrossRef] [PubMed]
10. Maheshwari, R.K.; Jagwani, Y. Mixed hydrotropy: Novel science of solubility enhancement. *Indian J. Pharm. Sci.* **2011**, *73*, 179–183. [CrossRef] [PubMed]
11. National Institute of Pharmacy and Nutrition. Available online: https://www.ogyei.gov.hu/gyogyszeradatbazis/ (accessed on 15 December 2016).
12. Melocchi, A.; Loreti, G.; Del Curto, M.D.; Maroni, A.; Gazzaniga, A.; Zema, L. Evaluation of hot-melt extrusion and injection molding for continuous manufacturing of immediate-release tablets. *J. Pharm. Sci.* **2015**, *104*, 1971–1980. [CrossRef] [PubMed]
13. Wei, X.; Gong, C.; Gou, M.; Fu, S.; Guo, Q.; Shi, S.; Luo, F.; Guo, G.; Qiu, L.; Qian, Z. Biodegradable poly(ε-caprolactone)-poly(ethylene glycol) copolymers as drug delivery system. *Int. J. Pharm.* **2009**, *381*, 1–18. [CrossRef] [PubMed]
14. Lvov, Y.; Abdullayev, E. Functional polymer–clay nanotube composites with sustained release of chemical agents. *Prog. Polym. Sci.* **2013**, *38*, 1690–1719. [CrossRef]
15. Sudhakar, Y.; Kuotsu, K.; Bandyopadhyay, A.K. Buccal bioadhesive drug delivery—A promising option for orally less efficient drugs. *J. Control. Release* **2006**, *114*, 15–40. [CrossRef] [PubMed]
16. Hearnden, V.; Sankar, V.; Hull, K.; Juras, D.V.; Greenberg, M.; Kerr, A.R.; Lockhart, P.B.; Patton, L.L.; Porter, S.; Thornhill, M.H. New developments and opportunities in oral mucosal drug delivery for local and systemic disease. *Adv. Drug Deliv. Rev.* **2012**, *64*, 16–28. [CrossRef] [PubMed]

17. Patel, V.F.; Liu, F.; Brown, M.B. Advances in oral transmucosal drug delivery. *J. Control. Release* **2011**, *153*, 106–116. [CrossRef] [PubMed]
18. Kapahi, H.; Khan, N.M.; Bhardwaj, A.; Mishra, N. Implication of nanofibers in oral drug delivery. *Curr. Pharm. Des.* **2015**, *21*, 2021–2036. [CrossRef] [PubMed]
19. Sebe, I.; Szabó, P.; Kállai-Szabó, B.; Zelkó, R. Incorporating small molecules or biologics into nanofibers for optimized drug release: A review. *Int. J. Pharm.* **2015**, *494*, 516–530. [CrossRef] [PubMed]
20. Kai, D.; Liow, S.S.; Loh, X.J. Biodegradable polymers for electrospinning: Towards biomedical applications. *Mater. Sci. Eng. C* **2014**, *45*, 659–670. [CrossRef] [PubMed]
21. Kazsoki, A.; Szabó, P.; Zelkó, R. Prediction of the hydroxypropyl cellulose-poly(vinyl alcohol) ratio in aqueous solution containing papaverine hydrochloride in terms of drug loaded electrospun fiber formation. *J. Pharm. Biomed. Anal.* **2017**, *138*, 357–362. [CrossRef] [PubMed]

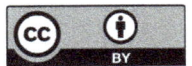

© 2017 by the authors. Licensee MDPI, Basel, Switzerland. This article is an open access article distributed under the terms and conditions of the Creative Commons Attribution (CC BY) license (http://creativecommons.org/licenses/by/4.0/).

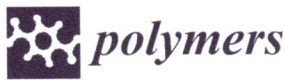

Review

Thiolated Hyaluronic Acid as Versatile Mucoadhesive Polymer: From the Chemistry Behind to Product Developments—What Are the Capabilities?

Janine Griesser [1], Gergely Hetényi [1] and Andreas Bernkop-Schnürch [1,2,*]

[1] Thiomatrix Forschungs-und Beratungs GmbH, Trientlgasse 65, 6020 Innsbruck, Austria; j.griesser@thiomatrix.com (J.G.); hetenyig@gmail.com (G.H.)
[2] Center for Chemistry and Biomedicine, Department of Pharmaceutical Technology, Institute of Pharmacy, University of Innsbruck, Innrain 80/82, 6020 Innsbruck, Austria
* Correspondence: andreas.bernkop@uibk.ac.at; Tel.: +43-512-507-58601

Received: 12 January 2018; Accepted: 24 February 2018; Published: 28 February 2018

Abstract: Within the last decade, intensive research work has been conducted on thiolated hyaluronic acids (HA-SH). By attaching sulfhydryl ligands onto naturally occurring hyaluronic acid various types of HA-SH can be designed. Due the ability of disulfide bond formation within the polymer itself as well as with biological materials, certain properties such as mucoadhesive, gelling, enzyme inhibitory, permeation enhancing and release controlling properties are improved. Besides the application in the field of drug delivery, HA-SH has been investigated as auxiliary material for wound healing. Within this review, the characteristics of novel drug delivery systems based on HA-SH are summarized and the versatility of this polymer for further applications is described by introducing numerous relevant studies in this field.

Keywords: thiolated hyaluronic acid; hydrogel; mucoadhesive; biocompatibility; controlled release; drug delivery; wound healing

1. Introduction

Hyaluronic acid (HA) is a polysaccharide exhibiting a linear molecular shape. The basic structure consists of two repeating saccharide units, namely D-glucuronic acid and N-acetyl glucosamine [1]. Over the years numerous modifications of HA have been introduced. Among them thiolated HA seems to be the most promising one. The attachment of ligands containing free thiol groups onto the polymeric backbone of HA has been the first time described by Bernkop-Schnürch [2] and opens wide possibilities for pharmaceutical applications by tailoring its function. Through thiolation of HA properties such as mucoadhesiveness, swelling capacity, stability and biocompatibility could be improved [3]. The protection of thiol groups via crosslinking or preactivation forming disulfide bonds generates more stable and effective drug delivery systems as the properties of thiomers are further improved [4]. Apart from drug delivery systems, thiolated HA is modified through crosslinkage leading to a scaffold structure and could be consequently applied for wound healing and tissue engineering. Within ocular regenerative medicine, for instance, an improved coronal and ocular wound care is highly on demand and the application of thiolated HA might be a promising approach [5].

It is the aim of this review to provide a comprehensive overview regarding the capabilities of thiolated HA starting with its properties—concretely, mucoadhesive properties, gelation properties, stability, enzyme inhibition properties, biocompatibility, permeation enhancing properties and controlled release. Moreover, further applications, various drug delivery systems (buccal, vaginal, and ocular) and finally product developments are discussed.

2. The Chemistry Behind

The linear polysaccharide HA consists of disaccharide units namely D-glucuronic acid and N-acetyl glucosamine linked via β(1,4) and β(1,3) glycosidic bonds, as illustrated in Figure 1. Due to the hydrophilicity of HA, it forms hydrogen bonds between water molecules and carboxyl- as well as acetyl-groups. As HA exhibits a high molecular weight and strong interactions with water, HA is highly viscous in aqueous solution [6,7]. Furthermore, HA naturally occurs in human body from the extracellular matrix of connective tissue, across the dermis of the skin and up to the vitreous body of the eye. Therefore, the major role of HA within the body is giving structure to tissues as well as hydration [8,9]. With a biological half-life of maximal 24 h, HA is continuously degraded within the organism by hyaluronidase enzymes as well as via HA cell internalization by CD44 cell surface receptors [10,11]. Apart from enzymatic degradation, HA could be cleaved through many ways such as via acidic or alkaline hydrolysis, thermal degradation and degradation by oxidants [12]. Due to high water solubility, the development of polymers used for tissue engineering represented a problem [13]. Hence, chemical modification and crosslinking is mandatory in order to expand the degradation time as well as to improve the mechanical stability in vivo [14]. Two chemical groups, namely carboxylic and hydroxyl groups, can be modified via different chemical reactions resulting in thiolated HA, as listed in Table 1. Moreover, Figure 1 illustrates the thiolation of carboxylic groups in the first step and subsequently the protection of this thiol group via preactivation utilizing 6-mercaptonicotinamide to provide just one example. Via this preactivation with 6-mercaptonicotinamide the free thiol groups are oxidized to disulfide bonds. As free thiol groups from thiolated HA are sensitive towards oxidation and rapidly react with the cysteine-rich domains in the mucus, S-protection (=preactivation) plays a major role in the improvement of mucoadhesiveness, cohesiveness as well as stability against degradation [4].

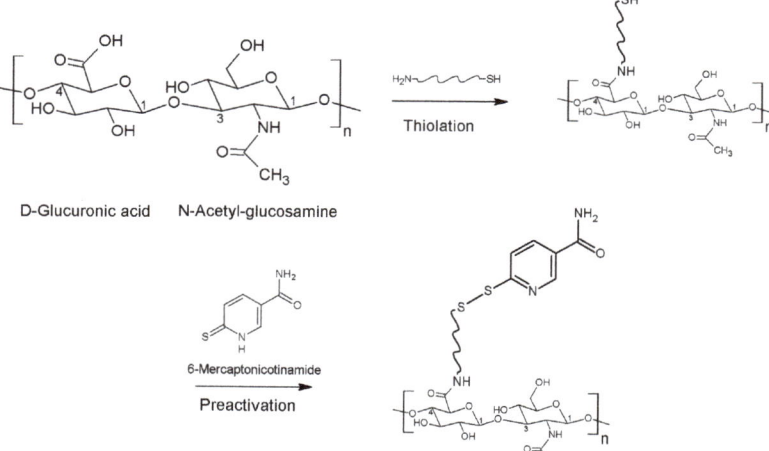

Figure 1. Chemical structure of disaccharide unit within the polysaccharide HA and schematic illustration of thiolation via amidation as well as preactivation with 6-mercaptonicotinamide as an example resulting in a disulfide bond.

Table 1. Overview various thiolated HAs including type of thiolated HA, targeted chemical group of HA, ligand and reaction type.

Type of thiolated HA	Targeted chemical group of HA	Ligand	Reaction type	Reference
HA-SH	Carboxylic	L-Cysteine	Amidation	[15–18]
HA-SH	Carboxylic	L-Cysteine ethyl ester	Amidation	[14,19–24]
HA-SH	Carboxylic	Cysteamine	Amidation	[25–28]
HA-SH	Carboxylic	Cysteamine	Amidation	[29–32]
HA(-ADH)-SH	Carboxylic	1. Adipic acid dihydrazide (ADH) 2. 2-Immoinothiolane	1. Amidation 2. Thiolation with Traut's reagent	[33,34]
Thiolated carboxymethyl HA	Carboxylic	5,5′-Dithiobis (2-nitrobenzoic acid)	Amidation	[35–38]
HA-DTPH	Carboxylic	Dithiobis (propanoic dihydrazide)	Amidation	[39–57]
HA-DTBH	Carboxylic	Dithiobis (butyric dihydrazide)	Amidation	[39]
HA-PDPH	Carboxylic	3-(2-pyridyldithio) propionyl hydrazide	Amidation	[58]
HA-SH	Hydroxyl	Ethylene sulfide	Ether formation	[59,60]
HA-SH	Hydroxyl	1. Divinyl sulfone 2. Dithiothreitol	1. Ether formation 2. Amidation	[61,62]

3. Properties of Thiolated Hyaluronic Acid

3.1. Mucoadhesive Properties

The improved mucoadhesive properties of thiolated hyaluronic acid (HA-SH) are primary based on the disulfide bonds between the sulfhydryl moieties of the polymer backbone and the cysteine-rich residues of the mucus. On the contrary, unmodified mucoadhesive polymers are only capable of forming ionic interactions, hydrogen bonds and electrostatic bonds with the mucosal surface [63]. In order to compare and evaluate in vitro mucoadhesiveness of unmodified and modified polymers, the rotating cylinder method represents one of the most studied and feasible methods [64]. For instance, Kafedjiiski et al. showed a 6.5-fold prolonged adhesion time comparing HA-cysteine ethyl ester (HA-Cys) with HA applying the rotating cylinder method (Figure 2) [14]. Recently, Laffleur et al. [23] demonstrated that thiolation of HA leads to an even 12-fold augmentation in mucoadhesion on buccal mucosa. Thiolated HA preactivated with 6-mercaptonicotinamide demonstrated a 4-fold improved adhesion time compared to thiolated HA [19]. These findings are based on the formation of covalent bonds between thiol groups of thiolated HA and cysteine-rich domains within the mucin glycoproteins [65,66]. Besides, Ding et al. [27] developed a delivery system for insulin, namely, multilayered mucoadhesive hydrogel films with thiolated HA and polyvinyl alcohol leading to unidirectional controlled insulin release.

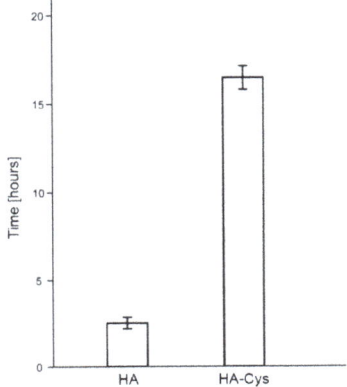

Figure 2. Adhesion time in hours of unmodified HA and HA-Cys on the rotating cylinder in 0.1 M phosphate buffer pH 6.8 with 1% NaCl at 37 °C. Indicated values are means of at least three experiments (±SD). Adapted from Kafedjiiski et al. [14].

3.2. Cohesive Properties

Swelling capacity has a major impact on adhesive and cohesive properties of thiolated HA. Generally, swelling capacity is determined by measuring the water uptake in function of time. Numerous research groups confirmed that HA-SH possesses superior properties over HA in terms of water uptake. For example, HA-cysteine ethyl ester exhibited 3.5-fold improved swelling capacity compared to the unmodified polymer [23]. Laffleur et al. [19] mentioned recently that it is not mandatory to reach the maximum swelling capacity in order to take the advantage of thiolated polymers. On the contrary, to overcome the worrying bottleneck of biodegradability, a balance between swelling and stability should be guaranteed. As through the rapid swelling the surface of the polymer increases and as a result, the degradable area for hyaluronidases grows. For instance, Figure 3 illustrates the close relation between swelling ratio and degradation rate. In brief, the more swelling of the polymer could be observed, the faster the hydrogel was degraded, as the hydrogel surface was increased through the swelling process. Thus, enzymes such as hyaluronidase could cleave HA into its fragments of D-glucuronic acid and N-acetyl-D-glucosamine in a faster manner [46].

As the gel stiffness also has an impact onto the cohesive properties, Vanderhooft et al. [47] performed rheological measurements of crosslinked thiolated HA gelatin hydrogels showing that the composition as well as the crosslinking rate plays a major role in the gel stiffness properties. This strategy might be useful to tailor polymer properties in consideration of application sites. Moreover, disulfide-crosslinked hyaluronan-gelatin sponges showed growth of fibrous tissue in mice representing high stiffness and a promising approach for tissue augmentation [40]. As gel stiffness represents an important parameter for tissue engineering in order to choose the appropriate composition considering the right tissue, Horkay et al. [51] investigated the structural, mechanical and osmotic properties of injectable hydrogels with respect of the polymer concentration and composition. The concentration of carboxymethylated thiolated HA showed a higher impact onto elasticity compared to the crosslinking density of the polymer backbone.

Overall, it could be discovered that the thermodynamic properties are mainly determined by the polymer concentration and other parameters such as interactions between the two polymeric compounds merely contribute to the thermodynamic behavior of the gels. Bian et al. [26] could verify that gelation time, swelling properties and controlled degradation behavior show correlation on the composition of HA-SH polymers.

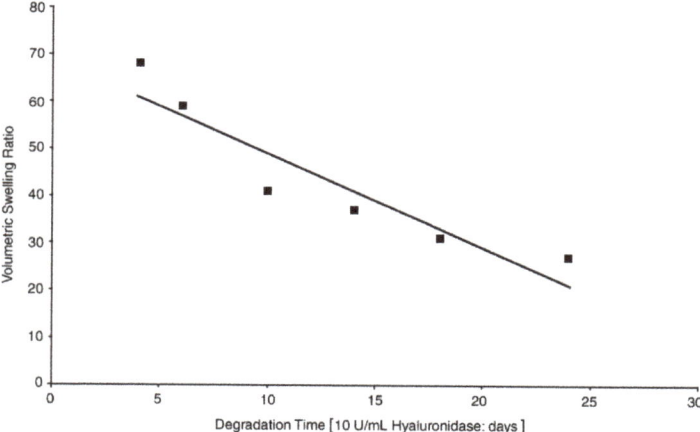

Figure 3. Comparison of swelling ratio and degradation time for six selected chemically modified thiolated HA variants. Increased swelling correlated with rapid degradation. Adapted from Orlandi et al. [46].

3.3. Stability against Degradation

As mentioned previously, swelling capacity is important for the mucoadhesiveness of thiolated HA. Nevertheless, its stability is negatively influenced by pronounced swelling, as the surface is more accessible towards hyaluronidases. Due to the sensitive application of hydrogels, in vivo studies regarding HA-SH stability and degradation of HA-SH hydrogels are from high interest. In general, chemical modification such as thiolation of HA should lead to a higher resistance against enzymatic degradation of the polymer [55]; however, biocompatibility of modified HA should not be impaired. Laffleur et al. [23] confirmed that chemical modification could have a great impact onto the stability as the thiolation process stabilized the polymer by intra- as well as inter-molecular disulfide bonds resulting in a higher resistance of the polymer towards degradation. Kafedjiiski et al. [14] investigated the viscous properties of different HA polymers (unmodified, thiolated and crosslinked thiolated) in presence of hyaluronidase as demonstrated in Figure 4. Within this study, it could be shown that HA is fastest degraded after addition of hyaluronidase, followed by thiolated HA with L-cysteine ethyl ester (HA-Cys), and finally, the crosslinked thiolated HA demonstrated only a minor decrease in viscosity due to the minimized excess of hyaluronidase onto HA. Moreover, Hahn et al. [33] found out that thiolated HA hydrogels are degraded only after 2 weeks in vivo. Additionally, HA hydrogels without disulfide bonds possessing other crosslinkage were tested resulting in a higher stability, which might be due to the absence of a thiol-exchange reaction between reduced glutathione presented in nearly all human cells and the disulfide bonds of polymers. Hence, it could be concluded that in vitro and in vivo data are not always correlating precisely, as many factors could have an additional influence in vivo. Degradation properties, viscosity and gelation time could be adjusted by varying the pH of the reaction mixture, the concentration of HA-SH and the stoichiometric ratio of thiol to acryloyl groups during the Michael addition [28]. Therefore, Dubbini et al. [52] examined gelation kinetic, mechanical properties and the swelling/degradation profile of vinyl sulfone thiolated HA hydrogels. Within this study, the degree of vinyl sulfonation and the degree of thiolation were shown to have an impact on the aforementioned properties. Another study from Li et al. [15] showed that HA-cysteine exhibited a protective effect for insulin against degradation by trypsin and α-chymotrypsin. This observation could be explained by the covalent attachment of the enzymes onto the polymer backbone by disulfide bond formation between the thiol moieties of HA-SH and the cysteine residues of the aforementioned proteases. This inhibitory effect could not be determined for unmodified hyaluronic acid. Furthermore, Liu et al. [31] synthesized thiolated HA in order to formulate a hydrogel with the ability of free radical scavenging and degradation resistance. Hence, (−)-epigallocatechin-3-O-gallate was attached to thiolated HA resulting in an inhibition of free radicals as well as the ability of inhibiting hyaluronidases.

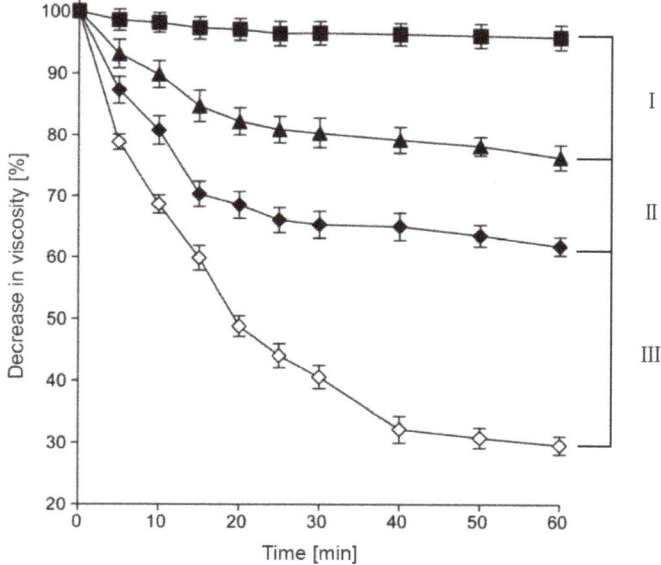

Figure 4. Decrease in viscosity of HA and HA-Cys by hyaluronidase (0.5 mg/mL) at pH 6.0; HA without hyaluronidase (■), HA-Cys (crosslinked) (▲), HA-Cys (♦) and HA (◊). Indicated values are means of at least three experiments (±SD); I and II differ from III, $p < 0.00001$; I, differs from II, $p < 0.0006$. Adapted from Kafedjiiski [14].

3.4. Biocompatibility

The biocompatibility represents an important issue within formulation development from the academic as well as the industrial point of view, as novel formulations should not cause adverse effects after administration. Within several studies from Laffleur and co-workers, thiolated HA did not affect cell viability of Caco-2 cells [16,19–23]. Moreover, other research groups demonstrated high cell viability on 3T3, RAW 264.7 and HMEC cells [67]. Thiolated HA did not show any cytotoxicity towards primary human fibroblasts either [59]. Moreover, another study showed an enhanced fibronectin absorption via increasing the degree of sulfonation [53]. This process allows more cells to adhere on the glycosaminoglycan surface. Additionally, the degree of thiolation was investigated illustrating that more thiolation is leading to a lower biocompatibility of glycosaminoglycans. Besides, metabolic activity and cell growth were found to be promoted up to a higher limit of thiolation degree. The importance of the chemical composition of hydrogels could be proven and additionally it is opening opportunities for a large field of applications. Nonetheless, it seems not to pose a problem finding the optimal composition for a biocompatible hydrogel, as Sabbieti et al. [54] verified the biocompatibility of vinyl sulfone thiolated HA hydrogels developed by Dubbini et al. [52] in vivo as well. Apart from that, biocompatibility could at the same time be improved via anti-fibronectin aptamer functionalization as studied by Galli et al. [68]. As lower molecular weight HA ensured maximum cell survival, the composition of hydrogels plays a crucial role in finding the right compounds for specific application.

3.5. Permeation Enhancing Properties

The permeation enhancement is mainly the result of reduced glutathione (GSH) mediated protein tyrosine phosphatase inhibition. In detail, the presence of GSH facilities the permeation of compounds across the mucosa. The thiol groups of the polymer convert the oxidized form of glutathione to reduced form after a thiol-exchange reaction [69]. In most cases, the permeation enhancement of HA-SH is the consequence of this aforementioned effect. The permeation rate of curcumin for instance was found to be 4.4-fold enhanced by utilizing thiolated HA compared to unmodified HA [24]. On the contrary, an insulin permeation study utilizing cell monolayer showed that the permeation rate of insulin from HA-SH gel was lower compared to the unmodified gel. In addition, an increasing amount of thiol groups on the polymer backbone led to slower permeation. Within this set-up, the formation of disulfide bonds between insulin and HA-SH outweighed the permeation enhancing effect of the thiolated polymer [15]. To prevent the oxidation of two free thiol groups, S-protection via 6-mercaptonicotinamide might be the key.

3.6. Controlled Release

The release of active pharmaceutical ingredients incorporated in thiolated HA systems could be controlled by different parameters such as structural changes and pH. Censi et al. [49] developed in situ forming hydrogels via Tandem thermal gelling and Michael addition reaction utilized as carrier system for controlled peptide (bradykinin) release. This thiolated HA system represented high potential for peptide as well as protein drug delivery, as the release kinetic of bovine serum albumin containing gel could be tailored by altering the chemical structure of the polymer. Furthermore, another study suggested biocompatible, biodegradable and thiolated HA hydrogels for gene delivery [29]. Small interfering RNA (siRNA) was entrapped into thiolated HA hydrogel and successfully transported into the cells via CD44 receptors located on the surface of the cell. To gain better knowledge about the influence of GSH onto the siRNA release out of the hydrogel, different GSH concentrations were examined. Figure 5 displays that the release rate of siRNA out of the hydrogel depends on the GSH concentration in the buffer solution. At a GSH concentration of 10 mM the whole siRNA was released after 60 min, which indicated that the thiolated HA hydrogels are degraded more rapidly through increasing GSH concentrations. It could be assumed that these hydrogels are stable in extracellular conditions, as the extracellular compartment exhibits lower GSH concentration as applied during the release studies. As soon as the hydrogels reach the intracellular compartment the drug is likely released. Thus, thiolated HA hydrogels can be assessed as potent gene delivery systems exhibiting GSH dependent controlled release rate, such as against genetic disorders or cancer [30]. Han et al. for instance [70] developed core-crosslinked thiolated HA micelle for doxorubicin as potential targeted cancer therapy. Within this study, the core-crosslinkage led to sustained doxorubicin release, however, in presence of 10 mM GSH the release increased. As tumor cells have a high level of GSH and drug is released at the desired area, a controlled release as well as an improved therapeutic efficiency directly at the tumor site could be guaranteed. Fu et al. [56] demonstrated a novel dual pH- and reduction-responsive release system utilizing doxorubicin hydrochloride. An accelerated doxorubicin release could be determined at acidic pH (pH 5) and in presence of increasing GSH concentrations. A novel hydrogel depot for protein release was formulated by Yu and Chau [61], which was based on the De Gennes' blob theory. This model represents concentrations by a sphere and the diameter is the average distance x between two chains. Furthermore, the diameter decreases as soon as the concertation increases. Altogether, the Gennes' blob model describes polymer solutions, crosslinked polymers (gels), polymer welds, interfaces and polymers at surfaces. Within this study, two problems for vinyl sulfonate-thiol in situ hydrogel systems such as fast release and protein binding could be solved via increasing degree of modification and concentration of SH polymers. In addition, this crosslinked thiolated HA hydrogel was injected into rabbit eyes in order to achieve controlled release of bevacizumab [62]. This study resulted in a 107 times higher bevacizumab concentration compared to the bolus injection 6 months after injection. Another study demonstrated the controlled release of ovalbumin from the matrix of thiolated HA [18]. Thereby, thiolated HA showed improved stability against hyaluronidase, further this controlled release system could be identified as tunable release system through varying molecular weight of HA. Apart from this, Fan et al. [17] incorporated cationic liposomes onto the surface of thiolated HA in order to form nanoparticles with thiolated polyethylene glycols (PEG). These nanoparticles exhibited improved colloidal stability as well as a prolonged release of antigens. Recently, a review article from Campani et al. [71] described the potential of these lipid-based core shell nanoparticles, especially hyaluronic acid-based core-shell nanoparticles, concluding that these drug delivery systems are opening new therapeutic possibilities.

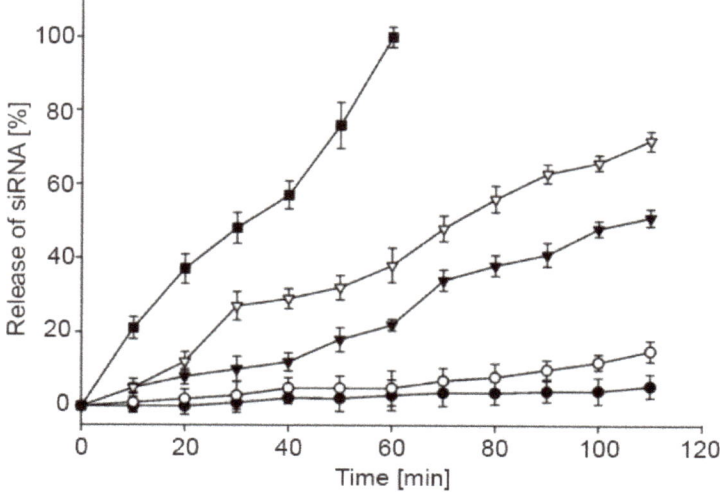

Figure 5. Release of siRNA from thiolated HA gels at various glutathione concentrations; (●) 0 mM GSH, (○) 0.1 mM GSH, (▼) 1 mM GSH, (▽) 5 mM GSH and (■) 10 mM GSH. Adapted from Lee et al. [29].

3.7. Further Applications of Thiolated HA

To accelerate the rejuvenation of tissues after injuries or damages, wound healing or regenerative medicine provides a tool for clinical practice. The combination of mucoadhesion and wound healing represents an interesting strategy. In particular, for healing of wounds on mucosal tissues the mucoadhesive properties of thiolated HA seem advantageous. Therefore, the adhesion of in vitro cultured and differentiated scaffold directly on the injured tissue with the ability of remaining at this area seems to highly on demand.

The utilization of thiolated HA offers numerous possibilities for engineering novel biomaterials. HA is present in the human body as the component of the extracellular matrix of the cartilage tissue or in the vitreous of the eye and it is part of the clinical practice for more than 35 years [72]. HA is the only non-sulfonated glycosaminoglycan and it is necessary for the stabilization of extracellular matrix, regulation of cell adhesion and mediation of cell proliferation. HA is continuously degraded within the body by hyaluronidase enzymes; thus, modifications of the polymer backbone such as thiolation are mandatory to obtain more mechanically and chemically robust materials [42]. For instance, Shu et al. [39] thiolated HA with dihydrazides generating HA-DTPH (dithiobis (propanoic dihydrazide)) and HA-DTBH (dithiobis (butyric dihydrazide)). The thiol groups were spontaneously oxidized on air and showed the ability to form hydrogel films via inter- and intramolecular disulfide bond formation. The use of these hydrogels with in vitro cultured fibroblasts led to proliferation even over 3 days. Moreover, HA-DTPH hydrogels were coupled to polyethylene glycols (PEG) to achieve an improved in situ crosslinkable HA hydrogel. The hydrogels with thiolated HA and PEGDA (PEG-diacrylate) demonstrated an in situ crosslinking and resulted in a 10-fold higher cell density over 4 weeks culture period compared to the initial cell density. Due to the in situ crosslinking of this polymer, hydrogel possessed high potential for wound healing and tissue repair. The same thiolated HA with PEGDA was modified utilizing peptides containing the Arg-Gly-Asp sequence to further endorse cell attachment, spreading and proliferation for novel injectable biomaterials. Due to the significant proliferation enhancement of Arg-Gly-Asp peptides, HA-DTPH-PEGDA hydrogels were identified as formulations with high potential for regenerative medicine in vivo [41]. Ouasti et al. [25] categorized HA/PEG hydrogels in the following groups: type I gels—HA dispersed in a PEGDA network, type II gels—HA-SH as chain transfer agent during PEGDA polymerization and type III gels—in situ preparation and polymerization of HA-SA/PEGDA macromolecules. Within this study, a relation for type II gel between fibroblast spreading and the mechanical properties was found out, which may open novel possibilities of cell and material fine tuning. As unmodified HA hydrogels are attached on the surface of cells and proliferate in a 2D model, the fabrication of 3D scaffolds based on electrospinning is of great interest. For instance, Ji et al. [43,44] demonstrated fibroblasts migrating and forming 3D dendritic morphology inside the HA-DTPH nanofibrous scaffold. These nanofibers possessed the potential for cell encapsulation and 3D cell culturing for tissue regeneration. Furthermore, these nanofibers exhibited the ability of controlling cell adhesion as well as cell morphology [73]. As previously mentioned, regenerative medicine for the treatment of neuronal injuries could revolutionize the medical therapy. In this field, Horn et al. [45] illustrated that HA-DTPH-PEGDA hydrogels might have a high potential for neurite outgrowth. A 50% increase in neurite length compared to the fibrin samples was achieved. In addition, regenerative medicine is of great importance in heart regeneration; namely, replacing cardiovascular implants with bioprinting of vessel-like constructs utilizing HA hydrogels can further improve the quality of life [50]. Besides, Young and Engel [58] demonstrated that hydrogels enhance the differentiation of cardiomyocytes in vitro. Thereby, pre-cardiac cells grown on collagen-coated HA showed 60% increased maturing muscle fibers as well as 3-fold higher number of cardiac-specific markers over a time period of 2 weeks.

The treatment or accelerated healing of corneal injuries as demonstrated by Yang et al. [48] illustrated the wound healing properties of a thiol-modified and crosslinked HA hydrogel by abrasion and alkali burning of the coronal epithelium from rabbits. Within this study, 1% of the thiolated HA hydrogel formulation was applied on the right eye four times per day resulting in a closure of coronal wound in the abrasion model. Furthermore, the closure rate as well as the thickness regarding the alkali burn model was greater compared to the control. Since more than 161 million people worldwide suffer from visual impairment and thereof 37 million are blind, an adequate treatment is of high interest [74]. Generally, coronial blindness can be surgical treated by transplantation of the corona. As 90% of visually impaired people live in low- or middle-income countries, a treatment such as Espandar et al. [75] demonstrated would be highly beneficial. Within this study, HyStem®—a hydrogel kit containing thiol-modified hyaluronan, thiol-reactive PEGDA crosslinker and thiol-modified collagen resulting in a semisynthetic extracellular matrix, which represents an affordable clinical product [76]—showed the highest yield of human adipose-driven stem cells (h-ADSCs) compared to other HA-derived synthetic extracellular matrix culture media [77]. Usually, h-ADSC, representing a derived synthetic extracellular matrix, are utilized to identify the capacity of proliferation and survival of cells [75]. More importantly, HyStem® hydrogels tested via h-ADSC can serve as carrier for stem cell-based therapy and for tissue engineering [78]. Moreover, HyStem® has an effect on controlling the retinal progenitor cell being part of the retinal repair, as it is forming a microenvironment for self-renewal and differentiation of retinal progenitor cell [79]. Zarembinski et al. [80] confirmed that hydrogels such as HyStem® are supporting the 3D culturing of h-ADSCs in vitro and especially in vivo demonstrating high biocompatibility. h-ADSCs were in situ encapsulated in PEG hyperbranched Hystem® hydrogels resulting in a high cell viability over 7 days, which might be a helpful tool for wound healing in the near future [81]. Besides, Yang et al. [35] utilized thiolated carboxymethyl HA films to test the efficiency of wound healing across multiple species, such as rats, dogs and horses. An increased keratinocyte proliferation resulting in thicker epidermis compared to the control could be observed. A significant ($p = 0.001$) difference between the wound area of the gel and the untreated control could be observed, as displayed in Figure 6. The wound area of the film treated group was smaller compared to the control (p = 0.01). Moreover, even vocal fold scars causing dysphonia could demonstrate significantly improved biomedical properties regarding elasticity and viscosity via a hydrogel kit containing equal ingredients such as Hystem® [57]. Walimbe et al. [82] recently summarized the advantages of thiolated HA hydrogels in order to engineer vocal fold tissue.

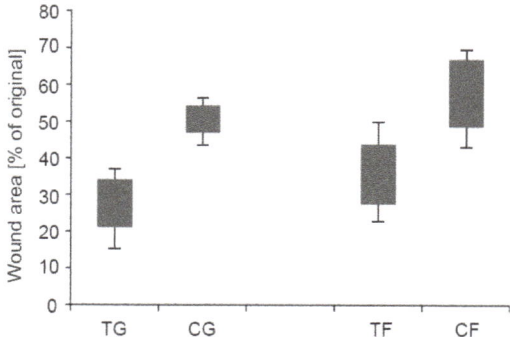

Figure 6. Overview of the wound area comparing thiolated carboxymethyl HA film and gel studied on rats. Wound area calculated in percent referring to the original wound area. Gel (TG) and film (TF) treatments compared with untreated controls (CG and CF) on day 7 after wounding. Bars represent 95% confidence intervals of the means; lines represent the range of values obtained. Adapted from Yang et al. [35].

4. Delivery Systems

4.1. Buccal Drug Delivery

Buccal drug delivery represents an appropriate alternative to the most common route namely the oral administration. Via the buccal route degradation in the stomach and small intestine can be avoided, as well the hepatic first-pass metabolism can be bypassed. The buccal mucosa is suitable for controlled drug delivery for extended time periods [83–86]. Nevertheless, lot of diseases could be treated in an improved way via the buccal route; just mentioning an example, patients suffering from Parkinson disease are confronted with dysphagia and therefore, the application of transmucosal buccal delivery systems might overcome this hindrance [23]. As for this administration high mucoadhesion is mandatory, thiolated or preactivated thiolated HA offers an effective tool to guarantee a prolonged residence time of the drug on the mucosa. For instance, our research group demonstrated a 4-fold improved mucoadhesion time of thiolated HA preactivated with 6-mercaptonicotinamide compared to unmodified HA that makes HA-SH as well as preactivated HA-SH a suitable polymer for buccal delivery [19]. Preactivated HA showed high stability as well as no cytotoxicity on Caco-2 cells. The preactivation or S-protection is of great importance in order to guarantee efficient stability against oxidation prior to administration and via preactivation of HA-SH an even longer residence time is predictable [16].

4.2. Vaginal Drug Delivery

Vaginal drug delivery is offering numerous of advantages, namely easy access, painlessness and prolonged retention of formulation, as no movements such as in the gastrointestinal tract are required [87]. The vagina possesses a highly beneficial permeation area, high vascularization, low enzymatic activity and most importantly, drugs applied on the vaginal site bypass the first-pass effect [88]. Through the application of mucoadhesive thiolated HA the retention time of drug delivery systems could be tremendously improved and subsequently the drug contact time at the target site is prolonged [89,90]. Nowak et al. [20] thiolated HA with L-cysteine ethyl ester followed by a preactivation with 6-mercaptonicotinamide. Preactivated HA demonstrated a 3.6-fold prolonged disintegration time compared to unmodified HA as well as a prolonged mucoadhesion time, presumably leading to an increased contact time of the drug with the adsorption sites in vivo. Moreover, these modified HAs were found to be biocompatible and therefore they are safe tools for vaginal application. Agrahari et al. [60] performed an interesting study based on nanofibers of thiolated HA loaded with tenofovir, which were further characterized in vitro and in vivo for topical intravaginal delivery of HIV/AIDS microbicides. Thereby, the nanofibers were found to be non-toxic and no damage on the genital tract of mice could be observed. Within the vaginal tissue, a significant bioavailability as well as retention improvement of tenofovir could be identified compared to the 1% tenofovir gel.

4.3. Ocular Drug Delivery

Due to its high biocompatibility, HA-SH might be applied onto the ocular surface as well. For example, Williams and Mann [36] demonstrated high effectiveness of crosslinked and thiolated HA hydrogels on dry eye syndrome in vivo. After application of the polymer in rabbits an increase in tear breakup time was found as well as the stabilization of the tear film was observed. In vivo studies on dogs suffering from keratoconjunctivitis sicca showed significantly reduces symptoms. Based on these results, Williams and Mann [37] performed a masked, randomized clinical study in dogs with keratoconjunctivitis sicca. Within this study, crosslinked and thiolated HA hydrogels showed significantly improved ocular surface health compared to HA-based iDrop® Vet Plus Eye Lubricant (ITRD; I-MED Animal Health). In another study, thiolated HA hydrogels were investigated regarding improved retention via 3D computational finite eye models. Simple geometrical modifications had an impact onto the hydrogel film retention [38]. The application of contact lenses generally contributes to the exacerbation of the symptoms associated to the dry eye syndrome. Reflexing to this, Korogiannaki et al. [32] formulated a thiolated HA hydrogel for the improvement of surface properties of contact lens, which improve a higher lens compatibility with the ocular environment. Apart from dry eye syndrome, improving the treatment of retinal attachment represents high industrial interest, as the current vitreous substitute such as silicone oils are not biodegradable and have to be removed via a second surgery. The efficiency of two artificial vitreous body substitutes (VBS) was evaluated and compared to silicone oil as gold standard. Therefore, the retina of rabbits was at first reattached via the injection of air and thereafter, the eye was filled with silicon oil or the corresponding number of hydrogels. Within the silicon oil group 87.5% demonstrated a recovered retinal attachment, whereas 73.3% of the hydrogel group exhibited intact retina. Therefore, biodegradable thiolated HA hydrogels show a comparable efficiency compared to the gold standard with the possibility of avoiding a second operation [91].

5. Product Development

As thiolated HA has great potential within the medical field, some products are already available on the market. For instance, Glycosil® [92] represents a thiol-modified hyaluronic acid and is utilized for 3D cell culturing and tissue engineering applications [93]. HyStem®, a hydrogel kit containing Glycosil® as a main component, could be applied for biomedical applications such as wound healing as mentioned previously [76]. Moreover, a fast-gelling thiolated HA was developed from Vornia Biomaterials in collaboration with the University College Dublin, Ireland. This thiolated HA possesses a purity of 98%, a gelation time of less than 30 min [94]. Apart from hydrogel kits, Croma-Pharma GmbH completed a Phase I study in April 2016 aiming the safety of implanting thiolated HA in patients suffering from primary open angle glaucoma [95]. In general, thiolated HA occupies an improved mucoadhesiveness and cohesive capacity on the ocular surface compared to not thiolated HA. The residence time is improved, and the administration interval is reduced. In addition, Eyegate Pharmaceuticals, Inc. has an ocular bandage gel consisting of thiolated carboxymethyl HA for ocular wound healing in its pipeline [96]. Therefore, it could be assumed that mucoadhesive thiolated HA will attract lots of attention in the imminent years.

6. Conclusions

The thiolation of hyaluronic acid leads to a higher stability and enhanced mucoadhesive properties of the polymeric backbone. Due to its versatility, thiolated hyaluronic acids can be utilized for wide ranges of pharmaceutical application. As exhibiting beneficial toxicological properties, it can be used beside oral application on sensitive target sites as well, such as vaginal or ocular surface. Furthermore, due to its in situ gelling properties it is a potent tool for mucoadhesive hydrogel films possessing controlled release properties. The properties of the forming gels may be easily tailored by adjusting the chemical properties, the density of the ligands and crosslinking rate. In addition, HA-SH is a promising excipient for wound healing, as it promotes the proliferation of cells by providing an appropriate 3D microenvironment. It is highly predictable, that within the next years HA-SH will gain more attention due to the rising relevance for targeted mucoadhesive drug delivery, cell-based therapy systems and wound healing. As thiolated HA is a biodegradable polymer, it has great potential for biomedical applications, for instance on eyes, to improve patient compliance and to save medical expenses. Finally, thiolated HA is in the pipeline of pharmaceutical industry, and therefore some highly innovative products will enter the market soon.

Conflicts of Interest: The authors declare no conflict of interest.

References

1. Schanté, C.E.; Zuber, G.; Herlin, C.; Vandamme, T.F. Chemical modifications of hyaluronic acid for the synthesis of derivatives for a broad range of biomedical applications. *Carbohydr. Polym.* **2011**, *85*, 469–489. [CrossRef]
2. Bernkop-Schnürch, A. Muco-Adhesive Polymers, Use Thereof and Method For Producing the Same. Patent Family WO0025823, 11 May 2000.
3. Prestwich, G.D. Hyaluronic acid-based clinical biomaterials derived for cell and molecule delivery in regenerative medicine. *J. Control. Release* **2011**, *155*, 193–199. [CrossRef] [PubMed]
4. Iqbal, J.; Shahnaz, G.; Dünnhaupt, S.; Müller, C.; Hintzen, F.; Bernkop-Schnürch, A. Preactivated thiomers as mucoadhesive polymers for drug delivery. *Biomaterials* **2012**, *33*, 1528–1535. [CrossRef] [PubMed]
5. Wirostko, B.; Mann, B.K.; Williams, D.L.; Prestwich, G.D. Ophthalmic Uses of a Thiol-Modified Hyaluronan-Based Hydrogel. *Adv. Wound Care (New Rochelle)* **2014**, *3*, 708–716. [CrossRef] [PubMed]
6. Nyström, B.; Kjøniksen, A.L.; Beheshti, N.; Maleki, A.; Zhu, K.; Knudsen, K.D.; Pamies, R.; Hernández Cifre, J.G.; García de la Torre, J. Characterization of polyelectrolyte features in polysaccharide systems and mucin. *Adv. Colloid Interface Sci.* **2010**, *158*, 108–118. [CrossRef] [PubMed]
7. Day, A.J.; Sheehan, J.K. Hyaluronan: Polysaccharide chaos to protein organisation. *Curr. Opin. Struct. Biol.* **2001**, *11*, 617–622. [CrossRef]
8. Fraser, J.R.; Laurent, T.C.; Laurent, U.B. Hyaluronan: Its nature, distribution, functions and turnover. *J. Intern. Med.* **1997**, *242*, 27–33. [CrossRef] [PubMed]
9. Robert, L.; Robert, A.M.; Renard, G. Biological effects of hyaluronan in connective tissues, eye, skin, venous wall. Role in aging. *Pathol. Biol. (Paris)* **2010**, *58*, 187–198. [CrossRef] [PubMed]
10. Brown, T.J.; Laurent, U.B.; Fraser, J.R. Turnover of hyaluronan in synovial joints: Elimination of labelled hyaluronan from the knee joint of the rabbit. *Exp. Physiol.* **1991**, *76*, 125–134. [CrossRef] [PubMed]
11. Aruffo, A.; Stamenkovic, I.; Melnick, M.; Underhill, C.B.; Seed, B. CD44 is the principal cell surface receptor for hyaluronate. *Cell* **1990**, *61*, 1303–1313. [CrossRef]
12. Stern, R.; Kogan, G.; Jedrzejas, M.J.; Soltés, L. The many ways to cleave hyaluronan. *Biotechnol. Adv.* **2007**, *25*, 537–557. [CrossRef] [PubMed]
13. Price, R.D.; Berry, M.G.; Navsaria, H.A. Hyaluronic acid: The scientific and clinical evidence. *J. Plast. Reconstr. Aesthet. Surg.* **2007**, *60*, 1110–1119. [CrossRef] [PubMed]
14. Kafedjiiski, K.; Jetti, R.K.; Föger, F.; Hoyer, H.; Werle, M.; Hoffer, M.; Bernkop-Schnürch, A. Synthesis and in vitro evaluation of thiolated hyaluronic acid for mucoadhesive drug delivery. *Int. J. Pharm.* **2007**, *343*, 48–58. [CrossRef] [PubMed]

15. Li, X.; Yu, G.; Jin, K.; Yin, Z. Hyaluronic acid L-cysteine conjugate exhibits controlled-release potential for mucoadhesive drug delivery. *Pharmazie* **2012**, *67*, 224–228. [PubMed]
16. Pereira de Sousa, I.; Suchaoin, W.; Zupančič, O.; Leichner, C.; Bernkop-Schnürch, A. Totally S-protected hyaluronic acid: Evaluation of stability and mucoadhesive properties as liquid dosage form. *Carbohydr. Polym.* **2016**, *152*, 632–638. [CrossRef] [PubMed]
17. Fan, Y.; Sahdev, P.; Ochyl, L.J.; Akerberg, J.J.; Moon, J.J. Cationic liposome-hyaluronic acid hybrid nanoparticles for intranasal vaccination with subunit antigens. *J. Control. Release* **2015**, *208*, 121–129. [CrossRef] [PubMed]
18. Du, J.; Fu, F.; Shi, X.; Yin, Z. Controlled release of a model protein drug ovalbumin from thiolated hyaluronic acid matrix. *J. Drug Deliv. Sci. Technol.* **2015**, *30*, 74–81. [CrossRef]
19. Laffleur, F.; Röggla, J.; Idrees, M.A.; Griessinger, J. Chemical modification of hyaluronic acid for intraoral application. *J. Pharm. Sci.* **2014**, *103*, 2414–2423. [CrossRef] [PubMed]
20. Nowak, J.; Laffleur, F.; Bernkop-Schnürch, A. Preactivated hyaluronic acid: A potential mucoadhesive polymer for vaginal delivery. *Int. J. Pharm.* **2015**, *478*, 383–389. [CrossRef] [PubMed]
21. Laffleur, F.; Wagner, J.; Mahmood, A. In vitro and ex vivo evaluation of biomaterials' distinctive properties as a result of thiolation. *Future Med. Chem.* **2015**, *7*, 449–457. [CrossRef] [PubMed]
22. Laffleur, F.; Psenner, J.; Suchaoin, W. Permeation enhancement via thiolation: In vitro and ex vivo evaluation of hyaluronic acid-cysteine ethyl ester. *J. Pharm. Sci.* **2015**, *104*, 2153–2160. [CrossRef] [PubMed]
23. Laffleur, F.; Wagner, J.; Barthelmes, J. A potential tailor-made hyaluronic acid buccal delivery system comprising rotigotine for Parkinson's disease? *Future Med. Chem.* **2015**, *7*, 1225–1232. [CrossRef] [PubMed]
24. Laffleur, F.; Schmelzle, F.; Ganner, A.; Vanicek, S. In Vitro and Ex Vivo Evaluation of Novel Curcumin-Loaded Excipient for Buccal Delivery. *AAPS PharmSciTech* **2017**, *18*, 2102–2109. [CrossRef] [PubMed]
25. Ouasti, S.; Donno, R.; Cellesi, F.; Sherratt, M.J.; Terenghi, G.; Tirelli, N. Network connectivity, mechanical properties and cell adhesion for hyaluronic acid/PEG hydrogels. *Biomaterials* **2011**, *32*, 6456–6470. [CrossRef] [PubMed]
26. Bian, S.; He, M.; Sui, J.; Cai, H.; Sun, Y.; Liang, J.; Fan, Y.; Zhang, X. The self-crosslinking smart hyaluronic acid hydrogels as injectable three-dimensional scaffolds for cells culture. *Colloids Surf. B Biointerfaces* **2016**, *140*, 392–402. [CrossRef] [PubMed]
27. Ding, J.; He, R.; Zhou, G.; Tang, C.; Yin, C. Multilayered mucoadhesive hydrogel films based on thiolated hyaluronic acid and polyvinylalcohol for insulin delivery. *Acta Biomater.* **2012**, *8*, 3643–3651. [CrossRef] [PubMed]
28. Liu, Y.; Zhang, F.; Ru, Y. Hyperbranched phosphoramidate-hyaluronan hybrid: A reduction-sensitive injectable hydrogel for controlled protein release. *Carbohydr. Polym.* **2015**, *117*, 304–311. [CrossRef] [PubMed]
29. Lee, H.; Mok, H.; Lee, S.; Oh, Y.K.; Park, T.G. Target-specific intracellular delivery of siRNA using degradable hyaluronic acid nanogels. *J. Control. Release* **2007**, *119*, 245–252. [CrossRef] [PubMed]
30. Yin, T.; Liu, J.; Zhao, Z.; Dong, L.; Cai, H.; Yin, L.; Zhou, J.; Huo, M. Smart nanoparticles with a detachable outer shell for maximized synergistic antitumor efficacy of therapeutics with varying physicochemical properties. *J. Control. Release* **2016**, *243*, 54–68. [CrossRef] [PubMed]
31. Liu, C.; Bae, K.H.; Yamashita, A.; Chung, J.E.; Kurisawa, M. Thiol-Mediated Synthesis of Hyaluronic Acid-Epigallocatechin-3-O-Gallate Conjugates for the Formation of Injectable Hydrogels with Free Radical Scavenging Property and Degradation Resistance. *Biomacromolecules* **2017**, *18*, 3143–3155. [CrossRef] [PubMed]
32. Korogiannaki, M.; Zhang, J.; Sheardown, H. Surface modification of model hydrogel contact lenses with hyaluronic acid via thiol-ene "click" chemistry for enhancing surface characteristics. *J. Biomater. Appl.* **2017**, *32*, 446–462. [CrossRef] [PubMed]
33. Hahn, S.K.; Park, J.K.; Tomimatsu, T.; Shimoboji, T. Synthesis and degradation test of hyaluronic acid hydrogels. *Int. J. Biol. Macromol.* **2007**, *40*, 374–380. [CrossRef] [PubMed]
34. Hahn, S.K.; Kim, J.S.; Shimobouji, T. Injectable hyaluronic acid microhydrogels for controlled release formulation of erythropoietin. *J. Biomed. Mater. Res. A* **2007**, *80*, 916–924. [CrossRef] [PubMed]
35. Yang, G.; Prestwich, G.D.; Mann, B.K. Thiolated carboxymethyl-hyaluronic-acid-based biomaterials enhance wound healing in rats, dogs, and horses. *ISRN Vet. Sci.* **2011**, *2011*, 851593. [CrossRef] [PubMed]

36. Williams, D.L.; Mann, B.K. A Crosslinked HA-Based Hydrogel Ameliorates Dry Eye Symptoms in Dogs. *Int. J. Biomater.* **2013**, *2013*, 460437. [CrossRef] [PubMed]
37. Williams, D.L.; Mann, B.K. Efficacy of a crosslinked hyaluronic acid-based hydrogel as a tear film supplement: A masked controlled study. *PLoS ONE* **2014**, *9*, e99766. [CrossRef] [PubMed]
38. Colter, J.; Wirostko, B.; Coats, B. Finite Element Design Optimization of a Hyaluronic Acid-Based Hydrogel Drug Delivery Device for Improved Retention. *Ann. Biomed. Eng.* **2018**, *46*, 211–221. [CrossRef] [PubMed]
39. Shu, X.Z.; Liu, Y.; Luo, Y.; Roberts, M.C.; Prestwich, G.D. Disulfide cross-linked hyaluronan hydrogels. *Biomacromolecules* **2002**, *3*, 1304–1311. [CrossRef] [PubMed]
40. Liu, Y.; Shu, X.Z.; Gray, S.D.; Prestwich, G.D. Disulfide-crosslinked hyaluronan-gelatin sponge: Growth of fibrous tissue in vivo. *J. Biomed. Mater. Res. A* **2004**, *68*, 142–149. [CrossRef] [PubMed]
41. Shu, X.Z.; Ghosh, K.; Liu, Y.; Palumbo, F.S.; Luo, Y.; Clark, R.A.; Prestwich, G.D. Attachment and spreading of fibroblasts on an RGD peptide-modified injectable hyaluronan hydrogel. *J. Biomed. Mater. Res. A* **2004**, *68*, 365–375. [CrossRef] [PubMed]
42. Shu, X.Z.; Ahmad, S.; Liu, Y.; Prestwich, G.D. Synthesis and evaluation of injectable, in situ crosslinkable synthetic extracellular matrices for tissue engineering. *J. Biomed. Mater. Res. A* **2006**, *79*, 902–912. [CrossRef] [PubMed]
43. Ji, Y.; Ghosh, K.; Shu, X.Z.; Li, B.; Sokolov, J.C.; Prestwich, G.D.; Clark, R.A.; Rafailovich, M.H. Electrospun three-dimensional hyaluronic acid nanofibrous scaffolds. *Biomaterials* **2006**, *27*, 3782–3792. [CrossRef] [PubMed]
44. Ji, Y.; Ghosh, K.; Li, B.; Sokolov, J.C.; Clark, R.A.; Rafailovich, M.H. Dual-syringe reactive electrospinning of cross-linked hyaluronic acid hydrogel nanofibers for tissue engineering applications. *Macromol. Biosci.* **2006**, *6*, 811–817. [CrossRef] [PubMed]
45. Horn, E.M.; Beaumont, M.; Shu, X.Z.; Harvey, A.; Prestwich, G.D.; Horn, K.M.; Gibson, A.R.; Preul, M.C.; Panitch, A. Influence of cross-linked hyaluronic acid hydrogels on neurite outgrowth and recovery from spinal cord injury. *J. Neurosurg. Spine* **2007**, *6*, 133–140. [CrossRef] [PubMed]
46. Orlandi, R.R.; Shu, X.Z.; McGill, L.; Petersen, E.; Prestwich, G.D. Structural variations in a single hyaluronan derivative significantly alter wound-healing effects in the rabbit maxillary sinus. *Laryngoscope* **2007**, *117*, 1288–1295. [CrossRef] [PubMed]
47. Vanderhooft, J.L.; Alcoutlabi, M.; Magda, J.J.; Prestwich, G.D. Rheological Properties of Cross-Linked Hyaluronan–Gelatin Hydrogels for Tissue Engineering. *Macromol. Biosci.* **2009**, *9*, 20–28. [CrossRef] [PubMed]
48. Yang, G.; Espandar, L.; Mamalis, N.; Prestwich, G.D. A cross-linked hyaluronan gel accelerates healing of corneal epithelial abrasion and alkali burn injuries in rabbits. *Vet. Ophthalmol.* **2010**, *13*, 144–150. [CrossRef] [PubMed]
49. Censi, R.; Fieten, P.J.; di Martino, P.; Hennink, W.E.; Vermonden, T. In situ forming hydrogels by tandem thermal gelling and Michael addition reaction between thermosensitive triblock copolymers and thiolated hyaluronan. *Macromolecules* **2010**, *43*, 5771–5778. [CrossRef]
50. Skardal, A.; Zhang, J.; Prestwich, G.D. Bioprinting vessel-like constructs using hyaluronan hydrogels crosslinked with tetrahedral polyethylene glycol tetracrylates. *Biomaterials* **2010**, *31*, 6173–6181. [CrossRef] [PubMed]
51. Horkay, F.; Magda, J.; Alcoutlabi, M.; Atzet, S.; Zarembinski, T. Structural, mechanical and osmotic properties of injectable hyaluronan-based composite hydrogels. *Polymer* **2010**, *51*, 4424–4430. [CrossRef] [PubMed]
52. Dubbini, A.; Censi, R.; Butini, M.E.; Sabbieti, M.G.; Agas, D.; Vermonden, T.; Di Martino, P. Injectable hyaluronic acid/PEG-p(HPMAm-lac)-based hydrogels dually cross-linked by thermal gelling and Michael addition. *Eur. Polym. J.* **2015**, *72*, 423–437. [CrossRef]
53. Köwitsch, A.; Niepel, M.S.; Michanetzis, G.P.; Missirlis, Y.F.; Groth, T. Effect of Immobilized Thiolated Glycosaminoglycans on Fibronectin Adsorption and Behavior of Fibroblasts. *Macromol. Biosci.* **2016**, *16*, 381–394. [CrossRef] [PubMed]
54. Sabbieti, M.G.; Dubbini, A.; Laus, F.; Paggi, E.; Marchegiani, A.; Capitani, M.; Marchetti, L.; Dini, F.; Vermonden, T.; Di Martino, P.; et al. In vivo biocompatibility of p(HPMAm-lac)-PEG hydrogels hybridized with hyaluronan. *J. Tissue Eng. Regen. Med.* **2016**, *11*, 3056–3067. [CrossRef] [PubMed]

55. Liu, Y.; Zheng, X.; Shu, G.D. Prestwich, Biocompatibility and stability of disulfide-crosslinked hyaluronan films. *Biomaterials* **2005**, *26*, 4737–4746. [CrossRef] [PubMed]
56. Fu, C.; Li, H.; Li, N.; Miao, X.; Xie, M.; Du, W.; Zhang, L.M. Conjugating an anticancer drug onto thiolated hyaluronic acid by acid liable hydrazone linkage for its gelation and dual stimuli-response release. *Carbohydr. Polym.* **2015**, *128*, 163–170. [CrossRef] [PubMed]
57. Thibeault, S.L.; Klemuk, S.A.; Chen, X.; Quinchia Johnson, B.H. In Vivo engineering of the vocal fold ECM with injectable HA hydrogels-late effects on tissue repair and biomechanics in a rabbit model. *J. Voice* **2011**, *25*, 249–253. [CrossRef] [PubMed]
58. Young, J.L.; Engler, A.J. Hydrogels with time-dependent material properties enhance cardiomyocyte differentiation in vitro. *Biomaterials* **2011**, *32*, 1002–1009. [CrossRef] [PubMed]
59. Serban, M.A.; Yang, G.; Prestwich, G.D. Synthesis, characterization and chondroprotective properties of a hyaluronan thioethyl ether derivative. *Biomaterials* **2008**, *29*, 1388–1399. [CrossRef] [PubMed]
60. Agrahari, V.; Meng, J.; Ezoulin, M.J.; Youm, I.; Dim, D.C.; Molteni, A.; Hung, W.T.; Christenson, L.K.; Youan, B.C. Stimuli-sensitive thiolated hyaluronic acid based nanofibers: Synthesis, preclinical safety and in vitro anti-HIV activity. *Nanomedicine* **2016**, *11*, 2935–2958. [CrossRef] [PubMed]
61. Yu, Y.; Chau, Y. Formulation of in situ chemically cross-linked hydrogel depots for protein release: From the blob model perspective. *Biomacromolecules* **2015**, *16*, 56–65. [CrossRef] [PubMed]
62. Yu, Y.; Lau, L.C.; Lo, A.C.; Chau, Y. Injectable Chemically Crosslinked Hydrogel for the Controlled Release of Bevacizumab in Vitreous: A 6-Month In Vivo Study. *Transl. Vis. Sci. Technol.* **2015**, *4*, 5. [CrossRef] [PubMed]
63. Oh, S.; Wilcox, M.; Pearson, J.P.; Borrós, S. Optimal design for studying mucoadhesive polymers interaction with gastric mucin using a quartz crystal microbalance with dissipation (QCM-D): Comparison of two different mucin origins. *Eur. J. Pharm. Biopharm.* **2015**, *96*, 477–483. [CrossRef] [PubMed]
64. Bernkop-Schnürch, A.; Hornof, M.; Zoidl, T. Thiolated polymers—Thiomers: Synthesis and in vitro evaluation of chitosan-2-iminothiolane conjugates. *Int. J. Pharm.* **2003**, *260*, 229–237. [CrossRef]
65. Salamat-Miller, N.; Chittchang, M.; Johnston, T.P. The use of mucoadhesive polymers in buccal drug delivery. *Adv. Drug Deliv. Rev.* **2005**, *57*, 1666–1691. [CrossRef] [PubMed]
66. Shinkar, D.M.; Dhake, A.S.; Setty, C.M. Drug delivery from the oral cavity: A focus on mucoadhesive buccal drug delivery systems. *PDA J. Pharm. Sci. Technol.* **2012**, *66*, 466–500. [CrossRef] [PubMed]
67. Pedrosa, S.S.; Pereira, P.; Correia, A.; Moreira, S.; Rocha, H.; Gama, F.M. Biocompatibility of a Self-Assembled Crosslinkable Hyaluronic Acid Nanogel. *Macromol. Biosci.* **2016**, *16*, 1610–1620. [CrossRef] [PubMed]
68. Galli, C.; Parisi, L.; Piergianni, M.; Smerieri, A.; Passeri, G.; Guizzardi, S.; Costa, F.; Lumetti, S.; Manfredi, E.; Macaluso, G.M. Improved scaffold biocompatibility through anti-Fibronectin aptamer functionalization. *Acta Biomater.* **2016**, *42*, 147–156. [CrossRef] [PubMed]
69. Clausen, A.E.; Kast, C.E.; Bernkop-Schnürch, A. The role of glutathione in the permeation enhancing effect of thiolated polymers. *Pharm. Res.* **2002**, *19*, 602–608. [CrossRef] [PubMed]
70. Han, H.S.; Choi, K.Y.; Ko, H.; Jeon, J.; Saravanakumar, G.; Suh, Y.D.; Lee, D.S.; Park, J.H. Bioreducible core-crosslinked hyaluronic acid micelle for targeted cancer therapy. *J. Control. Release* **2015**, *200*, 158–166. [CrossRef] [PubMed]
71. Campani, V.; Giarra, S.; de Rosa, G. Lipid-based core-shell nanoparticles: Evolution and potentialities in drug delivery. *OpenNano* **2018**, *3*, 5–17. [CrossRef]
72. Burdick, J.A.; Prestwich, G.D. Hyaluronic Acid Hydrogels for Biomedical Applications. *Adv. Mater.* **2011**, *23*, H41–H56. [CrossRef] [PubMed]
73. Wade, R.J.; Bassin, E.J.; Gramlich, W.M.; Burdick, J.A. Nanofibrous hydrogels with spatially patterned biochemical signals to control cell behavior. *Adv. Mater.* **2015**, *27*, 1356–1362. [CrossRef] [PubMed]
74. World Health Organization. Available online: http://www.who.int/features/factfiles/vision/01_en.html (accessed on 15 September 2017).
75. Espandar, L.; Bunnell, B.; Wang, G.Y.; Gregory, P.; McBride, C.; Moshirfar, M. Adipose-derived stem cells on hyaluronic acid-derived scaffold: A new horizon in bioengineered cornea. *Arch. Ophthalmol.* **2012**, *130*, 202–208. [CrossRef] [PubMed]
76. ESIBIO Stem Cell Solutions. Available online: http://www.esibio.com/index.php/products/product-category/hydrogels-kits/hystem-hydrogels/ (accessed on 2 January 2018).

77. Prestwich, G.D.; Erickson, I.E.; Zarembinski, T.I.; West, M.; Tew, W.P. The translational imperative: Making cell therapy simple and effective. *Acta Biomater.* **2012**, *8*, 4200–4207. [CrossRef] [PubMed]
78. Gwon, K.; Kim, E.; Tae, G. Heparin-hyaluronic acid hydrogel in support of cellular activities of 3D encapsulated adipose derived stem cells. *Acta Biomater.* **2017**, *49*, 284–295. [CrossRef] [PubMed]
79. Liu, Y.; Wang, R.; Zarembinski, T.I.; Doty, N.; Jiang, C.; Regatieri, C.; Zhang, X.; Young, M.J. The application of hyaluronic acid hydrogels to retinal progenitor cell transplantation. *Tissue Eng. Part A* **2013**, *19*, 135–142. [CrossRef] [PubMed]
80. Zarembinski, T.I.; Doty, N.J.; Erickson, I.E.; Srinivas, R.; Wirostko, B.M.; Tew, W.P. Thiolated hyaluronan-based hydrogels crosslinked using oxidized glutathione: An injectable matrix designed for ophthalmic applications. *Acta Biomater.* **2014**, *10*, 94–103. [CrossRef] [PubMed]
81. Hassan, W.; Dong, Y.; Wang, W. Encapsulation and 3D culture of human adipose-derived stem cells in an in-situ crosslinked hybrid hydrogel composed of PEG-based hyperbranched copolymer and hyaluronic acid. *Stem Cell Res. Ther.* **2013**, *4*, 32. [CrossRef] [PubMed]
82. Walimbe, T.; Panitch, A.; Sivasankar, P.M. A Review of Hyaluronic Acid and Hyaluronic Acid-based Hydrogels for Vocal Fold Tissue Engineering. *J. Voice* **2017**, *31*, 416–423. [CrossRef] [PubMed]
83. Bernkop-Schnürch, A.; Dünnhaupt, S. Chitosan-based drug delivery systems. *Eur. J. Pharm. Biopharm.* **2012**, *81*, 463–469. [CrossRef] [PubMed]
84. Hauptstein, S.; Hintzen, F.; Müller, C.; Ohm, M.; Bernkop-Schnürch, A. Development and in vitro evaluation of a buccal drug delivery system based on preactivated thiolated pectin. *Drug Dev. Ind. Pharm.* **2014**, *40*, 1530–1537. [CrossRef] [PubMed]
85. Laffleur, F.; Fischer, A.; Schmutzler, M.; Hintzen, F.; Bernkop-Schnürch, A. Evaluation of functional characteristics of preactivated thiolated chitosan as potential therapeutic agent for dry mouth syndrome. *Acta Biomater.* **2015**, *21*, 123–131. [CrossRef] [PubMed]
86. Laffleur, F.; Shahnaz, G.; Islambulchilar, Z.; Bernkop-Schnürch, A. Design and in vitro evaluation of a novel polymeric excipient for buccal applications. *Future Med. Chem.* **2013**, *5*, 511–522. [CrossRef] [PubMed]
87. Hombach, J.; Palmberger, T.F.; Bernkop-Schnürch, A. Development and in vitro evaluation of a mucoadhesive vaginal delivery system for nystatin. *J. Pharm. Sci.* **2009**, *98*, 555–564. [CrossRef] [PubMed]
88. Friedl, H.E.; Dünnhaupt, S.; Waldner, C.; Bernkop-Schnürch, A. Preactivated thiomers for vaginal drug delivery vehicles. *Biomaterials* **2013**, *34*, 7811–7818. [CrossRef] [PubMed]
89. Baloglu, E.; Ay Senyığıt, Z.; Karavana, S.Y.; Vetter, A.; Metın, D.Y.; Hilmioglu Polat, S.; Guneri, T.; Bernkop-Schnurch, A. In vitro evaluation of mucoadhesive vaginal tablets of antifungal drugs prepared with thiolated polymer and development of a new dissolution technique for vaginal formulations. *Chem. Pharm. Bull. (Tokyo)* **2011**, *59*, 952–958. [CrossRef] [PubMed]
90. Baloglu, E.; Senyigit, Z.A.; Karavana, S.Y.; Bernkop-Schnürch, A. Strategies to prolong the intravaginal residence time of drug delivery systems. *J. Pharm. Pharm. Sci.* **2009**, *12*, 312–336. [CrossRef] [PubMed]
91. Schnichels, S.; Schneider, N.; Hohenadl, C.; Hurst, J.; Schatz, A.; Januschowski, K.; Spitzer, M.S. Efficacy of two different thiol-modified crosslinked hyaluronate formulations as vitreous replacement compared to silicone oil in a model of retinal detachment. *PLoS ONE* **2017**, *12*, e0172895. [CrossRef] [PubMed]
92. ESIBIO Stem Cell Solutions. Available online: http://www.esibio.com/index.php/products/popular-brands/glycosil/glycosil-hyaluronic-acid/ (accessed on 2 January 2018).
93. Bi, X.; Liang, A.; Tan, Y.; Maturavongsadit, P.; Higginbothem, A.; Gado, T.; Gramling, A.; Bahn, H.; Wang, Q. Thiol-ene crosslinking polyamidoamine dendrimer-hyaluronic acid hydrogel system for biomedical applications. *J. Biomater. Sci. Polym. Ed.* **2016**, *27*, 743–757. [CrossRef] [PubMed]
94. VORNIA Biomaterials. Available online: http://www.vornia.com/products-page/functionalized-biopolymers/thiol-modified-hyaluronic-acid/ (accessed on 2 January 2018).
95. ClinicalTrials.gov. Available online: https://clinicaltrials.gov/ct2/show/NCT01887873?term=Croma+pharma&draw=2&rank=8 (accessed on 2 January 2018).
96. Eyegate Pharmaceuticals. Available online: http://www.eyegatepharma.com/pipeline/ocular-bandage-gel/ (accessed on 2 January 2018).

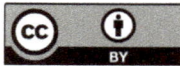

© 2018 by the authors. Licensee MDPI, Basel, Switzerland. This article is an open access article distributed under the terms and conditions of the Creative Commons Attribution (CC BY) license (http://creativecommons.org/licenses/by/4.0/).

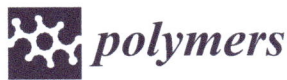

Article

Acrylated Chitosan Nanoparticles with Enhanced Mucoadhesion

Shaked Eliyahu [1], Anat Aharon [2,3] and Havazelet Bianco-Peled [1,4,*]

1. The Russell Berrie Nanotechnology Institute, Technion—Israel Institute of Technology, Haifa 3200003, Israel; shaked@campus.technion.ac.il
2. Bruce Rappaport Faculty of Medicine, Technion—Israel Institute of Technology, Haifa 3200003, Israel; a_aharon@technion.ac.il
3. Department of Hematology and Bone Marrow Transplantation, Rambam Health Care Campus, Haifa 3109601, Israel
4. Department of Chemical Engineering, Technion—Israel Institute of Technology, Haifa 3200003, Israel
* Correspondence: bianco@tx.technion.ac.il; Tel.: +972-4-829-3588

Received: 26 December 2017; Accepted: 19 January 2018; Published: 23 January 2018

Abstract: The aim of this study was to investigate the effect of acrylate modification on the mucoadhesion of chitosan at the nanoscale. Nanoparticles were fabricated from acrylated chitosan (ACS) via ionic gelation with tripolyphosphate and were characterized in terms of size, zeta potential, stability, and nanoparticle yield. Chitosan (CS) nanoparticles, serving as a control, were fabricated using the same procedure. The mucoadhesion of the nanoparticles was evaluated using the flow-through method after different incubation periods. The retention percentages of ACS nanoparticles were found to be significantly higher than those of CS nanoparticles, for all studied time intervals. An additional indication for the increased mucoadhesion of ACS nanoparticles was the increase in particle size obtained from the mucin particle method, in which mucin and nanoparticles are mixed at different ratios. NMR data verified the presence of free acrylate groups on the ACS nanoparticles. Thus, the improved mucoadhesion could be due to a Michael-type addition reaction between the nanoparticles and thiol groups present in mucin glycoprotein, in addition to entanglements and hydrogen bonding. Overall, ACS nanoparticles exhibit enhanced mucoadhesion properties as compared to CS nanoparticles and could be used as vehicles for drug delivery systems.

Keywords: chitosan; acrylated chitosan; nanoparticles; mucoadhesion; mucosal membranes; mucoadhesive polymers; retention

1. Introduction

The ability to adhere to mucosal surfaces, termed mucoadhesion, has attracted much attention in the last few decades. This adhesive property is considered valuable for pharmaceutical purposes, as mucosal drug delivery has great potential to provide improved drug absorption and bioavailability [1]. Drug residence time on mucosal surfaces can be prolonged using polymers designed to attach to mucosal membranes. Such mucoadhesive dosage forms are a useful tool for mucosal drug delivery. Polymeric nanoparticulate mucoadhesive carriers have even greater potential. Not only can they adhere to mucosal tissues, but they also offer increased surface area and enhanced bioavailability by protecting the drug from degradation [2].

Chitosan (CS) is a semisynthetic biocompatible polysaccharide derived from the deacetylation of the acetyl group in chitin [3]. CS has emerged as a promising vehicle for drug delivery, not only because of its mucoadhesion, but also because it can transiently open the tight junctions of epithelial tissues, increasing paracellular transport of drugs [4]. The mucoadhesive properties of CS arise from its ability to establish electrostatic interactions, hydrogen bonding, and hydrophobic interactions with mucin glycoprotein [5]. CS can be chemically or physically crosslinked, creating particles at the micro- or nanoscale [6,7]. The inherent mucoadhesion properties of CS nanoparticles can be further enhanced by thiolation, more specifically by grafting thiol-containing side groups to CS. Thiolated CS nanoparticles are capable of forming disulfide bridges with mucin's cysteine residues; as a result they demonstrate enhanced adhesion [8–12]. For example, the mucoadhesive force of nanoparticles composed of chitosan-4-thiobutylamidine was shown to be more than two-fold greater than that of CS nanoparticles [10].

Our group has pioneered the concept of acrylated polymers: hydrophilic macromolecules carrying acrylate end groups that covalently bind to mucin's thiol via a Michael-type addition reaction, which can take place in a physiological environment. We have established that acrylation of polymers, including polyethylene glycol (PEG) [13], alginate [14], poly(ethylene oxide)/poly (propylene oxide) blockcopolymer (Pluronic®127) [15], and chitosan [16], improves their mucoadhesive properties in comparison to the non-modified polymers. Previous studies have also demonstrated that acrylation does not cause any cytotoxic effect in neonatal human foreskin fibroblasts [14]. In particular, acrylated chitosan (ACS) was shown to be more mucoadhesive than both chitosan (CS) and thiolated chitosan [16]. The ability of ACS to form nanometric particles has not been explored before. Furthermore, it was not known whether the superior mucoadhesion properties of acrylated polymers are preserved at the nanoscale.

CS nanoparticles are commonly fabricated by ionic gelation using the multivalent ion tripolyphosphate (TPP) [17]. The formed nanoparticles are biodegradable, mucoadhesive, and nontoxic [18,19]. Even though methods for the formation of CS nanoparticles are well established, it is not straightforward to assume that TPP will react with modified CS in the same manner as with CS. Chemical modifications of CS typically consume its positively charged groups, hence affecting the ionic interactions between CS and TPP. In the specific case of acrylation, reducing electrostatic interaction could be accompanied by steric hindrance induced by the grafting of bulky PEG chains.

The current research had two main objectives. The first was to evaluate whether TPP can be utilized for fabrication of acrylated CS nanoparticles and investigate the conditions for their formation. The second was to investigate the influence of the chemical modification on the mucoadhesion of this nanometric system. Acrylated CS was previously shown to have superior mucoadhesive properties [16]. However, a recent review by das Neves et al. emphasized the possibility that bulk polymers will exhibit different behaviors to nanoscale particles [2].

Here, we report for the first time on the formation and characterization of acrylated CS nanoparticles. A procedure for the fabrication of ACS nanoparticles was developed, and the resulting nanoparticles were characterized in terms of size, stability, and particle yield. The mucoadhesive properties were studied with respect to the polymer-to-mucin ratio, by measuring the mucoadhesive index [20]. In addition, the flow-through method was used to measure the retention percentage of the nanoparticles on porcine intestine. The retention was examined with respect to the time of incubation with the mucosal tissue. CS nanoparticles served as a control in all measurements. We demonstrate that ACS nanoparticles exhibit enhanced mucoadhesion properties compared to CS nanoparticles and could be used as vehicles for drug delivery systems.

2. Materials and Methods

2.1. Materials

Low molecular mass chitosan (Mw 207 kDa, deacetylation degree 77.6%), mucin type II from porcine stomach, L-α-phosphatidylcholine, fluorescein isocyanate, and fluorescamine were obtained from Sigma Aldrich (Rehovot, Israel). Sodium tripolyphosphate was purchased from Alfa Aesar (Lancashire, UK). Sodium chloride, dichloromethane, and NaOH were obtained from Bio-Lab Ltd. (Jerusalem, Israel). Sodium taurocholate was purchased from Carbosynth (Berkshire, UK) and maleic acid from Arcos Organics (Geel, Belgium). Acetic acid glacial and dimethyl sulfoxide (DMSO) were purchased from Merck (Darmstadt, Germany). Polyethylene glycol diacrylate (PEGDA) with Mw of 10 kDa was obtained from the laboratory of biomaterials and regenerative medicine at the Department of Biomedical Engineering, Technion, Israel. Fresh porcine small intestine was obtained from the Pre-Clinical Research Authority, Technion, Israel. All research protocols involving live animals are subjected to the approval of the institute's ethical committee for animal experiments (IACUC). All procedures comply with the Animal Welfare Act of 1966 (P.L. 89–544), as amended by the Animal Welfare Act of 1970 (P.L. 91–579) and 1976 (P.L. 94–279). The protocol was approved by the Ethics Committee of the Technion (approval # IL-012-02-2016). The intestines were harvested immediately after the animals were euthanized. The porcine intestine was sliced shortly after removing it from the animal, and stored at $-20\ ^\circ$C until further use.

2.2. Synthesis of Acrylated Chitosan

Acrylated chitosan (Figure S1) was synthesized as described by Shitrit and Bianco-Peled [16]. We give a brief description of the process here. One g CS was dissolved in 100 mL 2 v/v % acetic acid at room temperature and stirred overnight. Then, 1 g PEGDA was added and stirred for 15 min. The reaction mixture was incubated for 3 h in the dark under shaking at the speed of 100 rpm at 60 $^\circ$C. Next, the reaction mixture was dialyzed in the dark against 5 L of double distilled water (DDW) for 3 days. After dialysis, the product was filtered with a Buchner funnel, lyophilized at 0.01 mbar and $-30\ ^\circ$C, and stored at $-20\ ^\circ$C until further use.

2.3. Synthesis of Fluorescein Isocyanate (FITC)-Labeled Polymers

Fluorescently labeled CS and ACS were synthesized by reacting the primary amino group of CS and the isothiocyanate group of fluorescein according to the procedure used by Tallury et al. [21] with minor modifications. One g of CS was dissolved in 100 mL of 2 v/v % acetic acid and stirred overnight. Fluorescein isocyanate (FITC) solution was prepared by dissolving 25 mg FITC in 100 mL methanol and adding it to the CS solution. The reaction was allowed to proceed under magnetic stirring in the dark at room temperature overnight. Next, 0.1 M NaOH was added, resulting in precipitation of the labeled CS that was then separated from the solution by filtration with a Buchner funnel. The product was washed with a mixture of ethanol/water (70:30) until no fluorescence was detected in the washing solution. The labeled CS was dissolved in 100 mL of 1 v/v % acetic acid and dialyzed against 5 L of the same solvent, followed by dialysis against DDW for 48 h. The final product was lyophilized at 0.01 mbar and $-30\ ^\circ$C and stored at $-20\ ^\circ$C until further use.

To prepare ACS-FITC, 500 mg of lyophilized CS-FITC was dissolved in 2 v/v % acetic acid. Then, 500 mg of PEGDA was added to the labeled CS solution under continuous stirring for 15 min. The reaction was allowed to proceed at 60 $^\circ$C under shaking for 3 h. The labeled ACS was dialyzed in the dark against 5 L DDW for 48 h. Finally, the labeled ACS was filtered, lyophilized at 0.01 mbar and $-30\ ^\circ$C, and stored at $-20\ ^\circ$C until further use.

2.4. Polymer Characterization

2.4.1. Nuclear Magnetic Resonance (NMR)

CS and ACS were dissolved in a mixture of 2 v/v % CD$_3$COOD and 98 v/v % D$_2$O and studied using a 400 MHz Bruker ARX400 (Bruker, Billerica, MA, USA) at ambient temperature. Lyophilized CS and ACS nanoparticles were redispersed in the same solvent prior to the NMR measurements.

2.4.2. Fluorescamine Test for Quantitative Determination of Acrylate Groups

To determine the acrylation percentage of ACS, we modified the method proposed by Shitrit and Bianco-Peled [16] by replacing ninhydrin with fluorescamine assay [22]. A series of CS or ACS solutions with decreasing concentrations was prepared using 2 v/v % acetic acid as a solvent. Samples of 140 µL of 0.1 M boric acid solution at pH 8 were placed in a black 96-well plate, and 10 µL of the polymer solution was added to each well. Then 50 µL of 1 mg/mL fluorescamine solution in DMSO was added to each well and mixed in the dark under shaking at 125 rpm for 10 min at room temperature. The fluorescence was measured using a UV–vis BioTek Synergy HT plate reader (BioTek Instruments, Winooski, VT, USA) with an excitation wave length of 360 ± 40 nm and an emission wave length of 460 ± 40 nm. Background fluorescence was determined using a solution of 2 v/v % acetic acid. The obtained fluorescence was plotted against the polymer concentration. The slope was used to calculate the acrylation percentage as follows:

$$Acrylation\ percentage = 100\% \cdot \left(1 - \frac{a_{pol}}{a_{CS}}\right), \tag{1}$$

where a_{pol} and a_{CS} are the slopes obtained from the a_{CS} curve and the CS curve, respectively.

2.5. Fabrication of Nanoparticles

CS and ACS nanoparticles were fabricated using the ionic gelation technique, where the positively charged amine residues of CS form electrostatic forces with the multivalent anion TPP [23]. A polymer to crosslinker ratio of 8:1 was chosen following preliminary experiments that yielded comparable particle size for both CS and ACS nanoparticles.

CS (0.1 w/v %) or ACS (0.2 w/v %) was dissolved in 0.1 v/v % acetic acid containing 0.1 M NaCl and stirred for 20 h. The mole excess of acetic acid, with respect to the amine groups of CS, is 300% for CS solutions and 2200% for ACS solutions. The pH was adjusted to 4, since at this value TPP possesses three negative charges that can physically crosslink the chitosan [24]. The concentration of NaCl was set to 0.1 M according to Huang and Lapitsky [25] and Antoniou et al. [26] to maintain stable particle size and low particle size distribution. A volume of 0.833 mL of TPP (0.025 w/v % in 0.1 M NaCl) aqueous solution was added dropwise to 1.667 mL of CS solution under magnetic stirring. Similarly, a volume of 0.5 mL of TPP (0.1 w/v % in 0.1 M NaCl) aqueous solution was added dropwise to 2 mL of ACS solution under magnetic stirring. The solutions were stirred for an additional 15 min at room temperature. FITC-labeled nanoparticles were created according to the same procedure using labeled polymers.

2.6. Nanoparticle Characterization

2.6.1. Size and Zeta Potential

Dynamic light scattering (DLS) was used to determine the average size, size distribution, and zeta potential of the nanoparticles. Measurements were performed in triplicate using a Zetasizer Nano ZSP (Malvern Instruments Ltd., Malvern, UK). A volume of 500 µL from the sample was placed in a polystyrene cuvette and measured at 25 °C.

2.6.2. Yield

A volume of 50 mL of nanoparticle solution was prepared in triplicate and the pH was adjusted to 5.9 using 5 M NaOH. The solution was centrifuged in a Heraeus Multifuge X3R centrifuge (ThermoFisher Scientific, Waltham, MA, USA) at 4 °C and 18,000 g for 1 h. Cycles of slow freezing at −20 °C and thawing at room temperature were performed in order to destabilize the nanoparticles and cause their aggregation, hence facilitating the precipitation. Nanoparticle pellets were lyophilized and weighed. The yield was calculated as follows:

$$Yield = \frac{M_{NPs}}{M_T} \times 100\% \tag{2}$$

where M_{NPs} is the mass of CS-TPP nanoparticles recovered and M_T is the combined total weight of CS and TPP used in the formulation.

2.7. Mucoadhesion Studies

2.7.1. Nanoparticle Retention Studies

Retention studies using porcine intestine as a substrate were performed as previously described by Eshel-Green et al. [27]. Portions of porcine intestine tissue (1.5 × 3 cm) were thawed for 5 min at 100% humidity and 37 °C. FITC-labeled nanoparticles in a volume of 50 µL (0.00135 mM) were placed on the mucosal side of the tissue and incubated at 37 °C and 100% humidity for different times in the dark. Then, the tissue was set in a trough made of half a pipe, placed at a 45 degree angle in relation to the table. Using a syringe pump, a flow of buffer simulating the fasted state condition in the upper small intestine (FaSSIF-V2, prepared according to [28]), was dripped onto the substrate at a constant rate of 2 mL/min. Small aliquots of 200 µL each were collected continuously and analyzed fluorescently using a UV–vis spectrophotometer (BioTek Instruments, Winooski, VT, USA) with excitation wave length of 485 ± 20 nm and emission wave length of 525 ± 20 nm. The aliquots were analyzed for their nanoparticle concentration using a calibration curve of the labeled nanoparticles in FaSSIF-V2 buffer. All measurements were performed in triplicate. At the end of the experiment, the tissues were observed under a Nikon Eclipse TS100 fluorescence microscope equipped with a Nikon digital sight DS-Fi2 camera.

2.7.2. Nanoparticle-Mucin Aggregation

The mucoadhesion of the nanoparticles was examined using the mucin solution method described by Raskin et al. [20], with minor modifications. First, a soluble fraction of mucin was obtained. A solution of 5 mg/mL was prepared by hydrating powdered mucin in DDW and employing magnetic stirring for 3 h at room temperature. The insoluble fraction was removed by centrifugation at 4000 g for 10 min. The supernatant was collected, lyophilized, and stored at 4 °C until further use. The lyophilized mucin was dissolved in DDW at predetermined mucin ratios f, defined as:

$$f = \frac{w_{mucin}}{w_{mucin} + w_{NPs}} \tag{3}$$

where w_{mucin} is the mass of mucin and w_{NPs} is the nanoparticle mass.

Solutions of soluble mucin were pre-incubated at 37 °C. Freshly prepared nanoparticle solutions were size measured by DLS before the experiment. The aggregation with mucin solutions was determined by adding 150 µL of nanoparticle solution to 1 mL mucin solution under magnetic stirring at 37 °C for 1 min. The final concentration of the nanoparticles in the solution was 0.0087 w/v %. The final size was measured by DLS immediately after the time noted. The mucoadhesive index, indicating the increase in particle size, was calculated according to:

$$MI = \frac{d}{d_0} \tag{4}$$

where d_0 and d denote the diameter of the particle before and after incubation with mucin, respectively. Measuring the size of nanoparticles mixed with a 1 mL of DDW served as a negative control. All measurements were performed in triplicate.

2.8. Statistical Data Analysis

Microsoft® Excel software was used for the statistical analysis of the data. Standard errors of the mean (SEM) were calculated and presented for each treatment group. Statistical analysis was performed using the one-way analysis of variance (ANOVA) for comparisons between multiple treatments, while the one-tailed Student's t-test was used for comparison between two treatments. A p-value of 0.05 was considered statistically significant.

3. Results and Discussion

3.1. Acrylation of Chitosan

Chitosan was covalently modified by grafting PEGDA with a molecular mass of 10 kDa. This molecular mass was selected following a previous study that demonstrated better mucoadhesion properties of CS modified with 10 kDa PEGDA compared to CS modified with 0.7 kDa PEGDA [16]. After the synthesis, the product was characterized using NMR spectra, and the presence of free acrylate end groups was verified (Figure S2). In order to quantify the acrylation percentage of the products, we modified the method developed by Shitrit and Bianco-Peled [16]. The ninhydrin reagent was replaced with fluorescamine, making the procedure easy to execute at room temperature with only one stage of mixing. Fluorescamine binds to primary amine groups, resulting in fluorescence that is proportional to the amine concentration. Simultaneously, the excess reagent undergoes hydrolysis [22]. To validate the method, the acrylation percentage was also determined using the ninhydrin assay and found to be identical for both methods. This percentage was calculated from Equation (1) and found to be 65%. The molecular mass of ACS was calculated from the acrylation percentage and was found to be 5.9×10^6 Da. The PEGDA grafting percentage is less than 100%, indicating that there are amine groups which are free to bind TPP to produce ionically crosslinked nanoparticles.

It is noted that grafting hydrophilic PEG chains improved the solubility of ACS in aqueous medium. Contrary to CS, which is soluble only in acidic solutions, ACS was found to be soluble also in neutral pH value.

3.2. Fabrication of Nanoparticles

Polymeric nanoparticles were prepared using the ionic gelation process with TPP, wherein the positively charged amine residues in CS or ACS form electrostatic forces with the multivalent anion TPP. To allow better comparison between CS and ACS, we attempted to formulate nanoparticles similar in size by screening several possible experimental variables. CS and ACS nanoparticles crosslinked with TPP were fabricated using different polymer to crosslinker mass ratios and a constant polymer concentration of 2 mg/mL, and their average size and polydispersity index (PDI) were then determined (Figure 1). Overall, the size of CS nanoparticles decreases significantly with an increase in polymer to crosslinker ratio (ANOVA, $p < 0.0001$), in agreement with previously published results [7,29,30]. The average diameter of CS nanoparticles fabricated using the lowest polymer to crosslinker mass ratio of 8:1 was 356.0 ± 4.5 nm, while at the highest mass ratio of 3:1 the average diameter was reduced to 244.2 ± 4.2 nm. The reason for this decrease in size was found to be the increase in particle compactness [7].

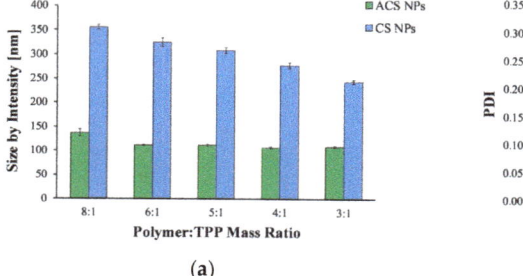 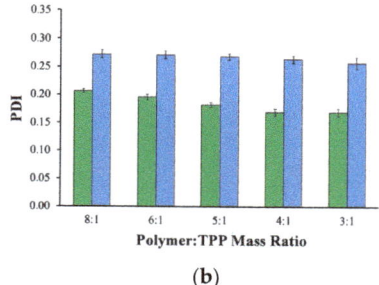

Figure 1. (a) Mean hydrodynamic diameter and (b) polydispersity index (PDI) value of acrylated chitosan (ACS) (green) and chitosan (CS) (blue) nanoparticles prepared at different polymer to crosslinker mass ratios.

Figure 1a shows that, in contrast to CS nanoparticles, the size of ACS nanoparticles did not change significantly with an increase of polymer to crosslinker ratio from 6:1 to 3:1 (ANOVA, $p > 0.05$). Only at a polymer to crosslinker ratio of 8:1 was the diameter significantly larger than it was at higher ratios ($p < 0.05$). This relatively minor influence of polymer to crosslinker ratio on ACS particle size may be attributed to the fact that 65% of the amine groups on the ACS backbone are conjugated to PEG, whereas only 35% are free to react with TPP. Therefore, fewer amine groups participate in the crosslinking. The ionic gelation process is mechanistically similar to the precipitation of colloids [25]. When TPP is added dropwise to a CS solution, every drop forms a nucleus, which is the source of the aggregation of polymer chains, forming a primary small nanoparticle. Primary nanoparticles aggregate into larger secondary colloids by bridges of TPP ions [31]. The balance between three processes—primary aggregation, secondary aggregation, and aggregate breakage due to stirring—determines the particle size. The grafting of acrylate groups on the CS backbone might weaken or interrupt the interactions of polymer chains via TPP ions. Consequently, the number of coagulation events (i.e., secondary aggregation) decreases, as does the rate of particle formation. Overall, the balance is tilted towards smaller particles, as secondary aggregation occurs less frequently, while TPP drops continue to form new particles.

Figure 1b displays the PDI values measured by DLS. PDI is a parameter calculated from a cumulants analysis of the DLS measured intensity autocorrelation function [32]. Low PDI values indicate homogeneous distribution, while high PDI points to polydispersity [26,33]. All nanoparticle formulations exhibit relatively low (mid-range) PDI values, over which the distribution algorithms best operate. For both CS and ACS nanoparticle formulations, as the polymer to crosslinker ratio increases, the PDI value decreases (ANOVA, $p < 0.0001$, $p < 0.0005$ respectively), indicating a narrow size distribution.

As evident from Figure 1, none of the tested polymer to crosslinker ratios could be used to obtain CS and ACS nanoparticles of similar size. Furthermore, many attempts to alter the size of ACS nanoparticles by varying the polymer and salt concentration were not successful since they all led to the formation of nanoparticles of about the same size (data not shown). Considering these results, we attempted to change the composition of the solutions used to create CS nanoparticles. This time, the polymer to crosslinker mass ratio was kept constant at 8:1, and the nanoparticles were created using different initial concentrations of polymer and crosslinker. DLS measurements were performed to determine the nanoparticle size (Table 1). Decreasing the initial TPP concentration from 1 mg/mL to 0.5 and 0.25 mg/mL resulted in smaller particles. A further decrease in the initial CS concentration from 2 mg/mL to 1 mg/mL led to the formation of particles of about 200 nm, a size comparable to that of the ACS nanoparticles. Therefore, CS nanoparticles for further study were prepared using 1 mg/mL of CS and 0.25 mg/mL of TPP at an 8:1 mass ratio of polymer to crosslinker.

Table 1. The effect of chitosan (CS) and tripolyphosphate (TPP) concentration on the nanoparticle size, at a constant CS to TPP mass ratio of 8:1.

CS Concentration (mg/mL)	TPP Concentration (mg/mL)	Size by Intensity (nm)
2	1	354.6 ± 4.5
2	0.5	317.0 ± 6.6
2	0.25	249.0 ± 3.4
1	0.5	228.6 ± 0.8
1	0.25	209.4 ± 3.0

3.3. Stability of the Nanoparticles

Particles are considered stable if their zeta potential value is between +30 mV and −30 mV [34]. The zeta potential of CS nanoparticles was found to be 27.7 ± 0.3 mV, while the zeta potential value obtained for ACS nanoparticles was 13.7 ± 0.2 mV. Since these values may indicate that the stability of the nanoparticles is less than optimal, we investigated particle stability by following the particle size and the PDI values as a function of time for a period of one month (Figure 2). The diameter of the nanoparticles, normalized to the initial size at the time of preparation, indicates that CS and ACS nanoparticle formulations display a similar pattern: the diameter slightly increases shortly after preparation with no further size changes after seven days (Figure 2a). The diameter of CS nanoparticles increased by 23% while that of ACS nanoparticles displayed a smaller increase of 12% over a long period of 30 days. Figure 2b displays the PDI values measured by DLS. As was mentioned before, low PDI values indicate homogeneous distribution, while high PDI points to polydispersity [26,33]. The formulations of the two nanoparticle types exhibit relatively low (mid-range) PDI values, over which the distribution algorithms best operate. The PDI of the CS nanoparticles gradually decreased during the first 14 days after preparation, with no further changes after this time. In contrast, the PDI of the ACS nanoparticles remained constant throughout the experiment. The smaller diameter change and constant PDI of the ACS nanoparticles support our hypothesis that they are more stable than CS nanoparticles. ACS nanoparticles possess bulky PEGDA chains that keep them from aggregating and maintain their stability, while primary CS nanoparticles aggregate into larger secondary colloids by bridges of TPP ions.

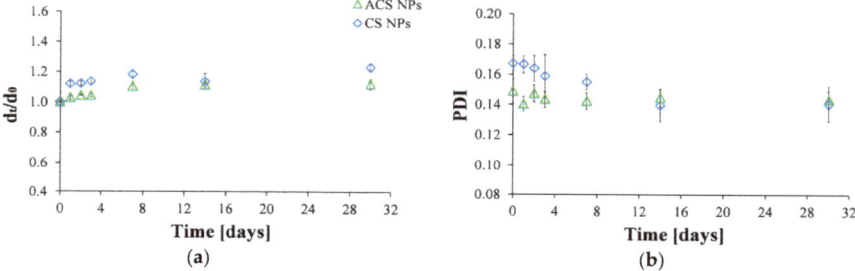

Figure 2. Size stability over time measured by: (**a**) Hydrodynamic diameter by intensity at time t divided by the initial diameter at time zero; (**b**) PDI values of ACS (green triangle) and CS (blue diamond) nanoparticles fabricated at an 8:1 mass ratio of polymer to crosslinker.

3.4. Nanoparticle Yield

To further investigate the differences between ACS and CS nanoparticle formulations, we determined the nanoparticle yield. Yield can be characterized by separating the nanoparticles with centrifugation, followed by either quantification of chitosan content in the supernatant or determining the weight of precipitated chitosan nanoparticles [35,36]. The downside of these approaches is that some of the smaller nanoparticles cannot undergo precipitation by centrifugation alone due to their light weight. A recent study by Rampino et al. showed that adding TPP to a CS nanoparticle suspension increases the amount of precipitated nanoparticles due to their flocculation, yet the final yield was still low, indicating that not all the nanoparticles precipitated [36]. Furthermore, if free chitosan chains coexist with the nanoparticles, TPP addition might nucleate new nanoparticles, hence increasing the measured yield to levels higher than the true value.

Here we suggest an improved method to measure the nanoparticle yield. Instead of centrifugation alone, or adding TPP prior to centrifugation, we conducted several cycles of freezing and thawing prior to centrifugation. This method is commonly used to assess solid content following emulsion polymerization. Slow freezing causes the formation of ice crystals, which force the particles to be in close proximity in a small volume. As a result, the particles aggregate and stay in this form even when they are re-thawed [37,38].

Figure 3 shows the precipitated mass after lyophilization, normalized to the total solid mass of polymer and crosslinker, as a function of the number of freeze/thaw cycles. Solutions of CS and ACS that were subjected to the same treatments—i.e., freeze/thaw cycles and centrifugation—were included in the study as controls. After one freeze/thaw cycle, the nanoparticle yield increased from 27.4 ± 0.01% to 55.4 ± 0.02% for CS and from 34.3 ± 0.02% to 39.0 ± 0.04% for ACS. These findings support the suggestion that some of the smallest nanoparticles cannot be separated by centrifugation alone and only disruption of their stability by freezing and thawing allows precipitation. Thus, after centrifugation, there is an increase in the precipitated nanoparticle mass. Adding another freeze/thaw cycle did not affect the CS nanoparticle yield, but it increased the ACS nanoparticle yield to 50.8 ± 0.01%.

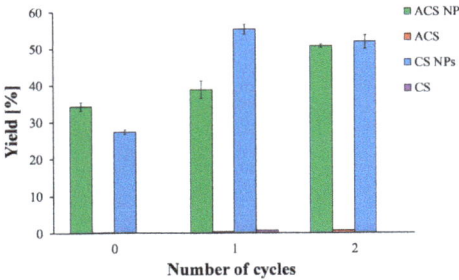

Figure 3. ACS (green) and CS (blue) nanoparticle yield as a function of the number of freeze/thaw cycles. ACS (purple) and CS (red) polymer solutions were examined as a control.

It is important to note that one or two cycles of freezing and thawing did not affect the solubility of the polymer solutions and resulted in a negligible precipitate. After three cycles of freezing and thawing, a sudden increase in the precipitate amount was observed for both nanoparticle formulations (data not shown). However, the amount of precipitate in the control experiment increased considerably as well, indicating an undesired effect of precipitation of free polymer chains. Therefore, the maximum yield is 55.4 ± 0.02% for CS nanoparticles and 50.8 ± 0.01% for ACS nanoparticles. These results revealed that CS and ACS nanoparticles with the same polymer to crosslinker ratio but different initial concentrations resulted in comparable nanoparticle yield. These yield values agree with the ones reported by Antoniou et al., who found a yield of 45% for CS-TPP nanoparticles prepared using a polymer to crosslinker ratio of 9:1 and CS concentration of 0.5 mg/mL [26].

3.5. Mucoadhesion Characterization

Many methods have been suggested to characterize mucoadhesion of nanoparticles [1]. Some of these methods are considered to give a direct measure of mucoadhesion as they assess the interactions of the nanoparticles with a mucus covered tissue. Others provide non-direct evidence for mucoadhesion by quantifying the interactions between mucins and nanoparticles. Out of these methods we chose flow-through as a representing direct method and nanoparticle-mucin aggregation as a representative non-direct method. The flow-through method allowed us to investigate for the first time the effect of incubation time on mucoadhesion. The nanoparticle-mucin aggregation method was used here to examine the influence of various mucin-polymer ratios.

3.5.1. Nanoparticle Retention on Mucosal Surfaces

The flow-through method was developed by Rao et al. to examine the mucoadhesion of polymers and coated microparticles [39]. Later, this technique was used to assess the adhesion of micro- and nanoparticles [40,41]. To quantify the ability to retain on the mucosa, a fluorescently labeled formulation is placed on a mucosal membrane. A flow of buffer, simulating the pH and salt content in the body, washes the polymer formulation off the tissue at a constant rate (Figure 4a). The mucosal membrane can be imaged for the remaining fluorescence [41], and the elution buffer can be analyzed to determine the polymer concentration washed away from the mucosa [27].

In the current study, we used this technique to evaluate and compare the retention of the two nanoparticle formulations on porcine small intestine. Fluorescent images were taken before and immediately after washing with 4 mL buffer, verifying the retention of FITC-labeled nanoparticles (green fluorescence) for both CS and ACS formulations after washing (Figure 4b). The dark fields in the images can be related to microscopic areas in the mucosal tissue with different affinity for the labeled particles.

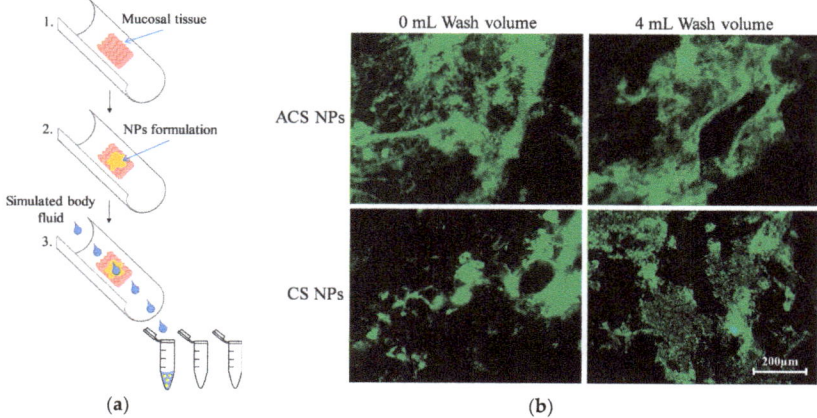

Figure 4. (a) Schematic representation of the flow-through method; (b) Fluorescent microphotographs of porcine intestine tissue samples with fluorescein isocyanate (FITC)-labeled ACS nanoparticles and CS nanoparticles, washed off with simulated intestinal fluid at a flow rate of 2 mL/min after incubation of 10 min.

Next, a quantitative evaluation was conducted by analyzing the nanoparticle concentration in the elution buffer and determining the nanoparticle mass retained on the mucosal surface and its dependence on the wash volume. The effect of different incubation times on the retention was also examined (Figure 5). When ACS nanoparticles were incubated for 1 min and washed at a flow rate of 2 mL/min, more particles were retained compared to the same experiment with no incubation stage (Figure 5a). After 10 min of incubation, nanoparticles were strongly bound to the mucosal membrane, and the retention percentages were higher than for 1 min incubation. The same trend was observed for CS nanoparticles (Figure 5b).

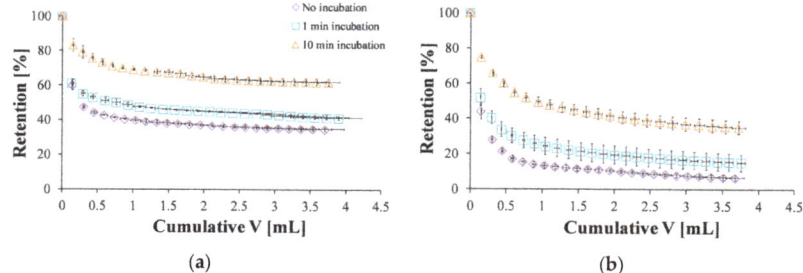

Figure 5. Retention profile of: (a) ACS nanoparticles without incubation (purple diamond), one minute of incubation (blue square), and ten minutes of incubation (orange triangle); (b) CS nanoparticles without incubation (purple diamond), one minute of incubation (blue square), and ten minutes of incubation (orange triangle).

The washing curves presented in Figure 5 were used to determine the retention at steady state, defined here as 95% of the final retention at the end of the experiment. Without incubation, ACS nanoparticles were initially washed away from the surface, reaching a steady state of 38% retention after 1.65 mL of wash volume (Figure 5a). CS nanoparticles, on the other hand, reached steady state at a lower value of 11% retention after 1.67 mL (Figure 5b). When the washing started after 1 min of incubation, a steady state of 44% retention was observed after 1.91 mL of wash volume for ACS nanoparticles, while CS nanoparticles reached a steady state of 19% retention after washing with 1.83 mL. Finally, after 10 min of incubation, the retention percentage of ACS nanoparticles leveled off to 64% after 2.17 mL of elution buffer, compared to 37% retention after washing with 2.90 mL for CS nanoparticles under the same conditions. These results indicate that the washing volume required to reach steady state is similar for both nanoparticle formulations, suggesting no great difference in the kinetics of reaching equilibrium. However, the steady state retention is lower for CS nanoparticles, indicating its lower mucoadhesion. Furthermore, the retention percentage at the end of the experiment, obtained after approximately 4 mL wash volume (Figure 6), demonstrates the differences in binding strength as well. A statistical analysis revealed that the retention values of both ACS and CS nanoparticles depends significantly on the incubation time (ANOVA, $p < 0.0001$, $n = 3$, $p < 0.05$, $n = 3$, respectively). The retention values of ACS nanoparticles at the end of the experiment were significantly higher than those of CS nanoparticles for all the examined incubation times (t-test, no incubation $p < 0.001$, 1 min incubation $p < 0.05$, 10 min incubation $p < 0.05$, $n = 3$).

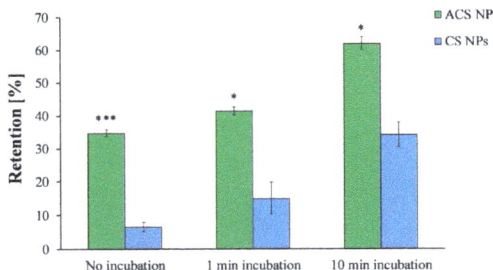

Figure 6. Final retention percentages of ACS nanoparticles (green) and CS nanoparticles (blue) obtained after different incubation time intervals (ANOVA, $p < 0.0001$, $n = 3$, $p < 0.05$, $n = 3$, respectively). (*) refers to statistically significant difference ($p < 0.05$), and (***) refers to statistically significant difference ($p < 0.001$).

The use of several theories of mucoadhesion can provide an explanation to the effect described. According to the diffusion theory of mucoadhesion, a liquid formulation interpenetrates via diffusion to the mucus layer. The interpenetration length depends directly on the contact time; as the contact time increases, so does the length [1]. The results displayed in Figures 5 and 6 imply that diffusion processes are involved in the studied system since the mucoadhesion increases with incubation time (i.e., contact time). Furthermore, the adsorption theory of mucoadhesion suggests that after an initial contact, the molecules form secondary bonds such as hydrogen bonds and Van der Waals forces across the interphase [42]. Chemisorption, which is a subsection of the adsorption theory, assumes that the interactions across the interface are related to strong covalent bonds [1].

A recent study by Shitrit and Bianco-Peled [16] found that acrylated CS presented improved mucoadhesion compared to unmodified CS. This improvement was attributed to the free acrylate group carried by PEGDA, associating with thiol end groups in mucin glycoprotein by a Michael-type addition reaction and form covalent bonds. To verify the presence of free acrylate end groups on the surface of ACS nanoparticles, we analyzed lyophilized CS and ACS nanoparticles, which were redispersed in D_2O, using NMR spectra. Figure 7 presents the chitosan spectrum (in blue) with peaks in the range of δ = 3 to δ = 4 ppm. The ACS nanoparticle spectrum (in green) contains new types of protons at δ = 3.59–4.06 ppm, representing the two methylene groups in PEG repeating units. The peaks at δ = 6–6.7 ppm represent the vinyl end group protons [43], thus verifying the existence of free acrylate groups. The peaks located at δ = 4.87 ppm and at δ = 2.13 ppm are assigned to water protons and acetic acid, respectively. The primary amine group in the CS nanoparticle spectrum is represented by the peak located at δ = 3.3 ppm. The appearance of this peak implies that even after crosslinking with TPP, some free amine groups remain. The same peak is observed in the ACS nanoparticle spectrum with a decrease in signal. Similar results were obtained in previous studies on ACS [16,44]. These results support our hypothesis that free acrylate end groups on ACS nanoparticles may associate covalently with thiol groups present on mucin. These nanoparticles also interact strongly with the mucus layer as a result of entanglements and hydrogen bonds between long PEGDA chains and mucin glycoprotein. CS nanoparticles, on the other hand, have fewer possibilities for entanglements, and can only interact with mucin via hydrogen bonding or electrostatic interactions [5]. It is noted that the kinetics of Michael-type addition between thiol and acrylate groups is in the order of minutes. A recent study by Eshel-Green et al. found that thiol-acrylate bonds in PEG-based hydrogels are formed after one min of mixing at room temperature [27]. Another study that used thiolated CS mixed with PEGDA reported a gelation time of 25 min at 37 °C [45]. These studies suggest that the reaction between thiol and acrylate starts immediately upon mixing but reaches equilibrium in a matter of minutes.

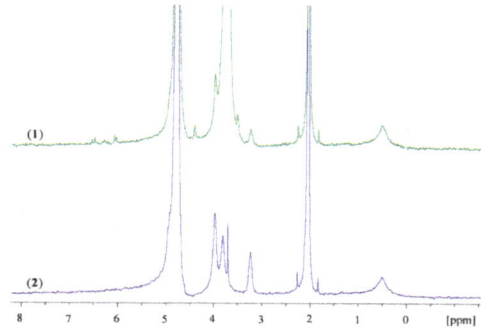

Figure 7. ^{1}H NMR spectra of (1) ACS nanoparticles; (2) CS nanoparticles in D_2O.

3.5.2. Nanoparticle-Mucin Aggregation

When a suspension of mucin is mixed with a solution of mucoadhesive polymer, the two components may aggregate due to covalent or electrostatic binding between the mucin and the polymer, supported by other forces such as hydrogen bonds and hydrophobic associations [46]. Similar association events occur between nanoparticles and mucin. Therefore, mucoadhesiveness can be evaluated by detecting the particle's diameter in the presence of soluble mucin [20]. The mucoadhesive index (MI) value is calculated by dividing the diameter of the aggregates formed after incubation with mucin by the initial diameter of the particle.

The use of dilute polymer solutions was proposed in previous studies of polysaccharide-polysaccharide interactions, because it renders the effects of polymer exclusion negligible [46]. For this reason, we examined the association between mucin glycoprotein and the nanoparticles in dilute solutions. A soluble mucin fraction was separated from porcine stomach mucin in order to reduce the effects of mucin gelation and self-aggregation [47].

A solution of nanoparticles with a fixed volume and concentration was incubated with soluble mucin solutions at increasing mucin ratio f (Equation (3)). Data in Figure 8a present the MI values against the mucin ratio f. It is noted that preliminary experiments with an incubation time of 5 h, as specified in a previous work [20], resulted in the same final diameter as incubation for just one min.

Figure 8a demonstrates that in most of the mucin ratio range, MI values of ACS nanoparticle-mucin mixtures were higher than those of CS nanoparticles and mucin. If we consider MI values to be an indication of mucoadhesion strength, we can deduce that ACS nanoparticles are more mucoadhesive than CS nanoparticles.

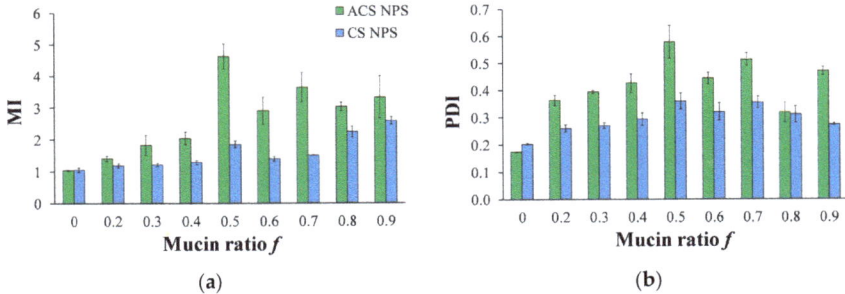

Figure 8. (a) MI values calculated for various compositions of mucin-ACS nanoparticle complexes (green) and mucin-CS nanoparticle complexes (blue) as measured by dynamic light scattering (DLS). (b) PDI for various compositions of mucin-ACS nanoparticle complexes (green) and mucin-CS nanoparticle complexes (blue) as measured by DLS.

The mucoadhesive strength (and thus the aggregate diameter) changes for different nanoparticle-mucin weight ratios (Figure 8a). For both ACS and CS nanoparticles, the MI ratio is significantly dependent on the mucin ratio f (ANOVA, $p < 0.00001$). For ACS nanoparticle-mucin mixtures in the range of $f < 0.5$, particle size increases with an increase in mucin fraction, from 152 ± 5 nm without mucin to 701 ± 0.4 at $f = 0.5$. When mucin is in excess, beyond the stoichiometric point, the MI values for ACS nanoparticles decrease from 4.9 ± 0.8 to 2.9 ± 0.4 at $f = 0.9$. A t-test for every two adjacent MI values confirmed the existence of a maximum in the MI vs. f curve ($p < 0.05$, $n = 3$), with the highest MI value obtained at the stoichiometric point ($f = 0.5$). As a control experiment, soluble mucin solutions were examined by DLS after dilution with buffer that does not contain nanoparticles. The results showed that the soluble mucin itself does not form measurable particles upon dilution. A similar test for CS nanoparticle-mucin mixtures did not detect a maximum in the MI vs. f curve: the MI values of CS nanoparticles grow with an increase in mucin fraction, from 1.0 ± 0.01 without mucin to 1.7 ± 0.14 at $f = 0.5$. MI values continue to rise when mucin is in excess, to 2.7 ± 0.11 at $f = 0.9$.

It was previously established by other methods that the binding between chitosan and mucin depends on the polymer to mucin ratio. Menchicchi et al. used an indirect colorimetric method to detect the amount of chitosan and mucin remaining in the solution after separating the polymer-mucin aggregates [46]. They found that the amount of mucin participating in the complex formation increased with the increase of polymer mucin ratio, up to a maximum value observed at the stoichiometric point. A similar effect was observed by Rossi et al., who calculated the rheological synergism parameter of polymer-mucin mixtures [48]. This study found a minimum value observed for 1:1 polymer to mucin weight ratio and suggested that the stoichiometry between chitosan hydrochloride and mucin is close to 1:1. To the best of our knowledge, this phenomenon is still unexplained, despite previous descriptions of an optimum in mucoadhesion for specific mucin-polymer ratios. We propose a possible mechanism to explain the complex formation and the observed optimal behavior (Figure 9).

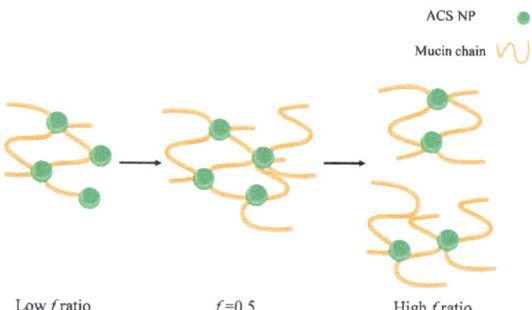

Figure 9. Schematic illustration of the proposed mechanism leading to the observed maximal complex diameter.

In our experiment, the particle concentration is constant, while the mucin concentration increases. In this case, the nanoparticles act as contact points between the mucin chains, leading to the complex formation (Figure 9). As the mucin ratio increases, the number of mucin chains sequestered into the complex increases, until the size of the aggregate reaches its critical value. Then, the aggregates disassociate into smaller complexes, in order to maximize the interactions between the nanoparticles and the mucin chains. In addition, large aggregates have more repulsion interactions between negatively charged mucin chains, destabilizing the complex and causing it to break under stirring. In light of the results in this experiment, it is possible that the decrease in the complex size might not indicate a decrease in mucoadhesion. Instead, at high f ratio, the large excess of mucin chains reorganizes between the nanoparticles in a specific arrangement to make the most of the interactions. CS nanoparticle-mucin complexes are originally smaller than ACS nanoparticle-mucin aggregates. Therefore, it is possible that they do not reach a critical size, and so do not disassociate.

To further support our results, we analyzed the PDI measured by DLS at increasing mucin ratio f (Figure 8b). As discussed above, the PDI value is a dimensionless measure of the broadness of the size distribution calculated from the cumulants analysis [32]. PDI values close to 1 indicate that the distribution is polydisperse. We hypothesize that the aggregation process of soluble mucin molecules with polymeric nanoparticles is likely to increase the polydispersity in solution. The results displayed in Figure 8b clearly show that the PDI values of mixtures of CS nanoparticles and soluble mucin are lower than those of ACS nanoparticles in the presence of mucin. The same maximum at $f = 0.5$ is observed in Figure 8a for mixtures of ACS nanoparticles and soluble mucin; however, this maximum is not statistically significant. These findings support the hypothesis that ACS nanoparticles have a greater tendency to associate with mucin than CS nanoparticles.

4. Conclusions

We demonstrate that ACS can be crosslinked with TPP to form a novel nanoparticulate system. These nanoparticles were characterized and compared to CS nanoparticles. The size of the CS nanoparticles was found to depend significantly on the polymer to crosslinker ratio. In contrast, ACS particles obtained at different polymer/TPP ratios had almost the same size. The stability of the ACS nanoparticles was evaluated over a period of 30 days and was found to be better than that of the CS nanoparticles, with a diameter increase of only 12% compared to 23% for the CS nanoparticles. The nanoparticle yield was measured using two cycles of slow freezing and thawing. The yield was similar for ACS and CS.

The nanoparticle retention on a mucosal surface increased with the increase in incubation time for both formulations, which is in line with the prediction of the diffusion and the adsorption theories of mucoadhesion. The ACS nanoparticles presented higher retention on the mucosal tissue for all examined incubation times. These results imply that ACS nanoparticles can form more entanglements, thanks to the bulky PEGDA chain, as well as covalent and hydrogen bonds with mucins. The mucin particle method was utilized to study the aggregation of nanoparticles in the presence of mucin. These measurements demonstrated that the size of the aggregates increased with the increase in the ratio of mucin to CS nanoparticles. In ACS nanoparticle-mucin mixtures, a peak was observed in the curve of aggregate size vs. mucin ratio. This observation was attributed to the breakage of aggregates larger than a critical value.

Supplementary Materials: The following are available online at www.mdpi.com/2073-4360/10/2/106/s1, Figure S1: The molecular structure of ACS, Figure S2: ^{1}H NMR spectra of (1) ACS, (2) PEGDA and (3) CS in D2O.

Acknowledgments: The generous financial support of the Technion EVPR Fund–Elias Fund for Medical Research is gratefully acknowledged. This research was supported in part by the Ministry of Science, Technology & Space, Israel (grant #3-11878).

Author Contributions: Shaked Eliyahu and Havazelet Bianco-Peled conceived and designed the experiments; Shaked Eliyahu performed the experiments and analyzed the data; Shaked Eliyahu, Anat Aharon and Havazelet Bianco-Peled wrote the paper.

Conflicts of Interest: The authors declare no conflict of interest.

References

1. Khutoryanskiy, V.V. Advances in Mucoadhesion and Mucoadhesive Polymers. *Macromol. Biosci.* **2011**, *11*, 748–764. [CrossRef] [PubMed]
2. Das Neves, J.; Bahia, M.F.; Amiji, M.M.; Sarmento, B. Mucoadhesive nanomedicines: Characterization and modulation of mucoadhesion at the nanoscale. *Expert Opin. Drug Deliv.* **2011**, *8*, 1085–1104. [CrossRef] [PubMed]
3. Andersen, T.; Mishchenko, E.; Flaten, G.E.; Sollid, J.U.E.; Mattsson, S.; Tho, I.; Škalko-Basnet, N. Chitosan-based nanomedicine to fight genital Candida Infections: Chitosomes. *Mar. Drugs* **2017**, *15*, 64. [CrossRef] [PubMed]
4. Yeh, T.-H.; Hsu, L.-W.; Tseng, M.T.; Lee, P.-L.; Sonjae, K.; Ho, Y.-C.; Sung, H.-W. Mechanism and consequence of chitosan-mediated reversible epithelial tight junction opening. *Biomaterials* **2011**, *32*, 6164–6173. [CrossRef] [PubMed]
5. Sogias, I.A.; Williams, A.C.; Khutoryanskiy, V.V. Why is chitosan mucoadhesive? *Biomacromolecules* **2008**, *9*, 1837–1842. [CrossRef] [PubMed]
6. Maciel, V.B.V.; Yoshida, C.M.P.; Pereira, S.M.S.S.; Goycoolea, F.M.; Franco, T.T. Electrostatic Self-Assembled Chitosan-Pectin Nano-and Microparticles for Insulin Delivery. *Molecules* **2017**, *22*, 1707. [CrossRef] [PubMed]
7. Jonassen, H.; Kjøniksen, A.L.; Hiorth, M. Effects of ionic strength on the size and compactness of chitosan nanoparticles. *Colloid Polym. Sci.* **2012**, *290*, 919–929. [CrossRef]
8. Bernkop-Schnürch, A.; Weithaler, A.; Albrecht, K.; Greimel, A. Thiomers: Preparation and in vitro evaluation of a mucoadhesive nanoparticulate drug delivery system. *Int. J. Pharm.* **2006**, *317*, 76–81. [CrossRef] [PubMed]
9. Chen, M.C.; Mi, F.L.; Liao, Z.X.; Hsiao, C.W.; Sonaje, K.; Chung, M.F.; Hsu, L.W.; Sung, H.W. Recent advances in chitosan-based nanoparticles for oral delivery of macromolecules. *Adv. Drug Deliv. Rev.* **2013**, *65*, 865–879. [CrossRef] [PubMed]
10. Alamdarnejad, G.; Sharif, A.; Taranejoo, S.; Janmaleki, M.; Kalaee, M.R.; Dadgar, M.; Khakpour, M. Synthesis and characterization of thiolated carboxymethyl chitosan-graft-cyclodextrin nanoparticles as a drug delivery vehicle for albendazole. *J. Mater. Sci. Mater. Med.* **2013**, *24*, 1939–1949. [CrossRef] [PubMed]
11. Dünnhaupt, S.; Barthelmes, J.; Köllner, S.; Sakloetsakun, D.; Shahnaz, G.; Düregger, A.; Bernkop-Schnürch, A. Thiolated nanocarriers for oral delivery of hydrophilic macromolecular drugs. *Carbohydr. Polym.* **2015**, *117*, 577–584. [CrossRef] [PubMed]
12. Sunena; Mishra, D.; Singh, S.K.; Kumar, A. Formulation and optimization of mucoadhesive galantamine loaded nanoparticles. *Pharm. Lett.* **2016**, *8*, 206–212.
13. Davidovich-Pinhas, M.; Bianco-Peled, H. Novel mucoadhesive system based on sulfhydryl-acrylate interactions. *J. Mater. Sci. Mater. Med.* **2010**, *21*, 2027–2034. [CrossRef] [PubMed]

14. Davidovich-Pinhas, M.; Bianco-Peled, H. Alginate–PEGAc: A new mucoadhesive polymer. *Acta Biomater.* **2011**, *7*, 625–633. [CrossRef] [PubMed]
15. Eshel-Green, T.; Bianco-Peled, H. Mucoadhesive acrylated block copolymers micelles for the delivery of hydrophobic drugs. *Colloids Surf. B Biointerfaces* **2016**, *139*, 42–51. [CrossRef] [PubMed]
16. Shitrit, Y.; Bianco-Peled, H. Acrylated chitosan for mucoadhesive drug delivery systems. *Int. J. Pharm.* **2017**, *517*, 247–255. [CrossRef] [PubMed]
17. Fwu-Long, M.I.; Shyu, S.S.; Lee, S.T.; Wong, T.B.I. Kinetic study of chitosan-tripolyphosphate complex reaction and acid-resistive properties of the chitosan-tripolyphosphate gel beads prepared by in-liquid curing method. *J. Polym. Sci. Part B Polym. Phys.* **1999**, *37*, 1551–1564. [CrossRef]
18. Zhang, H.; Oh, M.; Allen, C.; Kumacheva, E. Monodisperse chitosan nanoparticles for mucosal drug delivery. *Biomacromolecules* **2004**, *5*, 2461–2468. [CrossRef] [PubMed]
19. Dudhani, A.R.; Kosaraju, S.L. Bioadhesive chitosan nanoparticles: Preparation and characterization. *Carbohydr. Polym.* **2010**, *81*, 243–251. [CrossRef]
20. Raskin, M.M.; Schlachet, I.; Sosnik, A. Mucoadhesive nanogels by ionotropic crosslinking of chitosan-g-oligo(NiPAam) polymeric micelles as novel drug nanocarriers. *Nanomedicine (Lond.)* **2016**, *11*, 217–233. [CrossRef] [PubMed]
21. Tallury, P.; Kar, S.; Bamrungsap, S.; Huang, Y.-F.; Tan, W.; Santra, S. Ultra-small water-dispersible fluorescent chitosan nanoparticles: Synthesis, characterization and specific targeting. *Chem. Commun.* **2009**, 2347–2349. [CrossRef] [PubMed]
22. Udenfriend, S.; Stein, S.; Bohlen, P.; Dairman, W.; Leimgruber, W.; Weigele, M. Fluorescamine: A Reagent for Assay of Amino Acids, Peptides, Proteins, and Primary Amines in the Picomole Range. *Science* **1972**, *178*, 871–872. [CrossRef] [PubMed]
23. Nasti, A.; Zaki, N.M.; De Leonardis, P.; Ungphaiboon, S.; Sansongsak, P.; Rimoli, M.G.; Tirelli, N. Chitosan/TPP and chitosan/TPP-hyaluronic acid nanoparticles: Systematic optimisation of the preparative process and preliminary biological evaluation. *Pharm. Res.* **2009**, *26*, 1918–1930. [CrossRef] [PubMed]
24. Lim, S.; Seib, P.A. Preparation and Pasting Properties of Wheat and Corn Starch Phosphates. *Cereal Chem.* **1993**, *70*, 137–144. [CrossRef]
25. Huang, Y.; Lapitsky, Y. Salt-assisted mechanistic analysis of chitosan/tripolyphosphate micro- and nanogel formation. *Biomacromolecules* **2012**, *13*, 3868–3876. [CrossRef] [PubMed]
26. Antoniou, J.; Liu, F.; Majeed, H.; Qi, J.; Yokoyama, W.; Zhong, F. Physicochemical and morphological properties of size-controlled chitosan-tripolyphosphate nanoparticles. *Colloids Surf. A Physicochem. Eng. Asp.* **2015**, *465*, 137–146. [CrossRef]
27. Eshel-Green, T.; Eliyahu, S.; Avidan-Shlomovich, S.; Bianco-Peled, H. PEGDA hydrogels as a replacement for animal tissues in mucoadhesion testing. *Int. J. Pharm.* **2016**, *506*, 25–34. [CrossRef] [PubMed]
28. Jantratid, E.; Janssen, N.; Reppas, C.; Dressman, J.B. Dissolution media simulating conditions in the proximal human gastrointestinal tract: An update. *Pharm. Res.* **2008**, *25*, 1663–1676. [CrossRef] [PubMed]
29. Liu, H.; Gao, C. Preparation and properties of ionically cross-linked chitosan nanoparticles. *Polym. Adv. Technol.* **2009**, *20*, 613–619. [CrossRef]
30. Shah, S.; Pal, A.; Kaushik, V.K.; Devi, S. Preparation and characterization of venlafaxine hydrochloride-loaded chitosan nanoparticles and in vitro release of drug. *J. Appl. Polym. Sci.* **2009**, *112*, 2876–2887. [CrossRef]
31. Huang, Y.; Lapitsky, Y. Monovalent salt enhances colloidal stability during the formation of chitosan/tripolyphosphate microgels. *Langmuir* **2011**, *27*, 10392–10399. [CrossRef] [PubMed]
32. Arzenšek, D.; Podgornik, R.; Kuzman, D. Dynamic light scattering and application to proteins in solutions. In *Seminar*; University of Ljubljana: Ljubljana, Slovenia, 2010; pp. 1–18.
33. Masarudin, M.J.; Cutts, S.M.; Evison, B.J.; Phillips, D.R.; Pigram, P.J. Factors determining the stability, size distribution, and cellular accumulation of small, monodisperse chitosan nanoparticles as candidate vectors for anticancer drug delivery: Application to the passive encapsulation of [14C]-doxorubicin. *Nanotechnol. Sci. Appl.* **2015**, *8*, 67–80. [CrossRef] [PubMed]
34. Riddick, T.M. *Control of Colloid Stability through Zeta Potential*; Zeta-Meter: Staunton, VA, USA, 1968.
35. Hashad, R.A.; Ishak, R.A.H.; Fahmyb, S.; Mansour, S.; Geneidi, A.S. Chitosan-tripolyphosphate nanoparticles: Optimization of formulation parameters for improving process yield at a novel pH using artificial neural networks. *Int. J. Biol. Macromol.* **2016**, *86*, 50–58. [CrossRef] [PubMed]

36. Rampino, A.; Borgogna, M.; Blasi, P.; Bellich, B.; Cesàro, A. Chitosan nanoparticles: Preparation, size evolution and stability. *Int. J. Pharm.* **2013**, *455*, 219–228. [CrossRef] [PubMed]
37. Nakamura, A.; Okada, R. The coagulation of particles in suspension by freezing-thawing—I. Effect of freezing-thawing conditions and other factors on coagulation. *Colloid Polym. Sci.* **1976**, *254*, 718–725. [CrossRef]
38. Barb, W.G.; Mikucki, W. On the Coagulation of Polymer Latices by Freezing and Thawing. *J. Polym. Sci.* **1959**, *37*, 499–514. [CrossRef]
39. Rao, K.V.; Buri, P. A novel in situ method to test polymers and coated microparticles for bioadhesion. *Int. J. Pharm.* **1989**, *52*, 265–270. [CrossRef]
40. Albrecht, K.; Zirm, E.J.; Palmberger, T.F.; Schlocker, W.; Bernkop-Schnürch, A. Preparation of thiomer microparticles and in vitro evaluation of parameters influencing their mucoadhesive properties. *Drug Dev. Ind. Pharm.* **2006**, *32*, 1149–1157. [CrossRef] [PubMed]
41. Storha, A.; Mun, E.A.; Khutoryanskiy, V. V Synthesis of thiolated and acrylated nanoparticles using thiol-ene click chemistry: Towards novel mucoadhesive materials for drug delivery. *RSC Adv.* **2013**, *3*, 12275–12279. [CrossRef]
42. Shaikh, R.; Raj Singh, T.R.; Garland, M.J.; Woolfson, A.D.; Donnelly, R.F. Mucoadhesive drug delivery systems. *J. Pharm. Bioallied Sci.* **2011**, *3*, 89–100. [CrossRef] [PubMed]
43. Dust, J.M.; Fang, Z.H.; Harris, J.M. Proton NMR Characterization of Poly(ethylene Glycols) and Derivatives. *Macromolecules* **1990**, *23*, 3742–3746. [CrossRef]
44. Ma, G.; Zhang, X.; Han, J.; Song, G.; Nie, J. Photo-polymeriable chitosan derivative prepared by Michael reaction of chitosan and polyethylene glycol diacrylate (PEGDA). *Int. J. Biol. Macromol.* **2009**, *45*, 499–503. [CrossRef] [PubMed]
45. Teng, D.-Y.; Wu, Z.-M.; Zhang, X.-G.; Wang, Y.-X.; Zheng, C.; Wang, Z.; Li, C.-X. Synthesis and characterization of in situ cross-linked hydrogel based on self-assembly of thiol-modified chitosan with PEG diacrylate using Michael type addition. *Polymer* **2010**, *51*, 639–646. [CrossRef]
46. Menchicchi, B.; Fuenzalida, J.P.; Bobbili, K.B.; Hensel, A.; Swamy, M.J.; Goycoolea, F.M. Structure of Chitosan determines its interactions with mucin. *Biomacromolecules* **2014**, *15*, 3550–3558. [CrossRef] [PubMed]
47. Bansil, R.; Turner, B.S. Mucin structure, aggregation, physiological functions and biomedical applications. *Curr. Opin. Colloid Interface Sci.* **2006**, *11*, 164–170. [CrossRef]
48. Rossi, S.; Ferrari, F.; Bonferoni, M.C.; Caramella, C. Characterization of chitosan hydrochloride–mucin rheological interaction: Influence of polymer concentration and polymer: Mucin weight ratio. *Eur. J. Pharm. Sci.* **2001**, *12*, 479–485. [CrossRef]

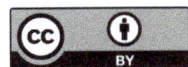

© 2018 by the authors. Licensee MDPI, Basel, Switzerland. This article is an open access article distributed under the terms and conditions of the Creative Commons Attribution (CC BY) license (http://creativecommons.org/licenses/by/4.0/).

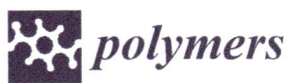

Review

Chitosan and Its Derivatives for Application in Mucoadhesive Drug Delivery Systems

Twana Mohammed M. Ways [1], Wing Man Lau [2] and Vitaliy V. Khutoryanskiy [1],*

[1] Reading School of Pharmacy, University of Reading, Whiteknights, Reading RG6 6AD, UK; t.m.m.ways@pgr.reading.ac.uk
[2] School of Pharmacy, Faculty of Medical Sciences, Newcastle University, Newcastle upon Tyne NE1 7RU, UK; wing.lau@newcastle.ac.uk
* Correspondence: v.khutoryanskiy@reading.ac.uk; Tel.: +44-(0)118-378-6119

Received: 12 January 2018; Accepted: 2 March 2018; Published: 5 March 2018

Abstract: Mucoadhesive drug delivery systems are desirable as they can increase the residence time of drugs at the site of absorption/action, provide sustained drug release and minimize the degradation of drugs in various body sites. Chitosan is a cationic polysaccharide that exhibits mucoadhesive properties and it has been widely used in the design of mucoadhesive dosage forms. However, its limited mucoadhesive strength and limited water-solubility at neutral and basic pHs are considered as two major drawbacks of its use. Chemical modification of chitosan has been exploited to tackle these two issues. In this review, we highlight the up-to-date studies involving the synthetic approaches and description of mucoadhesive properties of chitosan and chitosan derivatives. These derivatives include trimethyl chitosan, carboxymethyl chitosan, thiolated chitosan, chitosan-enzyme inhibitors, chitosan-ethylenediaminetetraacetic acid (chitosan-EDTA), half-acetylated chitosan, acrylated chitosan, glycol chitosan, chitosan-catechol, methyl pyrrolidinone-chitosan, cyclodextrin-chitosan and oleoyl-quaternised chitosan. We have particularly focused on the effect of chemical derivatization on the mucoadhesive properties of chitosan. Additionally, other important properties including water-solubility, stability, controlled release, permeation enhancing effect, and in vivo performance are also described.

Keywords: chitosan derivatives; mucosal drug delivery; mucoadhesion; trimethyl chitosan; thiolated chitosan; chitosan-catechol; acrylated chitosan

---

1. Introduction

Mucus is a viscoelastic gel lining the mucosal tissues exposed to the external environment including gastrointestinal, respiratory, and reproductive tracts and the eyes [1,2]. It is mainly composed of water (~90 to 98%), mucins (0.2–5% w/w), salts (~0.5 to 1.0% w/w), proteins (~0.5% w/v), cells and cellular debris, DNA, bacteria and lipids [1–7]. Mucins are the main component of the mucus, which are glycoproteins responsible for its gel-like characteristics. These glycoproteins are made of protein core to which carbohydrate side chains are covalently attached via O-glycosidic linkages [8,9].

Conventional (non-mucoadhesive) formulations lack the ability to withstand the strong involuntary muscular movement as well as the extensive washing effect by certain body fluids available, e.g., in the gastrointestinal lumen, ocular surface, urinary bladder and other mucosal surfaces. This limitation leads to the loss of a substantial amount of the administered drugs at the site of application/absorption. This may not only result in the overall increased cost of the treatment courses; it can also lead to the failure of therapy as effective drug concentration cannot be reached. This is especially more important in case of drugs such as antibiotics as amount lower than minimum inhibitory concentration probably leads to intractable complications including bacterial resistance. Mucoadhesive drug delivery systems are advantageous as they can adhere to the mucus layer of the mucous membrane. The adhesion of the delivery systems to mucosa (defined as mucoadhesion) increases the residence time of drugs, increases the concentration gradient, and protects the vulnerable small molecular weight drugs as well as peptide-based drugs. The overall effects could lead to controlled drug release, prolongation of therapeutic effects, enhancement in the bioavailability, cost-effective treatment, and improved patient compliance [2,9–12]. However, transmucosal drug delivery systems often have poor residence on mucosal surfaces, which justifies the need for novel mucoadhesive materials.

Various polymers have been used in the formulation of mucoadhesive delivery systems. Among them, chitosan and its derivatives are listed at the top [2,4,13–16]. Chitosan is a polysaccharide composed of N-acetyl-D-glucosamine and D-glucosamine and its units linked by 1-4-β-glycosidic bonds (Figure 1). It can be prepared by deacetylation of chitin in basic media [17,18]. Chitin is the second most abundant polysaccharide in nature, while cellulose is the most abundant [18]. Crustaceans produce chitin in their shells and plants produce cellulose in their cell walls. Therefore, these two polysaccharides impart structural integrity and protection to animals and plants [19].

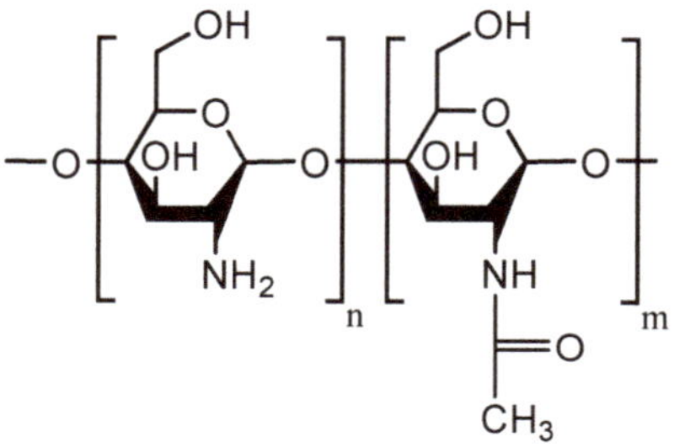

Figure 1. Chemical structure of chitosan.

Chitosan has –OH and –NH$_2$ groups leading to the capability of forming hydrogen and covalent bonding. This characteristic results in the possibilities of various chitosan chemical derivatization. These functional groups also play an essential role in the solubility character of chitosan macromolecules. At low pH, the amino groups undergo protonation, which makes chitosan macromolecules positively charged. This cationic nature provides strong electrostatic interaction with negatively charged components of mucus including sialic acid as well as epithelial surfaces [2,8,15,20–23]. Hydrogen bonding and hydrophobic interaction also play important role in the mucoadhesion of chitosan [15].

The derivatization of chitosan to improve its mucoadhesive properties has been considered in several publications (Figure 2). Some chitosan and its derivatives have shown potential in preclinical and clinical investigations for applications in transmucosal drug delivery (e.g., ChiSys® as a platform for nasal vaccination [24] and Lacrimera® eye drops [25]). However, there is still lack of review articles analyzing recent studies on the mucoadhesive applications of chitosan derivatives. In this review, we report various chitosan derivatives with potential applications as mucoadhesive materials. This review, however, does not consider any physical mixtures of chitosan or salt forms, which are discussed in several previous publications [26,27].

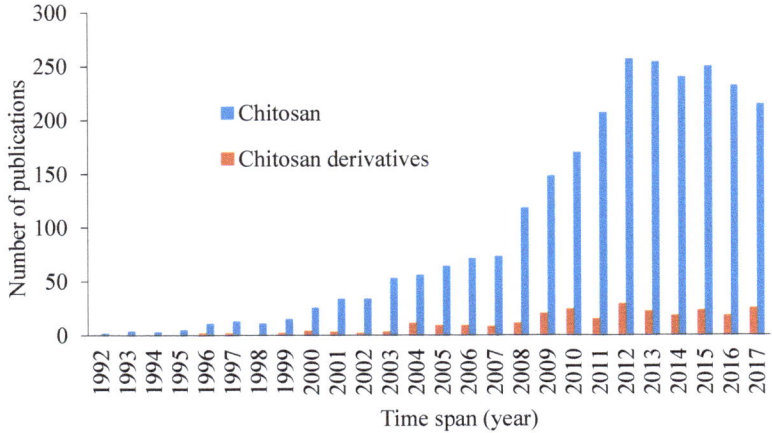

Figure 2. Number of publications related to mucoadhesive properties of chitosan and chitosan derivatives, source: SciFinder, keywords: chitosan or chitosan derivatives and mucoadhesion, retrieved on 24 November 2017.

2. Chitosan as a Mucoadhesive Material

Chitosan has been widely used in various biomedical and drug delivery areas because of its low toxicity, biocompatibility, antimicrobial activity, mucoadhesive properties and permeation enhancing effects [4,15,18,28–32]. It has been extensively studied as a potential excipient for the oral delivery of peptides [33]. Alonso and co-workers found that chitosan nanocapsules enhanced and prolonged intestinal absorption of salmon calcitonin because of their mucoadhesive properties and strong interactions with the intestinal barrier [34].

Our group has demonstrated the mucoadhesive character of chitosan in several studies. We have used a range of techniques including mucin-particle interaction [15], tensile strength [35] and most recently flow-through technique coupled with fluorescence microscopy [36,37]. In the latest case, fluorescein isothiocyanate-chitosan (FITC-chitosan) was used as a positive control and compared to other materials as well as FITC-dextran (non-mucoadhesive or negative control). Fluorescent samples were deposited onto ex vivo mucosal tissues (e.g., porcine urinary bladder or bovine eyes) and washed with bio-relevant fluids. Fluorescence images were taken after several wash cycles and the fluorescence intensity was used to compare the retention of each material on the mucosal tissues. We observed excellent mucoadhesive properties of chitosan in all cases, although some differences in the extent of its mucoadhesive potential in different mucosal tissues were noticed [37–39]. Figure 3 shows the result of mucoadhesion study of different silica nanoparticles in porcine urinary bladder ex vivo. The fluorescence signal of chitosan after washing was more intense compared to other materials and this indicated its excellent mucoadhesive properties. The rank of retention of materials was as follows: FITC-chitosan > thiolated silica nanoparticles > PEGylated (polyethylene glycol, 750 Da) silica nanoparticles > PEGylated (5000 Da) silica nanoparticles > FITC-dextran [37].

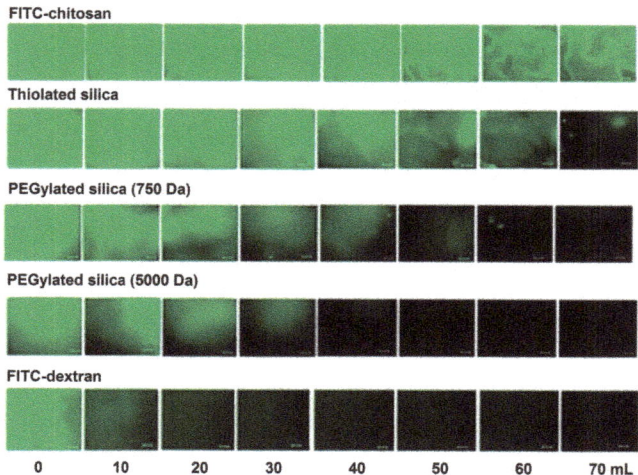

Figure 3. Representative microscopic fluorescence images of ex vivo porcine urinary bladder mucosa incubated with FITC-chitosan, thiolated silica, PEGylated silica (750 Da), PEGylated silica (5000 Da) and FITC-dextran and washed with different volumes of artificial urine solution. Scale bar = 200 μm. [37].

Behrens et al. [40] studied interactions of polystyrene, chitosan, polylactide (PLA)-PEG nanoparticles with two types of human intestinal cell lines, the enterocyte-like Caco-2 and mucus-secreting MTX-E12 cells. They revealed that the nanoparticles associated with Caco2 cells in the following order: polystyrene > chitosan > PEG-PLA. On the other hand, chitosan nanoparticles strongly bound to the mucus secreting cells and the binding of polystyrene nanoparticles was significantly decreased. PEG-PLA did not show any association with the mucus secreting cells. Intraduodenal administration of chitosan nanoparticles demonstrated that they could be internalized in both epithelial cells and Peyer's patches. The mechanism of the transport of chitosan and polystyrene nanoparticles was studied using Caco2 cells. It was found that chitosan nanoparticles were internalized by adsorptive endocytosis, whereas non-adsorptive endocytosis could be involved with polystyrene nanoparticles. Decreasing the temperature of incubation (4 °C) significantly decreased the transport of both types of nanoparticles. Addition of 1 mM protamine sulfate (inhibitor of active transport process) and pre-treatment of the cells with 10 U/mL heparinase II or 35 mM sodium chlorate (led to de-sulfation and the removal of anionic sites of mucus and cell membranes) significantly reduced the cellular transport of chitosan nanoparticles. However, the transport of polystyrene nanoparticles did not change with these factors. Chitosan endocytosis was saturable, i.e., cellular association increased linearly with concentration (31.25–1000 μg/mL) and reached a steady state at some point. Other studies have also reported the cellular uptake enhancing effect of chitosan, which could occur by adsorptive endocytosis, where a positively-charged coated nanoparticles adhere strongly to the negatively charged components of the cell membranes [41].

Thongborisute et al. [42] investigated the mucoadhesion and muco-penetration of chitosan solution, liposomes and chitosan-coated liposomes in rat small intestine in ex vivo and in vivo models. The systems were fluorescently labelled with FITC and administered orally to male Wistar rats or in the ex vivo model rats were sacrificed and the samples were incubated to interact with the mucosal tissues for 1 h at 37 °C. To visualize the penetration of these materials, cross-sections of 3 different regions of the small intestine (duodenum, jejunum, and ileum) were obtained and examined with confocal laser scanning microscopy (CLSM). They showed that chitosan, non-coated liposomes, and chitosan-coated liposomes could adhere and penetrate the mucosal tissues. However, the extent of adhesion and penetration of chitosan-coated liposomes was greater than for non-coated liposomes.

The authors related this behavior to firstly, the mucoadhesive properties of chitosan. Secondly, the presence of chitosan on the surface of liposomes could result in the formation of large aggregates due to the interactions of chitosan macromolecules leading to the large network of chitosan-coated liposomes adhering to the mucus layer. This phenomenon is not observed in the case of non-coated liposomes and only individual particles disperse in the suspension. Interestingly, although the authors did not discriminate the mucoadhesion and the mucosal penetration, they observed more mucosal penetration in the ileum region compared to both duodenum and jejunum, which they believe was due to the thicker nature of the ileum, which is also supported by other studies ([43–45]. Deacona et al. [46] also revealed the difference in the mucoadhesive interactions of chitosan in different regions of porcine stomach by sedimentation velocity technique using analytical ultracentrifuge equipped with conventional Philpott-Svensson Schlieren optical systems and coupled on-line to a charge-coupled device (CCD) camera. The cardiac region displayed the strongest interaction with chitosan compared to corpus and antrum.

3. Problems of Chitosan in Mucosal Drug Delivery

Being a basic polymer, chitosan is mucoadhesive only at limited pHs and is only soluble at acidic pH (pH < 6) [17,47]. The requirement of decreasing the pH of chitosan vehicles limits its applications in drug and gene delivery as many biomolecules including DNA, proteins and peptide-based drugs are not stable at low pH [48]. Additionally, even acidic chitosan formulations will encounter neutral to basic pHs once they administered into the human body either topically or systemically. High pH environment results in the precipitation of chitosan and can affect the performance of the carrier systems [17].

Chitosan-based mucosal drug delivery systems have been investigated to increase the residence time of drugs on the application/absorption sites [30,33,35]. The increase in the residence time is advantageous as it may prolong the action of drugs and provides sustained drug release. However, with unmodified chitosan, this is only possible to a certain degree. Therefore, there is an obvious need for further controlled drug release with subsequent prolongation of drug action [49].

Several modifications of chitosan have been investigated to enhance its mucoadhesive properties. In the next sections, we will discuss various chitosan derivatives with potential applications in transmucosal drug delivery.

4. Mucoadhesive Chitosan Derivatives

4.1. Trimethyl Chitosan (TMC)

TMC is a chitosan derivative which is always positively charged. This persistent cationic nature makes it one of the strongest mucoadhesive polymers. It has a much wider pH solubility range than unmodified chitosan due the presence of protonated groups ($-N^+(CH_3)_3$) [16]. TMC can be synthesized by three general methods: indirect trimethylation [50,51], direct trimethylation [52,53] and protection of chitosan hydroxyl groups (at C-3 and C-6 positions) by O-silylation [54]. The first method is usually a two-step process including the formation of an intermediate product (N,N-dimethyl chitosan) and can be conducted using two different reaction conditions. Whereas, the second method is a one-step process and does not contain any intermediate product, but it can also be conducted using two different reaction conditions. Using either indirect or direct trimethylation can often result in the formation of O-methylated TMC. However, using hydroxyl protection method by O-silylation, e.g., by employing tert-butyldimethylsilyl chloride, O-methylation can be avoided [16,50–55]. Verheul et al. [51] also claimed that their synthetic approach can result in O-methyl free TMC. The synthetic pathway for each method is illustrated in Figures 4–6. For the details of the experimental methods of TMC synthesis, readers are referred to two recent reviews by Wu et al. [55] and Kulkarni et al. [16].

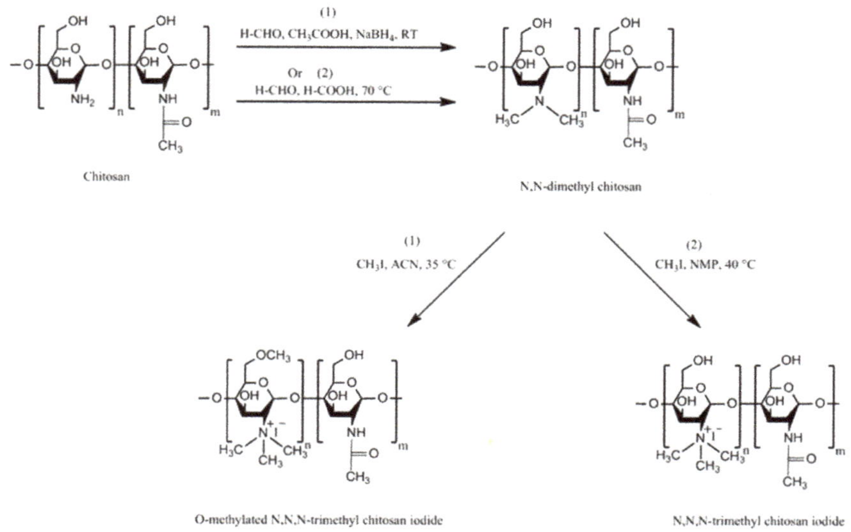

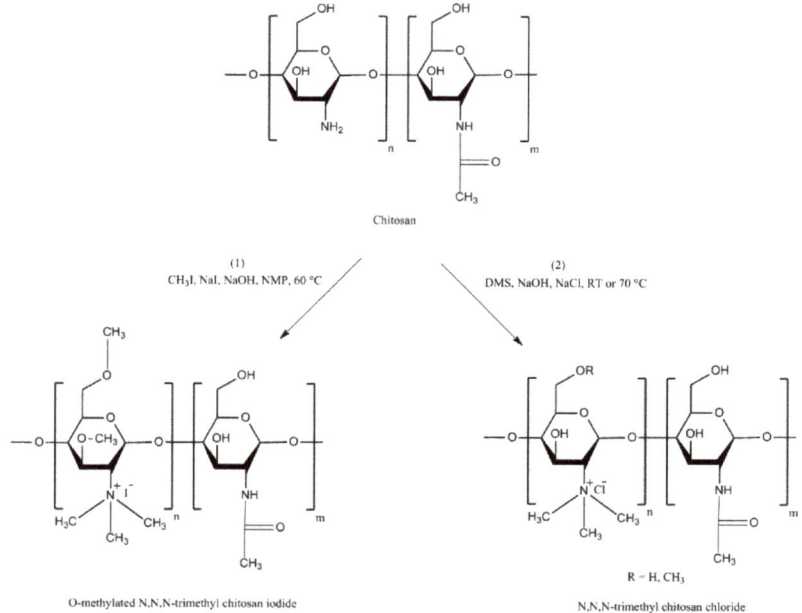

Figure 4. Synthetic pathway for preparation of TMC using indirect trimethylation approach according to (1) Muzzarelli and Tanfani [50], ACN = acetonitrile and (2) Verheul et al. [51] avoiding O-methylation, NMP = N-methyl-2-pyrrolidinone.

Figure 5. Synthetic pathway for preparation of TMC using direct trimethylation approach according to (1) Sieval et al. [52], NMP = N-methyl-2-pyrrolidinone and (2) de Britto and Assis [53], DMS = dimethyl sulfate.

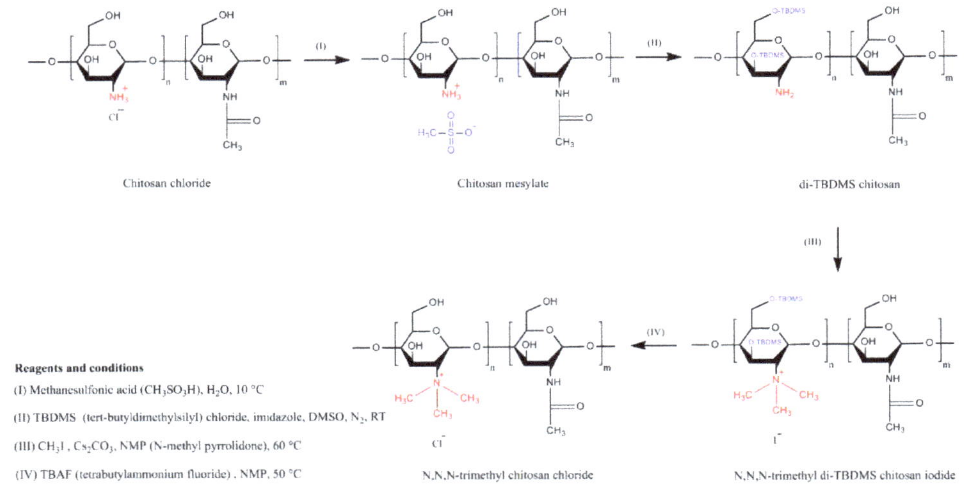

Figure 6. Synthetic pathway for preparation of TMC using hydroxyl groups protection approach by O-silylation according to Benediktsdóttir et al. [54].

TMC has been synthesized so as to enhance the water-solubility of chitosan with wider applications in drug delivery [56]. Subsequently, Sieval et al. [52] studied the effect of a few variables including the number of reaction steps, the duration of each reaction step and the amount of methyl iodide as a reagent. It was found that 2-step reaction resulted in products with high degree of substitution (40–80%). However, 3-step reaction led to even greater degree of substitution but at the same time water-solubility of the resulting product decreased.

Jintapattanakit et al. [57] synthesized TMC by reductive methylation of chitosan. TMC was then PEGylated. Both polymers were then fluorescently labelled using tetramethyl-rhodamine isothiocyanate (TRITC) and Oregon Green carboxylic acid succinimidyl ester (Oregon Green 448). The insulin-loaded nanoparticles were synthesized using self-assembly technique. The influence of TMC PEGylation and its positive charge density on mucoadhesive properties were assessed using a mucin assay and mucus-secreting HT29-MTX-E12 (E12) monolayers. It was found that introduction of PEG improved the mucoadhesive effect of TMC. This could be due to the interpenetration of PEG with mucus. In some other studies, PEGylation of chitosan also shown reduced toxicity and significantly increased the cellular permeation of hydrophilic macromolecules including FITC-dextran [23,58].

Hauptstein et al. [59] also studied the effect of PEGylation as well as thiolation (will be discussed in the next section) on adhesion of chitosan's compressed discs to porcine intestinal mucosa. They synthesized PEG-bearing thiolated chitosan by conjugating thiol-bearing polyoxyethylene ligand [O-(3-carboxylpropyl)-O′-[2-[3-mercaptopropionylamino)ethyl]-polyethyleneglycol] to amino groups of chitosan. The reaction was mediated by 1-ethyl-3-(3-dimethylaminopropyl)-carbodiimide hydrochloride (EDAC)/N-hydroxysuccinimide (NHS). In addition to its solubility in basic media, PEG-bearing thiolated chitosan showed greater mucoadhesive strength compared to unmodified chitosan. However, it was equally mucoadhesive as thiolated chitosan. Moreover, PEG-bearing thiolated chitosan enhanced the permeation of FITC-dextran through rat intestinal mucosa and Caco2 cells monolayer. The enhancement in mucoadhesion is based on the formation of disulfide bridges with mucus glycoproteins. The permeation enhancing effect could be due to the interaction of thiol groups of the thiolated chitosans with protein tyrosine phosphatase enzyme, which modulates the tight junction by a glutathione-dependent process.

Sayın et al. [60] demonstrated a novel approach for formation of nanoparticles via complexation between cationic TMC and polyampholytic N-carboxymethylchitosan without a crosslinker.

The nanoparticles were loaded with FITC-BSA (bovine serum albumin) and their cellular uptake was studied. A significant number of the nanoparticles was taken up by murine macrophage J774A.1 within 30 min of incubation. The authors believed that the mucoadhesive effect of TMC plays a major role in the enhancement of the cellular uptake. The nasal administration of tetanium toxiod-loaded 283 nm nanoparticles in mice, induced the mucosal and systemic immune responses.

Sajomsang et al. [61] synthesized two methylated N-aryl chitosan derivatives, methylated N-(4-N,N-dimethylaminocinnamyl) chitosan chloride and methylated N-(4-pyridylmethyl) chitosan chloride by reductive amination and methylation of chitosan. It was found that increasing the degree of quaternization led to a stronger mucin-particle interaction. Moreover, the cytotoxicity was dependent on the polymer structure, the location of the positive charge and the molecular weight after methylation.

On the other hand, some studies showed that TMC has greater potential to adhere to the epithelial tissue than to the mucin. For instance, Keely et al. [62] evaluated the adhesion of coumarin-labelled-poly(2-dimethylaminoethyl) methacrylate (pDMAEMA) with different levels of quaternization (0, 10, 24 and 32%) and TMC to human mucus-secreting and non-mucus-secreting intestinal cell monolayers (E12 and HT29, respectively) as well as freshly excised rat intestinal mucosa using non-everted intestinal sacs model. CLSM, light and fluorescence microscopy were used to quantify either mucoadhesion (adhesion to the mucus layer) or bioadhesion (adhesion to the epithelial tissue rather than mucosal surface). It was found that pDMAEMA, regardless of the degree of quaternization, was more mucoadhesive than bioadhesive, whereas TMC was found to be more bioadhesive and as mucoadhesive as unquaternized pDMAEMA and 24% quaternized pDMAEMA. When E12 cells and intestinal sacs were treated with mucolytic agent, N-acetylcysteine, for 15 min, the mucoadhesion of pDMAEMA polymers was significantly decreased, while the bioadhesion of TMC had not changed following this treatment. Additionally, the permeability of FITC-dextran through both E12 cells monolayer and intestinal sacs was significantly decreased in the presence of pDMAEMA, whereas the use of TMC led to a significant increase in the permeability. Although they did not study the interactions between the polymers and the mucus, the authors claimed that pDMAEMA perhaps increased the viscosity of the mucus gel as in case of carbopol [63] and thus impede the diffusion of FITC-dextran. However, chitosan and its derivatives can open the tight junctions [64–66] that could enhance the paracellular diffusion of FITC-dextran.

Liu et al. [67] developed core-shell nanoparticles based on TMC. The nanoparticles were coated with dissociable layer of N-(2-hydroxypropyl) methacrylamide copolymer (pHPMA). The diffusion of coated and uncoated nanoparticles in human cervicovaginal mucus was evaluated using multiple particle tracking technique and Ussing chamber. Cellular internalization and transport were evaluated using E12 cells. It was found that pHPMA coating could enhance the diffusion of TMC nanoparticles through both mucus and epithelial layer. Non-coated TMC nanoparticles were found to be less diffusive in both mucus and the cells. Liu et al. [67] indirectly demonstrated the mucoadhesive properties of TMC.

Generally, mucoadhesive properties of chitosan could be affected by both the degree of quaternization and its molecular weight. Nazar et al. [68] prepared TMC thermosensitive nasal gel from low, medium, and high molecular weight chitosan with quaternization of 25.6 to 61.3%. It was found that gels made from lower quaternization and medium molecular weight TMC had the greatest work of adhesion (252 ± 14 µJ) and the shortest sol-gel transition time (7 min) at 32.5 °C. This could be due to their great capacity to hydrate and absorb large amounts of water. Partially quaternized TMC has the advantage of having a better water solubility profile in neutral and basic environment than the native chitosan [69]. This is important since absorption of most drugs happens at slightly basic or neutral part of the gastrointestinal tract [70].

TMC has been used as an absorption enhancer for the delivery of buserelin and insulin across Caco-2 cells monolayers. Although at low concentrations TMC is a less active absorption enhancer than both chitosan hydrochloride and chitosan glutamate, increasing its concentration could increase its activity. Since it is more soluble than both chitosan salts, increasing TMC concentration is very unlikely to cause precipitation, however, it resulted in an increase in the transport rate of both buserelin and insulin across Caco-2 cell monolayers, which might be due to the decrease in transepithelial electrical resistance (TEER) [71]. TEER is a parameter, which determines the intercellular ion flux and indicates the tightness of paracellular "junctional complexes" of biological membranes [72].

4.2. Carboxymethyl Chitosans

Carboxymethyl chitosan is another derivative of chitosan with amphoteric properties, acting as both acid and base depending on the pH of its solution. The amphoteric properties originate from the presence of both amino (basic) and carboxylic (acidic) groups in its chemical structure [73–75]. The amino groups undergo protonation in acidic media and make carboxymethyl chitosan positively charged. On the other hand, in basic media carboxylic groups dissociate and impart carboxymethyl chitosan negative charged.

Chen and Park [76] studied the pH-solubility profile of various O-carboxymethyl chitosans synthesized at different reaction conditions (temperature and ratio of water/isopropanol). The resultant chitosans showed a pH-dependent water-solubility character. Based on the degree of substitution, carboxymethyl chitosans (0.2 mg/mL) were insoluble at pH ranges close to neutral. However, at highly acidic and basic pHs, they demonstrated complete water-solubility. It was found that using low temperature (0 and 10 °C, during the synthesis) resulted in completely water-soluble products but with low yield. Increasing the temperature and decreasing the water/isopropanol ratio resulted in more carboxymethylation, which subsequently shifted the region of insolubility towards the lower pH (~3). Vikhoreva and Gal'braikh [77] also reported that carboxymethyl chitosan was insoluble at pH range of 3.5–6.5, whereas it showed complete solubility at pH < 3.5 and > 6.5. The insolubility at those pH ranges could be due to the fact that the isoelectric point of carboxymethyl chitosan is 4.1 and therefore when the pH of the solution is near the isoelectric point, precipitation and aggregation could happen [73].

Generally, carboxymethyl chitosans can be prepared using two different approaches, which are reductive alkylation and direct alkylation. In case of reductive alkylation, the amino groups of chitosan react with aldehyde groups of glyoxylic acid to form an intermediate imine product, which then is hydrogenated using sodium borohydride or sodium cyanoborohydride. The ratio of glyoxylic acid to chitosan is important in determining whether mono- or di-carboxymethyl chitosan is formed. Direct alkylation can be performed by reacting chitosan with some alkyl halides, such as monochloroacetic acid, in the presence of inorganic bases including sodium bicarbonate and sodium carbonate to raise the pH to 8.0–8.5. The pH of the reaction mixture is considered to be one of the important factors in determining whether O-, N- or O, N-substitution takes place [74,78–80]. Also, the higher pH resulted in a greater degree of substitution [81]. Figure 7 shows the pathways for the synthesis of carboxymethyl chitosans.

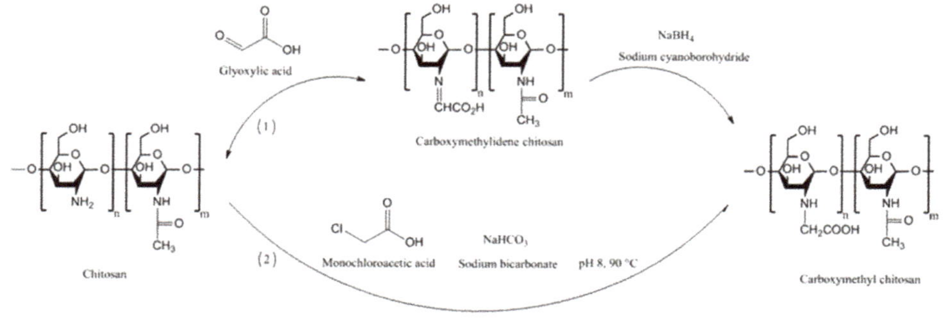

Figure 7. Schematic representation of the synthesis of carboxymethyl chitosans using reductive (1) [73] and direct (2) alkylation [79] methods.

Di Colo et al. [82] studied the effect of chitosan and N-carboxymethyl chitosan on the ocular pharmacokinetics of ofloxacin. Chitosan enhanced the penetration of the drug through the ocular tissue and its maximum concentration (C_{max}) in the aqueous humor was greater than in the case when conventional eye drops (Exocin® eye drops) and reference formulation (polyvinyl alcohol-based ofloxacin solution) were used. This may be due to the tight junction opening effect of chitosan. N-carboxymethyl chitosan did not significantly enhance the C_{max} of the drug in the aqueous humor. However, it resulted in a steady state drug concentration from 30–150 min post-ocular administration. The authors measured the viscosity of the three formulations and found that they were approximately similar. However, they still claimed that the viscosity enhancement is one of the reasons for the enhancement of pre-ocular drug residence time compared to the reference formulation. The binding of ofloxacin to N-carboxymethyl chitosan due to hydrogen bonding between amino groups of the drug and hydroxyl groups of the polymer, is also a reason for both the decrease in the ocular drug penetration and the increase in the residence time [82]. Although they did not evaluate the mucoadhesive properties of these polymers, they hypothesized that it could have an impact on the increased residence time in the ocular tissues. Clearly, the residence time of a formulation on the ocular tissues will be related to their mucoadhesive properties.

N-carboxymethyl chitosan has also been used as an intestinal absorption enhancer and proved to increase the in vitro and in vivo transmucosal absorption of low molecular weight heparin [73]. It has also showed potential in the oral delivery of small molecules. Prabaharan and Gong [83] synthesized thiolated carboxymethyl chitosan-g-β-cyclodextrin and showed its potential for the oral delivery of lipophilic drug ketoprofen. The modified chitosan resulted in 5-fold improvement in the adhesion to rat intestinal mucosa and slower drug release.

4.3. Thiolated Chitosans

Thiolation is one of the techniques used to functionalize various polymers including chitosan using thiolating agents bearing thiol groups. These include cysteine [84], thioglycolic acid (TGA) [85], 2-iminothiolane or 4-thiobutylamidine (TBA) [86], N-acetyl cysteine [87], isopropyl-S-acetylthioacetimidate [88] and glutathione [89]. This technique has been pioneered by Bernkop-Schnürch and co-workers [90] to enhance the mucoadhesion of polymers for pharmaceutical and biomedical applications. Thiolated chitosans are now one of the extensively studied mucoadhesive materials. Despite their superior mucoadhesive properties, they also have some permeation enhancing effects, ability to inhibit efflux pumps and in situ gelling properties [25]. Figure 8 shows the synthetic pathways to different thiolated chitosans.

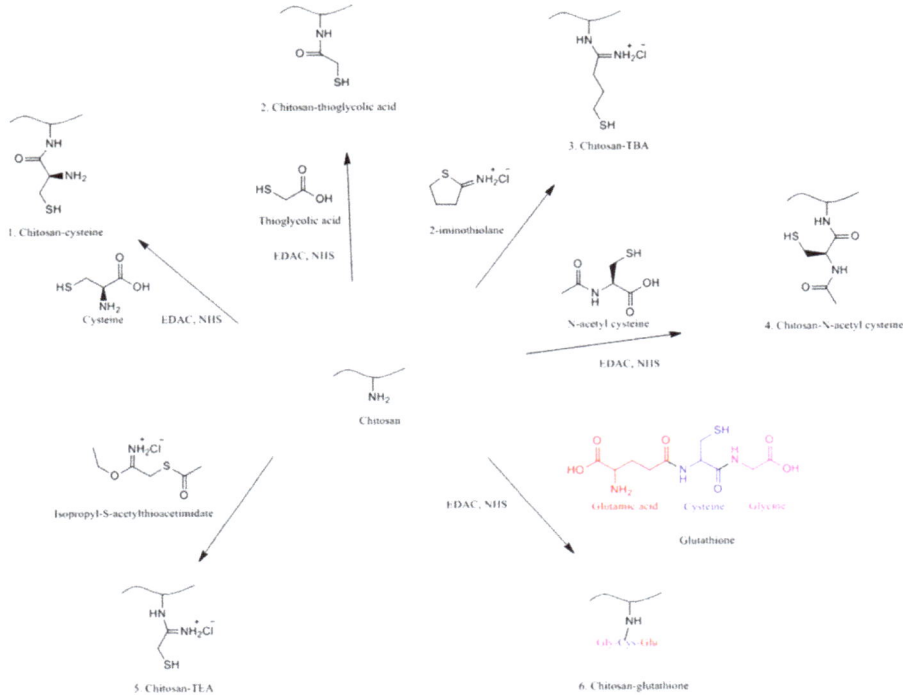

Figure 8. Synthetic pathways to different thiolated chitosan derivatives [14,84–89,91].

4.3.1. Chitosan-Cysteine

In 1999, Bernkop-Schnürch et al. [84] synthesized chitosan-cysteine conjugate by covalent attachment of cysteine to chitosan mediated by carbodiimide, where the amount of bound-cysteine was increased with an increase in the amount of the mediator reaching 1.2%. Subsequent mucoadhesion study revealed no significant difference between chitosan and thiolated chitosan. However, thiolated chitosan tablets showed superior cohesion over the chitosan tablets which could be due to the formation of intra/intermolecular disulfide bonds as a result of the oxidation of the thiol groups in thiolated chitosan. This improved cohesion is desirable not only for the mucoadhesion but also for the design of controlled release dosage forms [14,84].

TMC has also been thiolated by reacting with cysteine mediated with EDAC/N-NHS. Insulin-loaded nanoparticles were prepared using polyelectrolyte complexation method. The resultant TMC-cysteine showed significantly greater mucoadhesion capacity compared to unmodified TMC in both rat ileal loop and mucin adsorption models. This might be due firstly to the electrostatic interaction between positively charged chitosan and negatively charged sialic acid of mucin glycoproteins leads to the interpenetration of the polymer and mucin. Secondly, at neutral pH (pH of small intestine) the thiol groups of TMC-cysteine could be oxidized by reacting with cysteine-rich domains of mucin leads to the formation of disulfide bonds, which finally may immobilize more thiolated polymeric particles in the mucus layer than the unmodified polymer [92]. TMC-cysteine nanoparticles also showed greater permeability enhancement effect compared to unmodified TMC, which can be linked to the inhibition of protein tyrosine phosphatase which facilitates opening of tight junctions [14]. It might also be due to the greater mucoadhesion of TMC-cysteine than the native chitosan. Third possible reason is the inhibition of protease activities on insulin via shielding of enzymatic cutting sites after formation of self-assembled nanoparticles [92].

4.3.2. Chitosan-N-Acetyl-Cysteine

Schmitz et al. [87] synthesized chitosan-N-acetyl-cysteine conjugate via covalent attachment of N-acetyl-cysteine to chitosan using two different concentrations of EDAC as a mediator. They observed that this modification resulted in 50-fold increase in the retention of chitosan compressed discs on ex vivo porcine intestinal mucosa. The total work of adhesion required to detach the chitosan-N-acetyl-cysteine discs from the intestinal mucosa was 8.3-fold greater than unmodified chitosan. This may be due to the increase in the number of disulfide bonds between the polymers and the cysteine-rich domains of mucosa. They also revealed that increasing the concentration of EDAC resulted in products with greater amount of thiol groups. This is due to the activation of carboxylic groups of N-acetyl-cysteine, which resulted in immobilization of more thiol groups on the polymer. This eventually increased its mucoadhesive strength.

4.3.3. Chitosan-Thioglycolic Acid (Chitosan-TGA)

Chitosan-TGA has been synthesized by introducing TGA to chitosan using EDAC as a mediator. The resulting thiolated chitosan showed 4.3-fold increase in the viscosity, which is desirable for mucosal drug and gene delivery and scaffold materials in tissue engineering. This improvement in the viscosity may be related to the formation of disulfide bonds within the polymeric matrix [85]. The viscosity of this thiolated chitosan can be further improved by using different oxidizing agents including hydrogen peroxide, sodium periodate, ammonium persulfate and sodium hypochlorite. These agents accelerated the sol-gel transition to take place only within few min, while without them this transition requires 40 min. 25 nmol/L hydrogen peroxide has increased the dynamic viscosity of 1% chitosan-TGA solution by up to 16,500-fold. This may be due to the formation of more inter- and intra-chain disulfide bonds [93]. To assess the potential of chitosan-TGA for non-viral oral gene delivery, 100–200 nm nanoparticles with zeta potential of 5–6 mV have been formed by complex coacervation of plasmid DNA and the thiolated chitosan. These particles showed acceptable stability toward DNase and thus resulted in a 5-fold increase in the rate of transfection [94].

In another study, Barthelmes et al. [95] synthesized mucoadhesive nanoparticles based on chitosan-TGA using ionic gelation with sodium tripolyphosphate (TPP) for intravesical drug delivery. Two types of partially oxidized (different in their disulfide content, -SH groups oxidized to form -S-S- bonds) chitosan-TGA-TPP nanoparticles were also synthesized by the addition of H_2O_2 solution (0.5% v/v) to chitosan-TGA-TPP nanoparticles. Either fluorescein diacetate or trimethoprim were then loaded into the nanoparticles. Then, using a flow through technique, the amount of fluorescein diacetate adhered to the bladder mucosa was quantified using fluorescence spectrophotometry. It was found that using chitosan-TGA-TPP nanoparticles, 14.2 ± 7.2% of fluorescein diacetate remained on the surface of the mucosal tissues but in the case of unmodified chitosan-TPP nanoparticles, only 1.1 ± 0.1% fluorescein diacetate remained after washing with simulated artificial urine for 3 h with a flow rate of 2 mL/min. This improvement in the mucoadhesion was due to the covalent bonds formed between the thiol groups of the polymers and the cysteine-rich domains of the glycosaminoglycan layer of the mucus which is composed of proteoglycans and glycoproteins as in the case of adhesion to the intestinal mucosa [95,96]. To prove the concept, a quantitative analysis of free thiol groups of intestinal and urinary bladder mucus was performed and revealed no significant difference between the thiol contents of the two mucosal tissues. Interestingly, release study using artificial urine as a dissolution media shown that covalently crosslinked chitosan-TGA-TPP nanoparticles resulted in a slower and more controlled release of trimethoprim compared to ionically crosslinked chitosan-TGA-TPP and unmodified chitosan-TPP nanoparticles. The nanoparticles with greater content of disulfide bonds released the drug significantly slower than the nanoparticles with fewer disulfide bonds. The authors suggested that covalent crosslinking resulted in harder nanoparticles due to the formation of disulfide bridges within the matrix of the nanoparticles. This then increased the mechanical strength of the nanoparticles and thus made the artificial urine diffuse slowly into the nanoparticles. Consequently the dissolution of trimethoprim decreased and the nanoparticles released the drug slowly [95].

4.3.4. Chitosan-4-Thiobutylamidine

Chitosan-4-thiobutylamidine (chitosan-TBA) is another type of thiolated chitosan with mucoadhesive properties [97]. It remained on porcine small intestinal mucosa for 161 ± 7 h when tested using rotating cylinder method. In addition, the total work of adhesion was 740 ± 147 µJ. It has been reported that the mucoadhesive property of thiolated chitosans is pH dependent, and this point should be considered in the design of thiolated chitosan-based mucosal drug delivery systems [97].

Langoth et al. [98] designed mucoadhesive buccal delivery system of pituitary adenylate cyclase-activating polypeptide using chitosan-TBA as a promising treatment for type-2 diabetes mellitus. The in vivo buccal administration through porcine buccal mucosa resulted in a continuous rise in the plasma level of the enzyme over 6 h.

Dünnhaupt et al. [99] synthesized fluorescently-labelled nanoparticles of chitosan-TBA and polyacrylic acid-cysteine conjugate using ionotropic gelation technique. For the mucoadhesion study, fresh jejunum of rats was cut into 2 cm segments and filled with 0.1 mL nanoparticles. After fixation, the mucosal tissues were examined by fluorescence microscopy. The penetration study was performed using fresh "mucus-filled silicon tube" technique. It was found that nanoparticles of both modified chitosan (Figure 9) and polyacrylic acid exhibit greater mucoadhesive strength than unmodified nanoparticles. Chitosan particles showed 2-fold greater mucoadhesive property than polyacrylic acid particles. On the contrary, the muco-penetration ability of unmodified nanoparticles was greater than the thiolated nanoparticles.

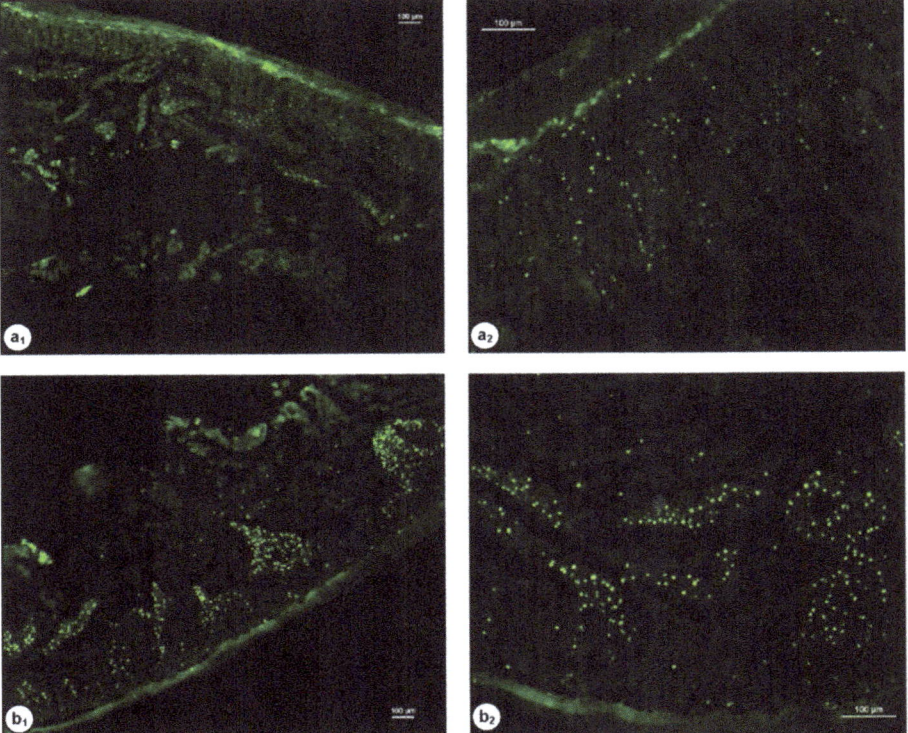

Figure 9. Fluorescent images of rat intestinal tissues after 2 h incubation with 100 µL (0.5% w/v) chitosan (**a**) and chitosan-TBA (**b**) nanoparticles labelled with Alexa Fluor 488, (a_1 and b_1, 40×; a_2 and b_2, 100× magnification). The scale bars = 100 µm. Reprinted from [99] with permission of Elsevier.

The combination of chitosan-TBA and chitosan-Bowman-Birk inhibitor in the design of 2 mg enteric coated microtablets showed a significant enhancement in the effect of oral salmon calcitonin on the level of plasma calcium when tested in rats [100]. The derivatization of chitosan with enzyme inhibitors will be discussed in a separate section.

4.3.5. Chitosan-Thioethylamidine

The use of 2-iminothiolane to synthesize thiolated chitosan resulted in a marked increase in the mucoadhesion. However, the resultant thiolated chitosan lacks sufficient stability leading to the reduction in the number of free thiol groups. One of the reasons for the instability could be the formation of N-chitosanyl-substituted 2-iminothiolane structures, which happens after modification of some amines using 2-iminothiolane. This intermediate product loses ammonia and results in the formation of re-cyclized N-substituted 2-iminothiolanes. To avoid this side reaction, Kafedjiiski et al. [88] synthesized thiolated chitosan using isopropyl-S-acetylthioacetimidate as a thiolating agent and an alternative to 2-iminothiolane. In contrast to chitosan-TBA (higher than unmodified chitosan) [101], the swelling property of chitosan-thioethylamidine was not significantly different from unmodified chitosan. However, the mucoadhesion was significantly improved. Using chitosan-thioethylamidine, the release of FITC-dextran was sustained over 3 h, which could be due to the presence of disulfide bonds in the structure of chitosan, which can slow the diffusion of FITC-dextran macromolecules down.

4.3.6. Chitosan-Glutathione

Several studies reported the use of glutathione for the synthesis of chitosan-glutathione conjugates [89,91,102,103]. Due to its permeation-enhancing effect, redox potential and safe toxicological profile, glutathione is a suitable thiolating agent for biomedical applications. Due to the presence of thiol groups in the glycine part of glutathione, it has strong electron donating property, acting as a reducing agent. Additionally, the stability of glutathione against cellular aminopeptidase is provided by the presence of γ-peptidic bond between glutamic acid and cysteine. Also, its conformational flexibility, makes glutathione a highly reactive ligand [89].

Similar to other thiolated chitosans, the synthetic approach is based on the formation of amide bonds between glycine carboxylic acid groups of glutathione and amino groups of chitosan. The reaction can be mediated by EDAC/NHS. The method was developed by Kafedjiiski et al. [89]. The resultant chitosan-glutathione exhibited acceptable cohesive properties and did not disintegrate in physiological solution (0.1 M phosphate buffer solution pH 6.8) for 48 h. However, unmodified chitosan was only stable for 9 h. Interestingly, both polymers showed the same swelling behavior, whereas chitosan glutathione had greater mucoadhesive properties (expressed as the total work of adhesion and tablets-intestinal detachment time) than unmodified chitosan. The apparent permeability of rhodamine 123 using chitosan-glutathione and unmodified chitosan were 2.06×10^{-7}, and 0.66×10^{-7} cm/s, respectively.

Jin et al. [104] demonstrated the application of chitosan-glutathione in the oral delivery of thymopentin (a synthetic pentapeptide with immune-regulatory action). They synthesized thymopentin-loaded poly(butyl cyanoacrylate) nanoparticles using emulsion polymerization technique. The particles were subsequently coated with either chitosan or chitosan-glutathione and orally administered to immunosuppressed rats. It was found that chitosan-glutathione-coated nanoparticles were able to normalize the immune function of rats, which is probably due to the enhanced mucoadhesive properties of chitosan-glutathione.

Chitosan-glutathione hydrogel was also found to be more effective in the reduction of oxidative stress in neonatal rat cardiomyocytes than unmodified chitosan hydrogel. The action possibly related to better cellular adhesion potential of chitosan-glutathione compared to unmodified chitosan as a result of the availability of the biocompatible glutathione promoting the cells survival [91].

4.3.7. Comparison of Chitosan, Trimethyl Chitosan and Thiolated Chitosan

In a comparative study, Mei et al. [105] investigated the mucoadhesion as well as the nasal absorption enhancing effect of chitosan, thiolated chitosan and trimethyl chitosan. Chitosans of different molecular weights were synthesized by depolymerization then the depolymerized samples were either trimethylated as reported in [106] or thiolated by reacting with cysteine using EDAC/NHS chemistry according to Bernkop-Schnürch and Steininger [107] with slight modification. The mucoadhesion of chitosan and thiolated chitosan was evaluated and the detachment time of 5 mm discs of the polymers from freshly excised porcine intestinal mucosa was evaluated. Discs of thiolated chitosan with greater degree of substitution (152 µmol/g) detached in a significantly longer time (about 12 h) than unmodified chitosan. The bioavailability of 2,3,5,6-tetramethylpyrazine phosphate through nasal route after its formulation with different chitosans was investigated. It was found that the use of any type of chitosan (unmodified, thiolated and trimethyl chitosan) resulted in a significantly improved absorption of 2,3,5,6-tetramethylpyrazine, however, no significant difference between thiolated chitosans (two different degrees of substitution) with unmodified chitosan was observed. The authors claimed that the permeation-enhancing effect is dose- and molecular weight-dependent and 100 kDa resulted in maximal absorption enhancement. On the other hand, trimethyl chitosan led to a significant enhancement in the nasal absorption of the drug. These results contradict those studies reporting the absorption enhancing effect of thiolated chitosan through intestinal mucosa. For example, Krauland et al. [101,108] demonstrated that chitosan-4-thiobulyamidine resulted in an increase in the oral and nasal absorption of insulin compared to unmodified chitosan. In Krauland et al. studies [101,108], the absorption enhancement could also be due to the inhibition of protein tyrosinase and P-glycoprotein efflux pump in the mucosal membranes [101,109].

4.3.8. Pre-Activated (S-Protected) Thiolated Chitosans

Vulnerability of thiolated chitosans to oxidation can be considered as one of the major limitations of their use as mucoadhesive polymers. Thiolated chitosans are generally stable in dry state. However, in solutions, they undergo rapid oxidation especially in the presence of oxidants such as oxygen and particularly at pH > 5 [86]. This, will not only lead to the formation of intra- and inter-molecular disulfide bonds, but also results in the reduction of the free thiol groups necessary for the formation of disulfide bridges with the cysteine-rich domains of the mucin. This will then lead to a significant reduction in the mucoadhesive potential of thiolated chitosans under physiological conditions of the gastrointestinal tract [86]. To prevent the unwanted oxidation of thiolated chitosans, pre-activated or S-protected thiolated chitosans have been developed by Bernkop-Schnürch and co-workers.

Generally, pre-activated thiolated chitosan can be synthesized by two steps. Firstly, thiolated chitosan is prepared using a thiolating agent and secondly thiol groups are protected by disulfide bond formation using ligands with mercaptopyridine substructure including mercaptonicotinamide, mercaptonicotinic acid and mercaptopyridine. Due to its toxicity profile mercaptopyridine is less commonly used [25]. Despite improvement of mucoadhesive properties, S-protection can also enhance the intestinal permeability of hydrophilic molecules such as FITC-dextran. In addition, S-protected thiolated chitosans have shown less cellular toxicity than the unprotected chitosans [110].

Dünnhaupt et al. [111] synthesized S-protected thiolated chitosan using a two-steps approach (Figure 10). First, thioglycolic acid was covalently attached to chitosan and resulted in the formation of amide bonds between the amino groups of chitosan and the carboxylic groups of thioglycolic acid. Secondly, aromatic ligand 6-mercaptonicotinamide (6-MNA) was synthesized by reacting 6-chloro-nicotinamide with thiourea, which was then oxidized using hydrogen peroxide to form 6,6'-dithionicotinamide (6,6'-DTNA). Both 6-MNA and 6,6'-DTNA were then reacted with thiolated chitosan to obtain S-protected thiolated chitosan. Tablets of unmodified, thiolated and S-protected thiolated chitosans were prepared. Using rotating cylinder method, it was found that S-protected thiolated chitosan with 660 µmol/g thiol groups remained attached to the intestinal mucosa for 90 h, whereas unprotected thiolated chitosan were only attached for 45 h. However, it seemed there was no significant difference between unprotected and S-protected thiolated chitosan with more thiol groups (980 µmol/g). Unmodified chitosan detached after only 10 h. Rheological studies also indicated that mixing S-protected thiolated chitosan with mucin resulted in a significant increase in the apparent viscosity of the mixture compared to both unmodified and unprotected thiolated chitosan. The authors believed that S-protected thiolated chitosan interacts more rapidly and quantitatively with mucus by thiol-disulfide exchange reaction between the thiol groups of mucus-cysteine and the pyridyl-thiol moiety of the S-protected thiolated chitosan. In the mucus, the amount of free thiol groups (-SH) is approximately two times greater than their oxidized form (-S–S-) [95] and this is in favor of thiol-disulfide exchange. Thus, more bonding between S-protected thiolated chitosan and the mucus can be achieved compared to unprotected thiolated chitosan [111].

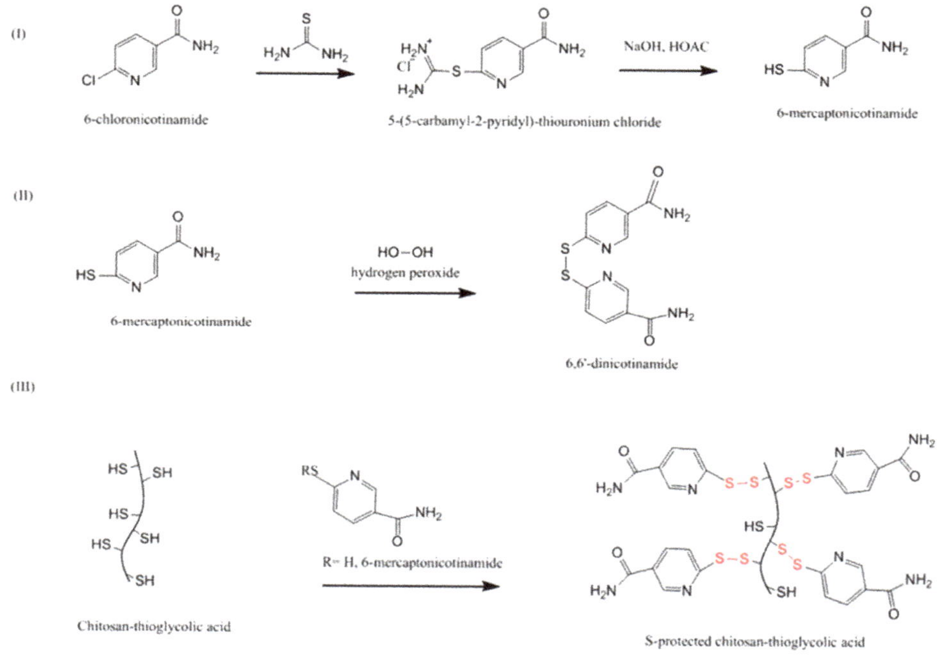

Figure 10. Synthetic pathway to S-protected chitosan-thioglycolic acid [111].

In another study, Dünnhaupt et al. [112] demonstrated the application of S-protected chitosan-TGA (chitosan-TGA-MNA) in the oral delivery of antide as tablets dosages forms. It was shown that hardness of chitosan-TGA-MNA tablets was significantly increased due to introduction of 6-MNA ligand and the presence of disulfide bonds within the polymeric network. Chitosan tablets swelled quickly and reached maximum within 2 h. However, chitosan-TGA tablets swelled slowly and continuously with greater extent than the unmodified chitosan. The presence of disulfide bonds might explain the enhanced water absorbing capacity of chitosan-TGA. On the other hand, chitosan-TGA-MNA tablets swelled to a lesser extent (1.5-fold) than chitosan-TGA tablets, which could be due to the presence of hydrophobic 6-MNA ligand. Additionally, chitosan-TGA-MNA resulted in a constant sustained release of antide and after 8 h, only 65% released. However, the% of antide released from chitosan-TGA and unmodified chitosan were 77 and 100%, respectively. The in vivo study in male Sprague Dawley rats, however, indicated only a slightly higher plasma concentration of antide, but not statistically significant ($p > 0.05$) using chitosan-TGA-MNA compared to chitosan-TGA. The authors claimed that this compromise in the oral bioavailability of antide could be due to the enhanced cohesiveness and controlled release of chitosan-TGA-MNA tablets. These two properties are essentially important in the design of mucoadhesive formulations as if the polymer is not cohesive enough it might collapse and therefore the peptide might not be protected and rapidly released into the lumen of the gastrointestinal tract and degraded and no longer contributes to the concentration gradient [112].

4.3.9. Other Thiolated Chitosans

Thiolated methylated dimethylaminobenzyl chitosan has been synthesized by Hakimi et al. [113]. Although the authors claimed that the modified chitosan had better water-solubility profile and potential for drug delivery, in their work, apart from cytotoxicity, they did not perform any studies related to the application of this type of thiolated chitosan as a mucoadhesive polymer. Clearly, this chitosan derivative will be of interest for evaluation of its mucoadhesive properties.

4.4. Acrylated Chitosan

The use of acrylate groups in the development of mucoadhesive materials was pioneered by Davidovich-Pinhas and Bianco-Peled [114]. The mechanism of mucoadhesion is believed to be due to Michael-type addition reaction between the acrylate vinyl groups of the polymers and the sulfhydryl groups of mucus glycoproteins. The nature of this interaction was proved by ^{1}H-NMR study, where the intensity of the peaks related to the vinyl groups of polyethylene glycol diacrylate hydrogels was decreased after their reactions with mucin dispersion [114]. Thus, the presence of covalent interactions with mucus is a common feature of acrylated and thiolated mucoadhesive materials [25,36,37,86,114–117]. The idea of acrylated chitosan synthesis was developed by Ma et al. [118]. However, they did not demonstrate any application in the mucosal drug delivery. This chitosan derivative is water-soluble, can be cross-linked under ultraviolet light using photoinitiator 2959 and has less antimicrobial activity compared to parent chitosan [118].

Shitrit and Bianco-Peled [119] synthesized acrylated chitosan by reacting chitosan solution (1% w/v in 2% v/v acetic acid, molecular weight 207 kDa, degree of deacetylation 77.6%) with poly(ethylene glycol) diacrylate (PEGDA) via Michael-type reaction (Figure 11). Two different molecular weight PEGDA (0.7 and 10 kDa) were used. The acrylated chitosan was characterized using ^{1}H-NMR spectroscopy and ninhydrin test. It was found that using smaller molecular weight (0.7 kDa PEGDA) at chitosan/PEGDA ratio of 1:4 resulted in more acrylation (98%) than using higher molecular weight PEGDA (10 kDa, 30%). The authors believed that this could be due the presence of greater molar amount of acrylate groups leading to a more efficient reaction. However, using chitosan/PEGDA 1:2 molar ratio led to the formation of a product with a lower degree of acrylation (45%).

The mucoadhesion was evaluated using tensile strength and rotating cylinder method using tablets of chitosan, thiolated and acrylated chitosan on porcine intestinal mucosa. The order of detachment force was the following: chitosan-PEGAc (10 kDa) > thiolated chitosan > chitosan = chitosan-PEGAc (0.7 kDa). Unexpectedly, the maximum detachment force of chitosan-PEGAc (0.7 kDa) was not significantly different from chitosan tablets. Both chitosan-PEGAc (10 kDa) and thiolated chitosan remained attached to the intestinal mucosa for more than 6 h, whereas chitosan-PEGAc (0.7 kDa) detached after 1 min. Chitosan tablets detached after 1.1 ± 0.2 h. The authors claimed that chitosan-PEGAc (0.7 kDa) has greater degree of acrylation than chitosan-PEGAc (10 kDa) and this means higher grafting density of PEG, which could result in the steric hindrance and preventing the covalent bonding with the cysteine-rich domain of mucus [119]. Similar trend with polyacrylic acid was observed; 450 kDa showed a stronger interaction with porcine gastric mucin whereas 2 kDa did not exert any effect [120]. Additionally, shorter PEG (smaller molecular weight) cannot deeply penetrate the mucosal tissues and results in a lower mucoadhesive strength, since mucoadhesive properties of polymers are proportional to the molecular weight [119]. Other studies reported that an optimum molecular weight of polymers is required to achieve maximal mucoadhesion. Small molecular weight polymers form weak gels and easily dissolve whereas high molecular weight polymers do not readily hydrate, thus the free binding groups are not available to interact with the mucus components. Therefore, in both cases, weak mucoadhesion can be observed [121].

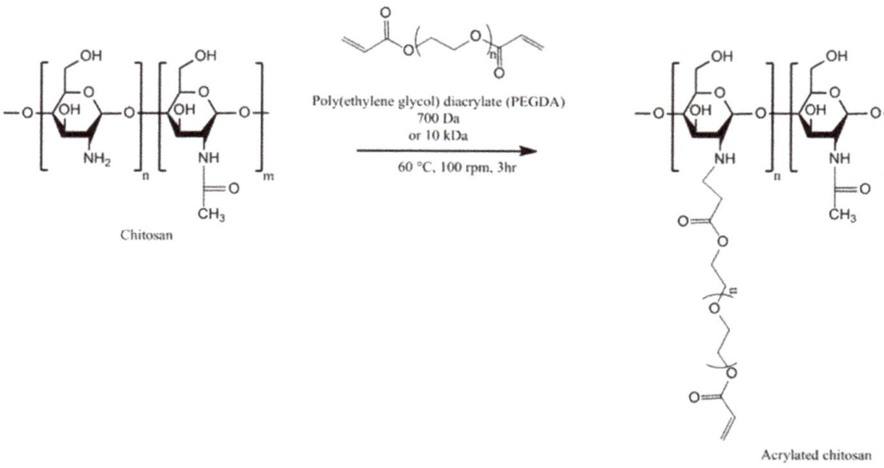

Figure 11. Synthetic pathway to acrylated chitosan [119].

4.5. Half-Acetylated Chitosan

Half-acetylated chitosan is another type of chitosan derivatives, which can be prepared by reacting chitosan with acetic anhydride. Several studies explored the solubility of half-acetylated chitosan and its subsequent effect on the antimicrobial and mucoadhesive properties of chitosan [15,17,35,122]. Qin et al. [122] found that half-acetylated chitosan had no antimicrobial activity against Staphylococcus aureus, Escherichia coli and Candida albicans. However, unmodified chitosan had antimicrobial effects against these microorganisms. They claimed that chitosan can interact with the components of the microorganism surfaces and thus be absorbed on their surfaces. Since the pH of bacterial and fungal cells is around 7, unmodified chitosan precipitates and forms an impermeable layer around the cells. This layer blocks the channels, which are essential for the cells survival. However, half-acetylated chitosan fully dissolved at neutral pH, thus did not form an impermeable layer, and led to a better survival of cells compared to unmodified chitosan.

Sogias et al. [17] demonstrated that half-acetylated chitosan (the degree of acetylation = 52 ± 4 mol %) was soluble over a broad pH range and did not precipitate below pH 7.4. This improved solubility profile of half-acetylated chitosan over unmodified chitosan was related to the reduced crystallinity (caused by disruption of inter- and intra-molecular hydrogen bonds) upon N-acetylation [15,17]. In another study, Sogias et al. [15] found that, at pH 2, half-acetylated chitosan interacted with porcine gastric mucin particles at a higher polymer/mucin ratio than unmodified chitosan, which was due to the decrease in the number of free amino groups in half-acetylated chitosan. At this pH, the amino groups undergone protonation and were responsible for the electrostatic interaction between chitosan macromolecules and mucin. They also revealed that at pH 7, where unmodified chitosan precipitates, half-acetylated chitosan was still able to interact with mucin particles. To explore the mechanisms of mucoadhesion, the polymer-mucin interaction was studied in the presence of sodium chloride (0.2 M), urea (8 M) and ethanol (10% v/v). These agents are known to disrupt the electrostatic interaction, hydrogen bonding and hydrophobic effects, respectively. The results indicated that all these forces were involved in the mucoadhesion of chitosan and half-acetylated chitosan. In case of half-acetylated chitosan, at pH 7, the electrostatic interaction was the major contributing force in the mucoadhesive interactions. This may be due to the higher negative charge density of mucin particles at pH 7 compared to pH 2 [15]. However, the mucoadhesive properties of unmodified chitosan at pH 7 were not evaluated, which could be due to its insolubility at this pH.

Sogias et al. [35] prepared microparticles containing ibuprofen and either chitosan or half-acetylated chitosan by two different techniques; spray-drying and co-grinding. 65 mg tablets were prepared from spray-dried chitosan and half-acetylated chitosan, spray-dried mixtures of chitosan or half-acetylated chitosan with ibuprofen and co-ground mixtures of the polymers and the drug. It was found that tablets of half-acetylated chitosan significantly enhanced ibuprofen release at pH 7. The force of detachment between unmodified chitosan tablets and porcine gastric mucosa was decreased when measured at very acidic (pH 1) and neutral (pH 7) media (Figure 12). However, the mucoadhesion of half-acetylated chitosan tablets was only decreased at low pH and increased linearly up to pH 7. Half-acetylated chitosan tablets were generally less mucoadhesive than chitosan tablets. This could be due to the reduction of cationic charge density upon acetylation, which diminished the electrostatic interaction with mucin [35]. Incorporation of ibuprofen in chitosans tablets resulted in a significant drop of mucoadhesion (Figure 12).

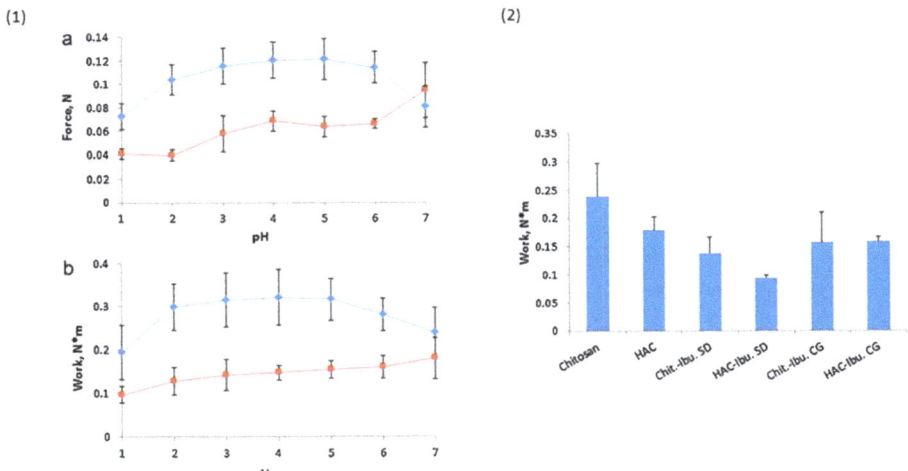

Figure 12. (**1**) Detachment force (**a**) and work of adhesion (**b**) for chitosan (♦) and half-acetylated chitosan (HACHI) (■) tablets as a function of pH on porcine gastric mucosal tissues at 37 ± 0.1 °C. Mean ± SD, n = 3. (**2**) Work of adhesion of tablets on porcine gastric mucosa at pH 7.0 and 37 ± 0.1 °C. Chit.: chitosan, Ibu.: ibuprofen, SD: spray-dried, CG: co-ground. Mean ± SD, n = 3. Reprinted from [35] with permission of Elsevier.

4.6. Glycol Chitosan

Glycol chitosan is a hydrophilic chitosan derivative, which can be prepared by adding ethylene glycol groups to chitosan backbone. It is soluble in water at any pHs [123,124]. It is commercially available from Sigma-Aldrich.

Glycol chitosan has been used in the design of nanoparticles for the delivery of poorly water-soluble drugs. Trapani et al. [124] prepared 6-coumarin-loaded glycol chitosan-TPP nanoparticles using ionic gelation method. Different cyclodextrins were used to form an inclusion complex with this dye. It was found that nanoparticles containing (2,6-di-O-methyl)-β-cyclodextrin could be internalized by Caco2 cells, which could be due to the mucoadhesive nature of chitosan.

Glycol chitosan has been modified to prepare amphiphilic chitosan derivatives. Below, we will discuss two examples of these amphiphilic glycol chitosan derivatives.

4.6.1. Palmitoyl Glycol Chitosan

Palmitoyl glycol chitosan is a hydrophobically-modified glycol chitosan. Its use in drug delivery started since the 1990s. The presence of both of hydrophilic and hydrophobic groups imparts it an amphiphilic character [125,126]. It has ability to self-assemble into vesicles suitable for delivery of water-soluble drugs such as bleomycin [126]. Its quaternized form (quaternary ammonium palmitoyl glycol chitosan) can self-assemble into micelles with a high drug loading capacity. It also facilitated transport of hydrophobic drugs including griseofulvin and propofol and hydrophilic drugs (but to a lower degree) including ranitidine through biological barriers such as intestinal and blood brain barriers, respectively, led to enhanced bioavailability [127,128]. It is conceivable that, the hydrophilic groups (–OH and –NH$_2$) of glycol chitosan located in the external shell of the micelles and the hydrophobic groups in the cores. Thus, the mucoadhesive property of glycol chitosan should be well maintained upon self-assembly as these groups are mainly responsible for the mucoadhesive nature of chitosan and its derivatives [15,129].

The hydrophobicity is one of the important factors affecting the mucoadhesive character of materials. Martin et al. [130] investigated this by synthesizing palmitoyl glycol chitosan with various degrees of palmitoylation (a hydrophobic group). First, glycol chitosan was dissolved in water before sodium bicarbonate and absolute ethanol were added. To this, ethanolic solution of palmitoyl-N-hydroxysuccinimide was added and then the mixture was stirred for 72 h in the dark (Figure 13). This was followed by dialysis and recovery of the product. The physically crosslinked gels were prepared by freeze drying the products and evaluated for their bioadhesive strength by measuring the force necessary to detach the gels from porcine buccal mucosa. It was found that by increasing the hydrophobicity (represented by the degree of palmitoylation), the hydration and erosion of the gels decreased. On the other hand, bioadhesion could be enhanced by increasing the hydrophobicity. Although no comparison with chitosan has been shown, palmitoyl glycol chitosans were found to be less bioadhesive than hydroxypropylmethyl cellulose/carbopol control. The most hydrophobic palmitoyl glycol chitosan gel (20.31 ± 2.22 mol % palmitoylation) resulted in the slowest controlled release of the model hydrophilic drug (FITC-dextran).

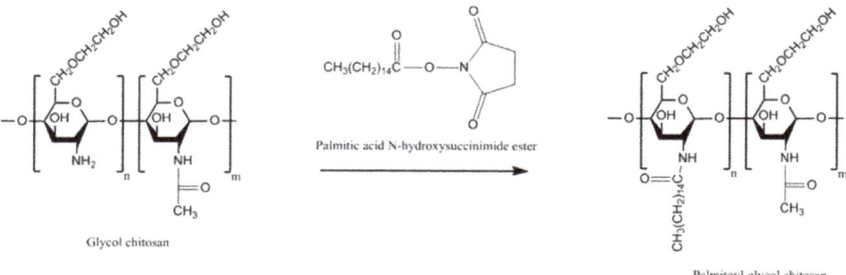

Figure 13. Synthetic pathway to palmitoyl glycol chitosan [130].

Siew et al. [127] developed nanoparticles based on quaternary ammonium palmitoyl glycol chitosan, which enhanced the oral absorption of both hydrophilic (ranitidine) and lipophilic drugs (griseofulvin and cyclosporine A). The bioavailability enhancement was believed to be due to a combination of increased drug dissolution rate (as a result of a great surface area of drug-loaded nanoparticles) and the mucoadhesive nature of chitosan, which increased the intestinal residence time of the nanoparticles, bringing them in close contact with the absorptive epithelial cells and thereby reducing the absorption barrier of the mucosal membrane [127]. This is because the established adhesion of the nanoparticles to the mucus layer provides some degree of penetration into the mucosal membranes [2].

4.6.2. Hexanoyl Glycol Chitosan

Cho et al. [131] synthesized hexanoyl glycol chitosan by *N*-acylation of glycol chitosan (Figure 14). To do that, glycol chitosan was dissolved in water and then diluted with methanol. Then, various amounts of hexanoic anhydride were added and the reaction mixture was continuously stirred for 24 h. The hexanoyl-glycol chitosan was precipitated by acetone and the product was recovered by lyophilization after been dialyzed against water.

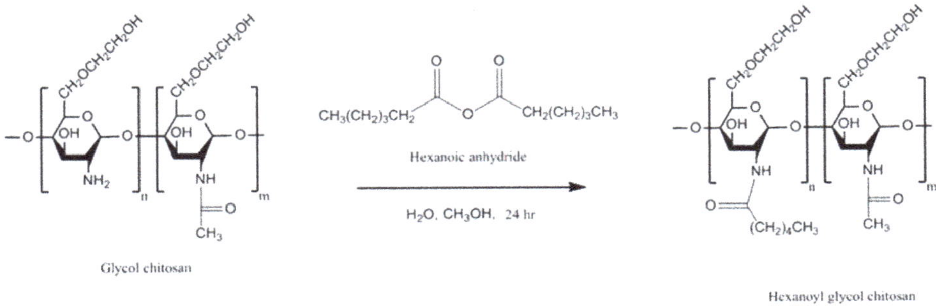

Figure 14. Synthetic pathway to hexanoyl glycol chitosan [131].

Interestingly, hexanoyl glycol chitosan with 39.5 ± 0.4% degree of hexanoylation had a thermosensitive gelling property as it underwent gelation at 37 °C. The in vitro release study showed no significant difference between brimonidine-loaded hexanoyl glycol chitosan-based formulation and the marketed eye drops (Alphagan P). However, the in vivo pre-ocular (inferior fornix of the eyes) retention study in rabbits revealed that hexanoyl glycol chitosan enhanced the retention of rhodamine in the pre-ocular tissues (Figure 15). The fluorescence signal from rhodamine was still strong after 60 min post administration, and became weak after 90 min. On the other hand, weak fluorescence signal was observed after only 10 min (and become weaker after 60 min) when both PBS (negative control) and unmodified glycol chitosan were used indicating their poor retention in pre-ocular tissues (Figure 15). Additionally, the intra-ocular pressure was significantly dropped and the therapeutic action was prolonged compared to unmodified glycol chitosan as well as conventional eye drops [131].

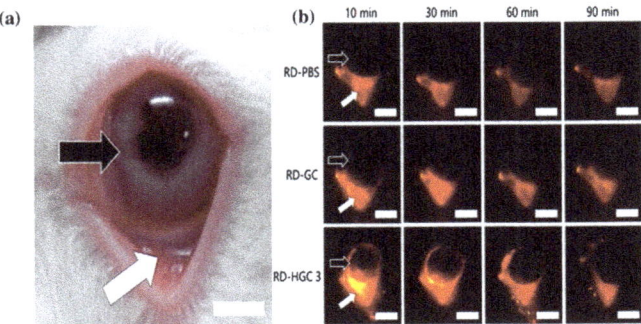

Figure 15. Photograph of rabbit eyes showing the eyeball and the inferior fornix (**a**). The fluorescence images of rabbit eyes at different time intervals after ocular administration of rhodamine-loaded PBS (RD-PBS), glycol chitosan (RD-GC) and hexanoyl glycol chitosan with 39.5 ± 0.4% degree of hexanoylation (RD-HGC 3). The eyeball and the inferior fornix (into which the formulations were administered) were shown by the black and white arrows, respectively (**b**). Scale bars = 5 mm. Reprinted from [131] with permission of Elsevier.

Subsequently, Cho et al. [132] have further modified hexanoyl glycol chitosan by reacting it with glycidyl methacrylate (Figure 16) to form methacrylated hexanoyl glycol chitosan, which demonstrated a thermo-reversible sol–gel transition behavior in aqueous solutions. Moreover, the thermally-induced hydrogels could be chemically crosslinked by photo-crosslinking under UV-radiation. Although no studies, to our knowledge, reported the mucoadhesive potential of methacrylated hexanoyl glycol chitosan, the presence of a methacrylated part within this polymer can potentially lead to a strong interaction with the mucin because of the covalent bonding between methacrylate part of methacrylated hexanoyl glycol chitosan and the thiol groups of the mucin components.

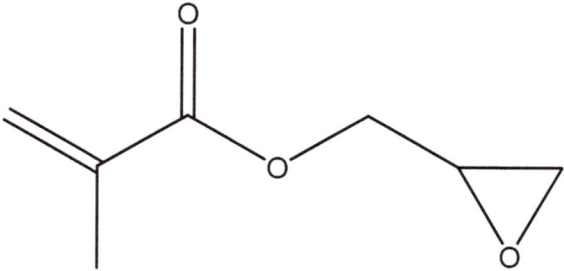

Figure 16. Chemical structure of glycidyl methacrylate.

4.7. Chitosan Conjugates

4.7.1. Chitosan-Enzyme Inhibitors

These systems have been developed to protect orally administered peptide-based drugs from enzymatic degradation in the gastrointestinal lumen. Some mucoadhesive polymers including carbomer could also act as weak enzyme inhibitors [133], however, chitosan lacks this property. Examples of enzyme inhibitors include antipain, chymostatin, elastatinal and Bowman-Birk inhibitor [134]. It has been shown that enzyme inhibitors are toxic to certain types of cells. They also could induce pancreatic secretion of secretin and cholecystokinin in rats [135]. These characters could limit the application of free enzyme inhibitors in the formulation of peptide-based drugs. However, covalent attachment of enzyme inhibitors to mucoadhesive polymers such as chitosan could reduce the unwanted effects as their absorption can be reduced. Bernkop-Schnürch et al. [13] synthesized chitosan-antipain conjugate. The synthetic approach based on the formation of amide bond between carboxylic acid groups of enzyme inhibitors and the primary amino groups of chitosan which was mediated with EDAC and sulfo-N-hydroxysuccinimide. Chitosan-antipain conjugate not only showed mucoadhesive properties similar to unmodified chitosan, it also inhibited the action of trypsin. Tablets containing 5% chitosan conjugate protected insulin from trypsin inactivating effect. A sustained insulin release for 6 h was also achieved.

4.7.2. Chitosan-Complexing Agent

Ethylenediaminetetraacetic acid (EDTA) is a potent chelating agent and has US FDA approval for the treatment of heavy metal poisoning since 1950s [136]. Removal of ions has been shown to enhance the permeation of antiviral drugs such as dolutegravir across Caco2 cells monolayer and rat intestinal mucosa ex vivo [137]. EDTA is also able to decrease pre-systemic metabolism of peptide-based drugs by inhibiting brush border membrane bound enzymes by their deprivation of ions such as Zn^{2+} in the mucous membrane [134,138]. However, the rapid biodistribution of EDTA limits this application. Thus, chitosan-based EDTA system has been developed which has mucoadhesive properties on one side and metal chelating ability on the other side [138,139].

Compared to unmodified chitosan, chitosan-EDTA tablets showed better retention on porcine intestinal mucosa. The mucoadhesive strength decreased with the reduction of the % of EDTA attached to chitosan. It also inhibited Zn- and Co-dependent proteases including carboxypeptidase A and aminopeptidase N. This is because chitosan-EDTA conjugate strongly bound to Zn and Co. [140].

S-protected thiolated chitosan-EDTA has also been synthesized to combine the advantages of EDTA, thiolation and pre-activation or protection of thiol groups. The synthetic pathway is shown in Figure 17 [138]. The multifunctional thiolated chitosan exhibited 5.6- and 3.6-fold longer residence time on porcine intestinal mucosa compared to chitosan-EDTA and chitosan-EDTA-cysteine, respectively (Figure 18).

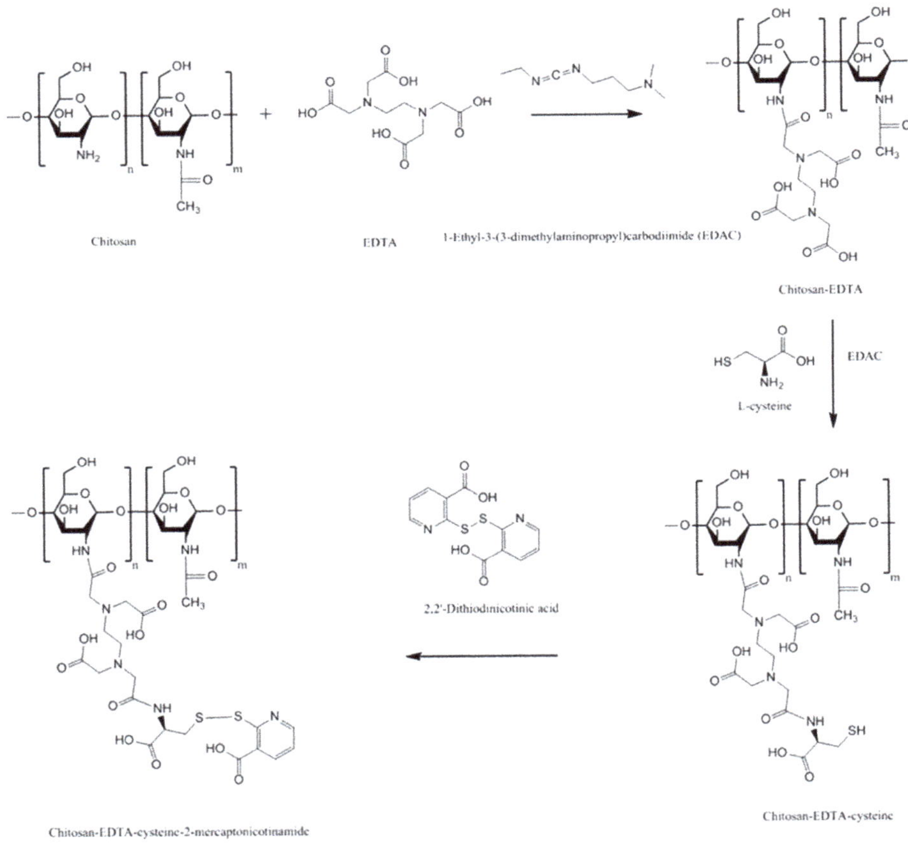

Figure 17. Synthetic pathway to chitosan-EDTA-cysteine-2-mercaptonicotinamide [138].

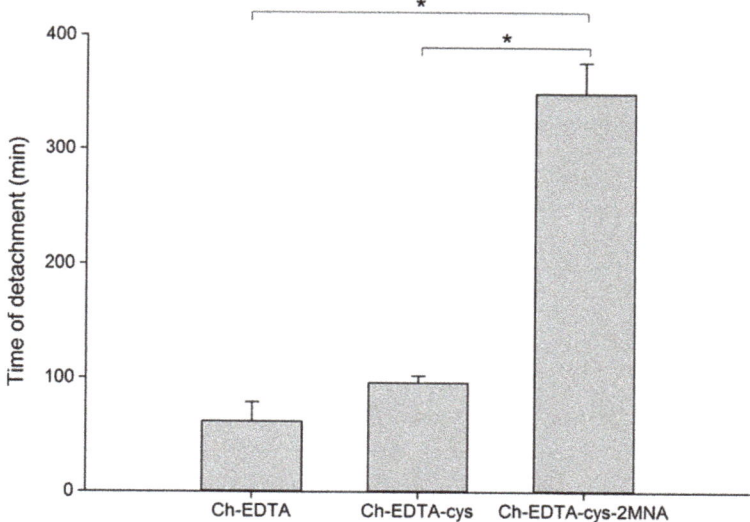

Figure 18. Mucoadhesion time of mini-tablets containing 30 mg of Ch-EDTA, Ch-EDTA-cys or Ch-EDTA-cys-2MNA studied by rotating cylinder method using porcine intestinal mucosa. Ch: chitosan, cys: cysteine, 2MNA: 2-mercaptonicotinamide. (Mean ± SD, $n = 5$, * denotes statistical significant difference at $p < 0.05$). Reprinted from [138] with permission of Elsevier.

4.7.3. Chitosan-EDTA-Enzyme Inhibitors

By combining enzyme inhibitors and complexing agents coupled with chitosan, the degradation of peptide-based drugs by the gut luminal enzymes could be significantly minimized [139]. Additionally, as EDTA could bind to ions such as Zn^{2+} and Ca^{2+}, the concentration of free forms of these ions can be reduced. This decreases the formation of non-absorbable complexes between some drugs and these ions leading to enhanced drug permeation [136,137]. Thus, chitosan-EDTA-serine protease inhibitors were synthesized using a two-step approach. First, to form chitosan-serine protease inhibitors, covalent attachment of antipain, chymostatin and elastatinal to chitosan was performed. Second, chitosan-enzyme inhibitors were bound to EDTA. Tensile study using porcine intestinal mucosa demonstrated that the mucoadhesive strength of the chitosan-EDTA-serine inhibitor was lower than both chitosan-EDTA and chitosan. The reduction of the mucoadhesion of chitosan-EDTA-serine protease inhibitors could be due to the substitution of the free amino groups of chitosan or chitosan-EDTA upon covalent attachment to the enzyme inhibitors [139].

4.8. Chitosan-Catechol (Chi-C)

Catechol is a naturally occurring compound. It is an essential component of L-3,4-dihydroxyphenylalanine (L-DOPA), which is an amino acid secreted by certain marine mussels (e.g., Mytilus edulis), which have ability to adhere to various substrates under wet conditions [141]. This adhesive property is mainly linked to the ability of catechol to form covalent and non-covalent bonds to different organic, inorganic, and metallic surfaces [142,143]. Generally, chitosan-catechol can be synthesized by chemical, electrochemical and enzymatic methods. The chemical method includes three main approaches: amide bond formation using carbodiimide chemistry (Figure 19), reductive amination using aldehyde-terminated catechol and reducing agents such as $NaCNBH_3$ or $NaBH_4$, and formation of catechol-amine adducts using oxidizing agents such as $NaIO_4$ [141,144].

Inspired by mussel adhesion to surfaces, Kim et al. [141] synthesized chitosan-catechol conjugate by reacting chitosan with 3,4-dihydroxy hydrocinnamic acid mediated with EDAC (Figure 19).

Mucoadhesion was evaluated in vitro using mucin-particle interaction, turbidimetry, surface plasmon resonance (SPR) spectroscopy and rheological characterization as well as in vivo fluorescence imaging technique and fluorescence measurement in various organs of mice. Chitosan-catechol conjugate showed superior mucoadhesion than both unmodified chitosan and polyacrylic acid. The in vivo study explored the difference in the retention of different polymers in different body sites. No fluorescence was detected in organs lacking mucosal tissues including liver, spleen, and kidney (Figure 20). However, at 3 h post-oral administration, strong fluorescence signal from chitosan-catechol conjugate in intestinal tissues was observed (Figure 20). This could be due to the formation of strong covalent bonds via Michael-type addition reaction upon the reaction of oxidized form of catechol (quinone) and amine or thiol functionalities of mucins or Schiff base formation reaction [141]. The electrostatic attractive interaction between the positively charged groups of chitosan and negatively charged carboxyl and sulfate groups of mucin could lead to an initial contact stage and the adsorption of chitosan-catechol macromolecules on the mucosal surfaces. This was then followed by an established consolidation stage via the covalent interaction [121,141]. Unmodified chitosan and polyacrylic acid showed poor fluorescence signal. The retention of chitosan-catechol conjugate decreased significantly in both stomach and esophagus. The authors claimed that chitosan-catechol conjugate-mucin interaction was stronger when the pH of mucin solution was 7 compared to pH 2 [141]. This might explain better retention in small intestine, where pH is near neutral compared to poor retention in stomach (highly acidic) and esophagus (slightly acidic, pH 4–6) [141]. The oxidation of catechol to quinone in alkaline environment is more likely than in acidic environment, which could provide additional adhesive interactions [141,142,145]. On the other hand, polyacrylic acid showed slightly greater mucoadhesion to esophagus than stomach and intestine (Figure 20C). The difference in the pH of these organs might explain this observation as it may affect the structures of both polyacrylic acid and the mucus layer resulting in a different nature and extent of mucoadhesive interactions at different pHs [146]. Some studies reported that the mucoadhesive nature of polyacrylic acid may be due to its ability to form hydrogen bonds with the mucus components [120,141,146,147], which is strongest at slightly acidic pHs, depending on the type of the polymer [147,148]. However, Kim et al. [141] suggested further studies to investigate the organ-specific mucoadhesive properties of chitosan, chitosan-catechol and polyacrylic acid. Chitosan-catechol conjugate also enhanced the oral bioavailability of insulin and C_{max} reached after 2 h compared to unmodified chitosan which was 30 min (Figure 20D).

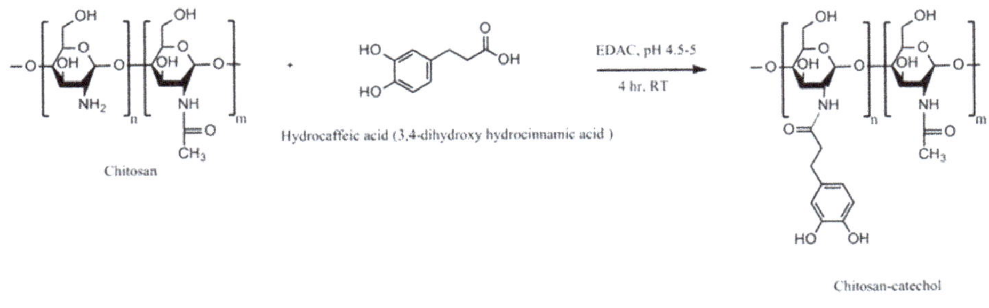

Figure 19. Synthetic pathway to chitosan-catechol using carbodiimide chemistry [141].

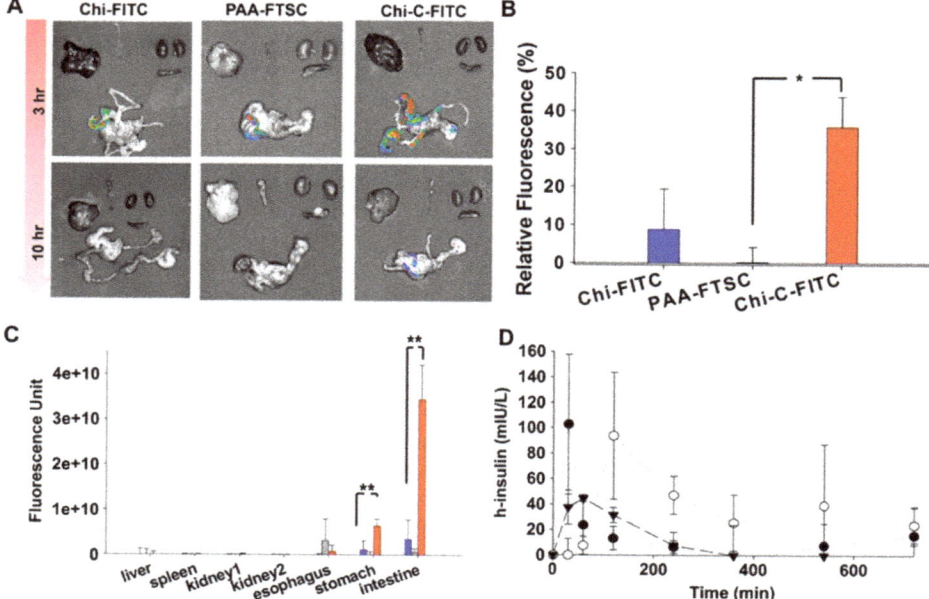

Figure 20. Chitosan-fluorescein isothiocyanate (Chi-FITC), polyacrylic acid-fluorescein-5-thiosemicarbazide (PAA-FTSC) and chitosan-catechol-fluorescein isothiocyanate (Chi-C-FITC) were orally administered to BALB/c mice and the animals were euthanized after 3 or 10 h. (**A**) The extracted organs were imaged using in vivo imaging system. (**B**) The relative fluorescence intensity of Chi-FITC, PAA-FTSC and Chi-C-FITC in the gastrointestinal tract (esophagus, stomach and intestine) at 10 h after administration. (**C**) The fluorescence in the liver, spleen, kidneys, esophagus, stomach, and small/large intestine at 10 h after administration are shown (mean $\pm$ SD, n = 3 mice/time point). (* denotes statistical significant difference at $p < 0.05$, ** indicates $p < 0.005$). (**D**) The human (h)-insulin (closed triangle), h-insulin/chitosan (closed circle) and h-insulin/chitosan-catechol (open circle) were orally administered to Wistar rats and blood insulin concentration was measured using enzyme-linked immunosorbent assay (ELISA) (n = 4 rats/time point). Reprinted from [141] with permission of Elsevier.

4.9. Methyl Pyrrolidinone Chitosan

Methyl pyrrolidinone chitosan can be synthesized by reacting chitosan with levulinic acid (Figure 21) [149,150]. Specific experimental conditions including pH of the reaction mixture, type and the rate of addition of reducing agents (NaCNBH$_3$ or NaBH$_4$), molar ratio of levulinic acid/chitosan/reducing agents are required to obtain methyl pyrrolidinone chitosan and not N-carboxybutylchitosan derivatives [151,152]. Sandri et al. [153] studied the mucoadhesive and penetration enhancing properties of various chitosans including 5-methyl pyrrolidinone chitosan, low molecular weight chitosan, a partially re-acetylated chitosan and chitosan HCl using buccal or submaxillary bovine mucin dispersion, vaginal mucosa or porcine gastric mucin dispersion. It was found that different chitosans behaved differently in different substrates. In submaxillary mucin dispersion, chitosan·HCl was the most mucoadhesive. However, 5-methyl pyrrolidinone chitosan showed the greatest mucoadhesion among other polymers in all other studied substrates and provided the greatest permeation of acyclovir through porcine cheek mucosa and deepest penetration into the vaginal mucosa. This could be due to the penetration enhancing effect of 5-methyl pyrrolidinone, which has been demonstrated in other studies [154,155].

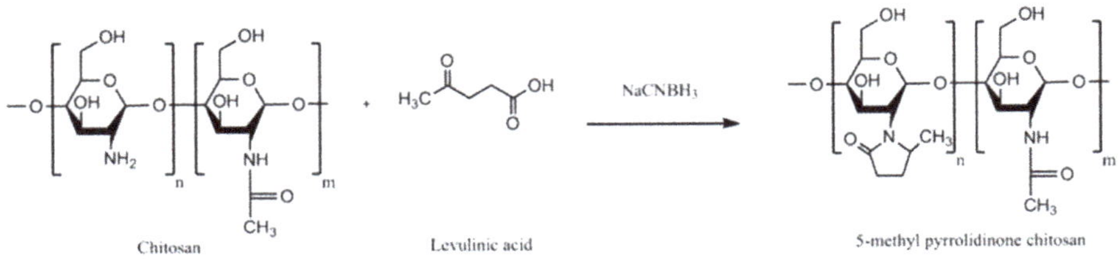

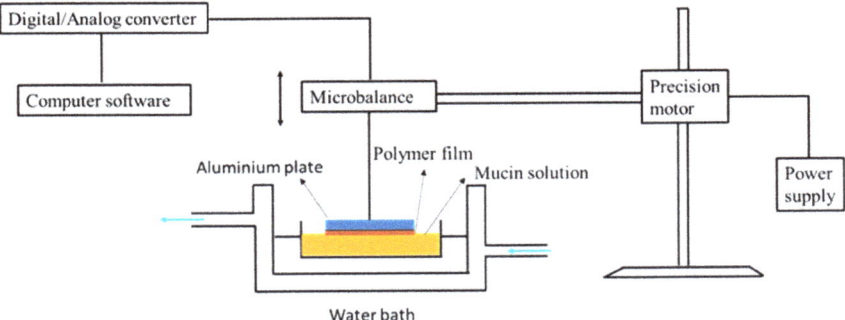

Figure 21. Synthetic pathway to 5-methyl pyrrolidinone chitosan.

4.10. Cyclodextrin-Chitosan

Cyclodextrins can enhance solubility and dissolution of poorly water-soluble drugs by forming inclusion complexes. In 2001, the idea of grafting cyclodextrin to chitosan was adopted by Auzély-Velty and Rinaudo [156], who used a reductive amination approach, where a solution of chitosan in acetic acid/methanol was reacted with aldehyde-containing cyclodextrin derivative in the presence of sodium cyanoborohydride (NaCNBH$_3$). The reaction was mediated with EDAC. The inclusion ability of the grafted-cyclodextrin was studied using NMR spectroscopy and found that it could form inclusion complexes with two model compounds tert-butylbenzoic acid and (+)-catechin.

In 2006, Venter et al. [157] studied the mucoadhesion of this cyclodextrin-chitosan derivative by tensile separation test (microbalance method) using partially purified porcine gastric mucin type III (Sigma, UK) as a substrate. Figure 22 shows the experimental set-up for the mucoadhesion study. Briefly, the aluminum plates of the apparatus were coated with the polymer solution (1% w/v) and left to dry until polymeric films formed. Mucin solution (30% w/v) was prepared and placed in a water bath (25 °C). The polymer-coated plate was lowered to contact with the mucin solution for 2 min. Then, the maximum detachment force to separate the polymeric films from the mucin solution was measured using a computerized system. It was found that upon derivatization, chitosan lost its mucoadhesive properties by 13.5%, but, it was 12% stronger than pectin.

In another study, Chaleawlert-umpon et al. [158] synthesized citrated cyclodextrin-g-chitosan. In this study, citric acid was used to facilitate cyclodextrin mobility. Glycidyl trimethylammonium chloride was also used to quaternize chitosan. The mucoadhesion study using mucin-particle interaction method and SPR revealed that combination of quaternization and citrate modification led to a significant enhancement in the mucoadhesive interactions. This could be due to an increase in the cationic charge of chitosan as well as hydrogen bonding between carboxyl and hydroxyl groups of the spacer and the mucus components.

Figure 22. Experimental set-up for evaluation of mucoadhesion using microbalance method according to Venter et al. [157] with some modifications.

4.11. Oleoyl-Quaternised Chitosan

Yostawonkul et al. [159] developed a nanostructure lipid carrier for the delivery of lipophilic drug molecules using high-pressure homogenization technique. They found coating of these carriers with oleoyl-quaternised chitosan enhanced carcinoma Caco-2 cellular uptake of the model drug (alpha-mangostin). This enhancement could be due to the mucoadhesive properties of oleoyl-quaternised chitosan, which was evaluated by mucin-particle interaction method. However, cytotoxicity of the carriers was also increased and thus the authors suggested careful optimization of the drug loading to target cancer cells for chemotherapy.

5. Comparison of Different Chitosan Derivatives

Table 1 illustrates the advantages and disadvantages of different chitosan-based systems reported in the literature together with the drug model, administration routes and mucus substrates types that were used to evaluate them.

Table 1. A summary of chitosan derivatives properties with examples of drug candidates used in the mucoadhesive drug delivery evaluation.

Chitosan Derivatives	Advantages	Disadvantages	Drug	Route of Administration/ Substrate	References
Trimethyl chitosan	Soluble at broad range of pHs (2–12), strong mucoadhesion; decreased TEER; increased paracellular permeability of basic or neutral macromolecules	Strong aggregation with anionic macromolecules such as heparin	Buserelin, ropinirole·HCl	Oral, small intestine, cattle nasal mucosa	[52,160,161]
N-carboxymethyl chitosan	Decreased TEER; increased paracellular permeability of anionic macromolecules	Insoluble at pH 3–7 (depending on the degree of substitution) due to its polyampholytic character	Low molecular weight heparin; Ofloxacin	Oral, rat small intestine; Ocular, rabbit eyes, in vivo	[73,76,82]
Chitosan-cysteine	Same mucoadhesion as unmodified chitosan, improved cohesion compared to unmodified chitosan, permeation enhancing effect	Susceptible to premature oxidation, undesirable side reactions led to the formation of (chitosan-cysteine-cysteine)$_n$ side chains	-	Oral, porcine intestinal mucosa	[25,84]
Chitosan-N-acetylcysteine	50-fold longer retention time than unmodified chitosan, biodegradability as indicated by the reduction of its solution viscosity after addition of hen white egg	Susceptible to premature oxidation	-	Oral, flat faced-discs, porcine intestinal mucosa	[87]
Chitosan-TGA	Controlled drug release, longer disintegration time (up to 100-fold) and 26-fold longer mucoadhesion time against unmodified chitosan	Need of mediator such as EDAC	Clotrimazole	Vaginal, tablets, bovine vaginal mucosa	[162]
Chitosan-TBA	Strong mucoadhesion, permeation enhancing effect, controlled release, no need for mediator	Prone to oxidation. In addition, unintended cyclisation side reactions	Insulin, cefadroxil	Oral, tablets, porcine and rat intestinal mucosa	[108,163]
Chitosan-thioethylamidine	Much quicker synthetic reaction rate than chitosan-TBA (1.5 h vs. 24 h), 8.9-fold longer mucosal detachment time than unmodified chitosan, controlled release, no cyclisation side reactions as in chitosan-TBA	Stability issues	FITC-dextran	Oral, tablets, porcine intestinal mucosa	[88]

Table 1. Cont.

Chitosan Derivatives	Advantages	Disadvantages	Drug	Route of Administration/ Substrate	References
Chitosan-glutathione	Improved stability compared to unmodified chitosan, enhanced mucoadhesion (9.9-fold increased adhesion force and 55-fold longer adhesion time), 4.9-fold higher permeation-enhancing effect against unmodified chitosan, used as oxidative stress suppressant	Stability issues	Thymopentin	Oral, tablets, in vitro porcine rat intestinal mucosa; Oral nanoparticles, in vivo rats; Injectable hydrogels	[89,91,104]
Pre-activated (S-protected) thiolated chitosan	Improved stability and mucoadhesion compared to unmodified chitosan and unprotected thiolated chitosan	2-fold less swelling than unmodified chitosan	Leuprolide; Antide	Oral, tablets, porcine intestinal mucosa Oral, rat intestinal mucosa	[111,112]
Acrylated chitosan	Strong mucoadhesion, water-soluble	Use of low molecular weight PEGDA results in a weaker mucoadhesion	-	Oral, porcine intestinal mucosa	[119]
Half-acetylated chitosan	Better solubility at higher pHs (up to 7.4) compared to unmodified chitosan, sustained drug release	Less mucoadhesive compared to unmodified chitosan	Ibuprofen	Oral, porcine gastric mucosa	[35]
Palmitoyl glycol chitosan	Amphiphilic property, diminished erosion and slow hydration led to controlled release, control bioadhesive strength by changing the degree of palmitoylation	Potential problems with reproducibility with the degrees of substitution related to insolubility of the final product	FITC-dextran	Buccal/disc shaped gels, porcine buccal mucosa	[130]
Hexanoyl glycol chitosan	In situ gelling property, in vivo ocular retention, longer duration of action	-	Rhodamine, brimonidine	Ocular, rabbit, in vivo ocular tissues	[131]
Chitosan-enzyme inhibitors	Protects drugs from enzymatic degradation. Controlled antipain release over 6 h, mucoadhesive properties preserved	Potential stability issues	Insulin	Oral, flat-faced discs, porcine intestinal mucosa	[13]
Chitosan-EDTA	Better mucoadhesion than unmodified chitosan Inhibits Zn and Co-dependent proteases including carboxypeptidase A and aminopeptidase N	No Ca-dependent serine proteases inhibition	-	Oral, flat-faced discs, porcine intestinal mucosa	[140]
Chitosan-enzyme inhibitors-EDTA	Strong inhibitory action against serine proteases, Zn-dependent exopeptidases including carboxypeptidase A and B, aminopeptidase N	Less mucoadhesive than unmodified chitosan and chitosan-EDTA	-	Oral, flat-faced discs, porcine intestinal mucosa	[139]
Chitosan-catechol conjugate	Strong mucoadhesion, higher solubility at neutral pH, sustained drug release, improved therapeutic effect in vivo compared to unmodified chitosan	Poor mucoadhesion in acidic environment, optimum degree of substitution (7.2%) is required to achieve water-soluble product and formation of large gel-like aggregates has been observed for greater degree of substitution (12.7%)	Lidocaine; Sulfasalazine	Oral, mice gastrointestinal tract, porcine gastric mucin type II; Buccal, hydrogels, porcine and rabbit buccal mucosa; Rectal, hydrogels, mice rectal mucosa in vivo	[141,143, 164,165]
Methyl pyrrolidinone chitosan	Greater mucoadhesion and penetration enhancing effect than unmodified chitosan	-	Acyclovir	Buccal and vaginal, porcine cheek or submaxillary bovine mucin, vaginal mucosa, or porcine gastric mucin	[153]
Chitosan-cyclodextrin	Inclusion ability, sustained release	Weaker mucoadhesion than the parent chitosan	-	Porcine gastric mucin	[156,157]

6. Conclusions

In this review, general methods of synthesis of potential mucoadhesive chitosan derivatives have been highlighted. Some properties of chitosan and chitosan derivatives have been discussed. These include solubility profile, stability, mucoadhesive and permeation enhancing effects. The mucoadhesive properties of the derivatives have been particularly considered. It was shown that the mucoadhesive properties of some derivatives have been significantly increased compared to unmodified chitosan. In the majority of cases, this resulted in an enhancement in the bioavailability and a significant improvement of the therapeutic efficacy of several candidate drugs compared to unmodified chitosan. In some others, the mucoadhesive character either did not change or slightly decreased. This however, was compensated with an improvement of other important chitosan properties including solubility in physiological pH and cohesiveness, which are crucial parameters in mucoadhesion. Therefore, improvement in the properties of chitosan derivatives discussed in this review clearly demonstrate that its chemical modification could potentially lead to further advances in transmucosal drug delivery. However, chemical modification of chitosan has limitations. These include low reproducibility, especially with hydrophobically-modified chitosans, poor solubility of chitosan in organic solvents used for the synthesis and changes with the degree of acetylation during chemical modification.

Acknowledgments: We are thankful to HCED-Iraq for funding this research.

Conflicts of Interest: The authors declare no conflict of interest.

References

1. Lai, S.K.; Wang, Y.Y.; Hanes, J. Mucus-penetrating nanoparticles for drug and gene delivery to mucosal tissues. *Adv. Drug Deliv. Rev.* **2009**, *61*, 158–171. [CrossRef] [PubMed]
2. Khutoryanskiy, V.V. Advances in mucoadhesion and mucoadhesive polymers. *Macromol. Biosci.* **2011**, *11*, 748–764. [CrossRef] [PubMed]
3. Leal, J.; Smyth, H.D.C.; Ghosh, D. Physicochemical properties of mucus and their impact on transmucosal drug delivery. *Int. J. Pharm.* **2017**, *532*, 555–572. [CrossRef] [PubMed]
4. Peppas, N.A.; Huang, Y. Nanoscale technology of mucoadhesive interactions. *Adv. Drug Deliv. Rev.* **2004**, *56*, 1675–1687. [CrossRef] [PubMed]
5. Lai, S.K.; Wang, Y.Y.; Wirtz, D.; Hanes, J. Micro- and macrorheology of mucus. *Adv. Drug Deliv. Rev.* **2009**, *61*, 86–100. [CrossRef] [PubMed]
6. Boegh, M.; Nielsen, H.M. Mucus as a barrier to drug delivery—Understanding and mimicking the barrier properties. *Basic Clin. Pharmacol. Toxicol.* **2015**, *116*, 179–186. [CrossRef] [PubMed]
7. Bansil, R.; Turner, B.S. Mucin structure, aggregation, physiological functions and biomedical applications. *Curr. Opin. Colloid Interface Sci.* **2006**, *11*, 164–170. [CrossRef]
8. Peppas, N.A.; Buri, P.A. Surface, interfacial and molecular aspects of polymer bioadhesion on soft tissues. *J. Control. Release* **1985**, *2*, 257–275. [CrossRef]
9. Serra, L.; Domenech, J.; Peppas, N.A. Engineering design and molecular dynamics of mucoadhesive drug delivery systems as targeting agents. *Eur. J. Pharm. Biopharm.* **2009**, *71*, 519–528. [CrossRef] [PubMed]
10. Date, A.A.; Hanes, J.; Ensign, L.M. Nanoparticles for oral delivery: Design, evaluation and state-of-the-art. *J. Control. Release* **2016**, *240*, 504–526. [CrossRef] [PubMed]
11. Gullberg, E.; Cao, S.; Berg, O.G.; Ilback, C.; Sandegren, L.; Hughes, D.; Andersson, D.I. Selection of resistant bacteria at very low antibiotic concentrations. *PLoS Pathog.* **2011**, *7*, e1002158. [CrossRef] [PubMed]
12. Lee, C.R.; Cho, I.H.; Jeong, B.C.; Lee, S.H. Strategies to minimize antibiotic resistance. *Int. J. Environ. Res. Public Health* **2013**, *10*, 4274–4305. [CrossRef] [PubMed]
13. Bernkop-Schnürch, A.; Bratengeyer, I.; Valenta, C. Development and in vitro evaluation of a drug delivery system protecting from trypsinic degradation. *Int. J. Pharm.* **1997**, *157*, 17–25. [CrossRef]
14. Bernkop-Schnürch, A.; Hornof, M.; Guggi, D. Thiolated chitosans. *Eur. J. Pharm. Biopharm.* **2004**, *57*, 9–17. [CrossRef]
15. Sogias, I.A.; Williams, A.C.; Khutoryanskiy, V.V. Why is chitosan mucoadhesive? *Biomacromolecules* **2008**, *9*, 1837–1842. [CrossRef] [PubMed]

16. Kulkarni, A.D.; Patel, H.M.; Surana, S.J.; Vanjari, Y.H.; Belgamwar, V.S.; Pardeshi, C.V. N,N,N-Trimethyl chitosan: An advanced polymer with myriad of opportunities in nanomedicine. *Carbohydr. Polym.* **2017**, *157*, 875–902. [CrossRef] [PubMed]
17. Sogias, I.A.; Khutoryanskiy, V.V.; Williams, A.C. Exploring the factors affecting the solubility of chitosan in water. *Macromol. Chem. Phys.* **2010**, *211*, 426–433. [CrossRef]
18. Hejazi, R.; Amiji, M. Chitosan-based gastrointestinal delivery systems. *J. Control. Release* **2003**, *89*, 151–165. [CrossRef]
19. Pillai, C.K.S.; Paul, W.; Sharma, C.P. Chitin and chitosan polymers: Chemistry, solubility and fiber formation. *Prog. Polym. Sci.* **2009**, *34*, 641–678. [CrossRef]
20. Robinson, J.R.; Longer, M.A.; Veillard, M. Bioadhesive polymers for controlled drug delivery. *Ann. N. Y. Acad. Sci.* **1987**, *507*, 307–314. [CrossRef] [PubMed]
21. Smart, J.D.; Kellaway, I.W.; Worthington, H.E.C. An in vitro investigation of mucosa-adhesive materials for use in controlled drug delivery. *J. Pharm. Pharmacol.* **1984**, *36*, 295–299. [CrossRef] [PubMed]
22. Robinson, J.R.; Mlynek, G.M. Bioadhesive and phase-change polymers for ocular drug delivery. *Adv. Drug Deliv. Rev.* **1995**, *16*, 45–50. [CrossRef]
23. Casettari, L.; Vllasaliu, D.; Castagnino, E.; Stolnik, S.; Howdle, S.; Illum, L. PEGylated chitosan derivatives: Synthesis, characterisations and pharmaceutical applications. *Prog. Polym. Sci.* **2012**, *37*, 659–685. [CrossRef]
24. Watts, P.; Smith, A.; Hinchcliffe, M. ChiSys® as a chitosan-based delivery platform for nasal vaccination. In *Mucosal Delivery of Biopharmaceuticals: Biology, Challenges and Strategies*; das Neves, J., Sarmento, B., Eds.; Springer: Boston, MA, USA, 2014; pp. 499–516, ISBN 978-1-4614-9524-6.
25. Bonengel, S.; Bernkop-Schnürch, A. Thiomers-from bench to market. *J. Control. Release* **2014**, *195*, 120–129. [CrossRef] [PubMed]
26. Bonferoni, M.C.; Sandri, G.; Rossi, S.; Ferrari, F.; Caramella, C. Chitosan and its salts for mucosal and transmucosal delivery. *Expert Opin. Drug Deliv.* **2009**, *6*, 923–939. [CrossRef] [PubMed]
27. Ganguly, S.; Dash, A.K. A novel in situ gel for sustained drug delivery and targeting. *Int. J. Pharm.* **2004**, *276*, 83–92. [CrossRef] [PubMed]
28. Rabea, E.I.; Badawy, M.E.-T.; Stevens, C.V.; Smagghe, G.; Steurbaut, W. Chitosan as antimicrobial agent: Applications and mode of action. *Biomacromolecules* **2003**, *4*, 1457–1465. [CrossRef] [PubMed]
29. Agnihotri, S.A.; Mallikarjuna, N.N.; Aminabhavi, T.M. Recent advances on chitosan-based micro- and nanoparticles in drug delivery. *J. Control. Release* **2004**, *100*, 5–28. [CrossRef] [PubMed]
30. Illum, L.; Farraj, N.F.; Davis, S.S. Chitosan as a novel nasal delivery system for peptide drugs. *Pharm. Res.* **1994**, *11*, 1186–1189. [CrossRef] [PubMed]
31. Illum, L.; Jabbal-Gill, I.; Hinchcliffe, M.; Fisher, A.N.; Davis, S.S. Chitosan as a novel nasal delivery system for vaccines. *Adv. Drug Deliv. Rev.* **2001**, *51*, 81–96. [CrossRef]
32. Issa, M.M.; Köping-Höggård, M.; Artursson, P. Chitosan and the mucosal delivery of biotechnology drugs. *Drug Discov. Today Technol.* **2005**, *2*, 1–6. [CrossRef] [PubMed]
33. Bernkop-Schnürch, A.; Scholler, S.; Biebel, R.G. Development of controlled drug release systems based on thiolated polymers. *J. Control. Release* **2000**, *66*, 39–48. [CrossRef]
34. Prego, C.; Fabre, M.; Torres, D.; Alonso, M.J. Efficacy and mechanism of action of chitosan nanocapsules for oral peptide delivery. *Pharm. Res.* **2006**, *23*, 549–556. [CrossRef] [PubMed]
35. Sogias, I.A.; Williams, A.C.; Khutoryanskiy, V.V. Chitosan-based mucoadhesive tablets for oral delivery of ibuprofen. *Int. J. Pharm.* **2012**, *436*, 602–610. [CrossRef] [PubMed]
36. Irmukhametova, G.S.; Mun, G.A.; Khutoryanskiy, V.V. Thiolated mucoadhesive and PEGylated nonmucoadhesive organosilica nanoparticles from 3-mercaptopropyltrimethoxysilane. *Langmuir* **2011**, *27*, 9551–9556. [CrossRef] [PubMed]
37. Mun, E.A.; Williams, A.C.; Khutoryanskiy, V.V. Adhesion of thiolated silica nanoparticles to urinary bladder mucosa: Effects of PEGylation, thiol content and particle size. *Int. J. Pharm.* **2016**, *512*, 32–38. [CrossRef] [PubMed]
38. Tonglairoum, P.; Brannigan, R.P.; Opanasopit, P.; Khutoryanskiy, V.V. Maleimide-bearing nanogels as novel mucoadhesive materials for drug delivery. *J. Mater. Chem. B* **2016**, *4*, 6581–6587. [CrossRef]
39. Kaldybekov, D.B.; Tonglairoum, P.; Opanasopit, P.; Khutoryanskiy, V.V. Mucoadhesive maleimide-functionalised liposomes for drug delivery to urinary bladder. *Eur. J. Pharm. Sci.* **2018**, *111*, 83–90. [CrossRef] [PubMed]

40. Behrens, I.; Pena, A.I.; Alonso, M.J.; Kissel, T. Comparative uptake studies of bioadhesive and non-bioadhesive nanoparticles in human intestinal cell lines and rats: The effect of mucus on particle adsorption and transport. *Pharm. Res.* **2002**, *19*, 1185–1193. [CrossRef] [PubMed]
41. Kim, B.-S.; Kim, C.-S.; Lee, K.-M. The intracellular uptake ability of chitosan-coated Poly (D,L-lactide-*co*-glycolide) nanoparticles. *Arch. Pharm. Res.* **2008**, *31*, 1050–1054. [CrossRef] [PubMed]
42. Thongborisute, J.; Takeuchi, H.; Yamamoto, H.; Kawashima, Y. Visualization of the penetrative and mucoadhesive properties of chitosan and chitosan-coated liposomes through the rat intestine. *J. Liposome Res.* **2006**, *16*, 127–141. [CrossRef] [PubMed]
43. Atuma, C.; Strugala, V.; Allen, A.; Holm, L. The adherent gastrointestinal mucus gel layer: Thickness and physical state in vivo. *Am. J. Physiol. Gastrointest. Liver Physiol.* **2001**, *280*, G922–G929. [CrossRef] [PubMed]
44. Varum, F.J.O.; Veiga, F.; Sousa, J.S.; Basit, A.W. An investigation into the role of mucus thickness on mucoadhesion in the gastrointestinal tract of pig. *Eur. J. Pharm. Sci.* **2010**, *40*, 335–341. [CrossRef] [PubMed]
45. Varum, F.J.O.; Veiga, F.; Sousa, J.S.; Basit, A.W. Mucus thickness in the gastrointestinal tract of laboratory animals. *J. Pharm. Pharmacol.* **2012**, *64*, 218–227. [CrossRef] [PubMed]
46. Deacona, M.P.; Davis, S.S.; White, R.J.; Nordman, H.; Carlstedt, I.; Errington, N.; Rowe, A.J.; Harding, S.E. Are chitosan–mucin interactions specific to different regions of the stomach? Velocity ultracentrifugation offers a clue. *Carbohydr. Polym.* **1999**, *38*, 235–238. [CrossRef]
47. Caramella, C.; Ferrari, F.; Bonferoni, M.C.; Rossi, S.; Sandri, G. Chitosan and its derivatives as drug penetration enhancers. *J. Drug Deliv. Sci. Technol.* **2010**, *20*, 5–13. [CrossRef]
48. Jeong, Y.-I.; Kim, D.-G.; Jang, M.-K.; Nah, J.-W. Preparation and spectroscopic characterization of methoxy poly(ethylene glycol)-grafted water-soluble chitosan. *Carbohydr. Res.* **2008**, *343*, 282–289. [CrossRef] [PubMed]
49. Bernkop-Schnürch, A. Chitosan and its derivatives: Potential excipients for peroral peptide delivery systems. *Int. J. Pharm.* **2000**, *194*, 1–13. [CrossRef]
50. Muzzarelli, R.A.A.; Tanfani, F. The *N*-permethylation of chitosan and the preparation of *N*-trimethyl chitosan iodide. *Carbohydr. Polym.* **1985**, *5*, 297–307. [CrossRef]
51. Verheul, R.J.; Amidi, M.; van der Wal, S.; van Riet, E.; Jiskoot, W.; Hennink, W.E. Synthesis, characterization and in vitro biological properties of *O*-methyl free *N,N,N*-trimethylated chitosan. *Biomaterials* **2008**, *29*, 3642–3649. [CrossRef] [PubMed]
52. Sieval, A.B.; Thanou, M.; Kotzé, A.F.; Verhoef, J.C.; Brussee, J.; Junginger, H.E. Preparation and NMR characterization of highly substituted *N*-trimethyl chitosan chloride. *Carbohydr. Polym.* **1998**, *36*, 157–165. [CrossRef]
53. De Britto, D.; Assis, O.B.G. A novel method for obtaining a quaternary salt of chitosan. *Carbohydr. Polym.* **2007**, *69*, 305–310. [CrossRef]
54. Benediktsdóttir, B.E.; Gaware, V.S.; Rúnarsson, Ö.V.; Jónsdóttir, S.; Jensen, K.J.; Másson, M. Synthesis of *N,N,N*-trimethyl chitosan homopolymer and highly substituted *N*-alkyl-*N,N*-dimethyl chitosan derivatives with the aid of di-*tert*-butyldimethylsilyl chitosan. *Carbohydr. Polym.* **2011**, *86*, 1451–1460. [CrossRef]
55. Wu, M.; Long, Z.; Xiao, H.; Dong, C. Recent research progress on preparation and application of *N,N,N*-trimethyl chitosan. *Carbohydr. Res.* **2016**, *434*, 27–32. [CrossRef] [PubMed]
56. Dung, P.L.; Milas, M.; Rinaudo, M.; Desbrières, J. Water soluble derivatives obtained by controlled chemical modifications of chitosan. *Carbohydr. Polym.* **1994**, *24*, 209–214. [CrossRef]
57. Jintapattanakit, A.; Junyaprasert, V.B.; Kissel, T. The role of mucoadhesion of trimethyl chitosan and PEGylated trimethyl chitosan nanocomplexes in insulin uptake. *J. Pharm. Sci.* **2009**, *98*, 4818–4830. [CrossRef] [PubMed]
58. Casettari, L.; Vllasaliu, D.; Mantovani, G.; Howdle, S.M.; Stolnik, S.; Illum, L. Effect of PEGylation on the toxicity and permeability enhancement of chitosan. *Biomacromolecules* **2010**, *11*, 2854–2865. [CrossRef] [PubMed]
59. Hauptstein, S.; Boengel, S.; Griessinger, J.; Bernkop-Schnürch, A. Synthesis and characterization of pH tolerant and mucoadhesive (thiol–polyethylene glycol) chitosan graft polymer for drug delivery. *J. Pharm. Sci.* **2014**, *103*, 594–601. [CrossRef] [PubMed]
60. Sayin, B.; Somavarapu, S.; Li, X.W.; Sesardic, D.; Şenel, S.; Alpar, O.H. TMC-MCC (*N*-trimethyl chitosan-mono-*N*-carboxymethyl chitosan) nanocomplexes for mucosal delivery of vaccines. *Eur. J. Pharm. Sci.* **2009**, *38*, 362–369. [CrossRef] [PubMed]

61. Sajomsang, W.; Ruktanonchai, U.R.; Gonil, P.; Nuchuchua, O. Mucoadhesive property and biocompatibility of methylated N-aryl chitosan derivatives. *Carbohydr. Polym.* **2009**, *78*, 945–952. [CrossRef]
62. Keely, S.; Rullay, A.; Wilson, C.; Carmichael, A.; Carrington, S.; Corfield, A.; Haddleton, D.M.; Brayden, D.J. In vitro and ex vivo intestinal tissue models to measure mucoadhesion of poly(methacrylate) and N-trimethylated chitosan polymers. *Pharm. Res.* **2005**, *22*, 38–49. [CrossRef] [PubMed]
63. Foster, S.N.E.; Pearson, J.P.; Huton, D.A.; Allen, A.; Detmar, P.W. Interaction of polyacrylates with porcine pepsin and the gastric mucus barrier: A mechanism for mucosal protection. *Clin. Sci.* **1994**, *87*, 719–726. [CrossRef] [PubMed]
64. Jonker, C.; Hamman, J.H.; Kotzé, A.F. Intestinal paracellular permeation enhancement with quaternised chitosan: In situ and in vitro evaluation. *Int. J. Pharm.* **2002**, *238*, 205–213. [CrossRef]
65. Smith, J.; Wood, E.; Dornish, M. Effect of chitosan on epithelial cell tight junctions. *Pharm. Res.* **2004**, *21*, 43–49. [CrossRef] [PubMed]
66. Hamman, J.H.; Schultz, C.M.; Kotzé, A.F. N-trimethyl chitosan chloride: Optimum degree of quaternization for drug absorption enhancement across epithelial cells. *Drug Dev. Ind. Pharm.* **2003**, *29*, 161–172. [CrossRef] [PubMed]
67. Liu, M.; Zhang, J.; Zhu, X.; Shan, W.; Li, L.; Zhong, J.; Zhang, Z.; Huang, Y. Efficient mucus permeation and tight junction opening by dissociable "mucus-inert" agent coated trimethyl chitosan nanoparticles for oral insulin delivery. *J. Control. Release* **2016**, *222*, 67–77. [CrossRef] [PubMed]
68. Nazar, H.; Fatouros, D.G.; van der Merwe, S.M.; Bouropoulos, N.; Avgouropoulos, G.; Tsiboukis, J.; Roldo, M. Thermosensitive hydrogels for nasal drug delivery: The formulation and characterization of systems based on N-trimethyl chitosan chloride. *Eur. J. Pharm. Biopharm.* **2011**, *77*, 225–232. [CrossRef] [PubMed]
69. Van der Merwe, S.M.; Verhoef, J.C.; Verheijden, J.H.M.; Kotzé, A.F.; Junginger, H.E. Trimethylated chitosan as polymeric absorption enhancer for improved peroral delivery of peptide drugs. *Eur. J. Pharm. Biopharm.* **2004**, *58*, 225–235. [CrossRef] [PubMed]
70. DeSesso, J.M.; Jacobson, C.F. Anatomical and physiological parameters affecting gastrointestinal absorption in humans and rats. *Food Chem. Toxicol.* **2001**, *39*, 209–228. [CrossRef]
71. Kotzé, A.F.; de Leeuw, B.J.; Lueßen, H.L.; de Boer, A.G.; Verhoef, J.C.; Junginger, H.E. Chitosans for enhanced delivery of therapeutic peptides across intestinal epithelia: In vitro evaluation in Caco-2 cell monolayers. *Int. J. Pharm.* **1997**, *159*, 243–253. [CrossRef]
72. Deli, M.A. Potential use of tight junction modulators to reversibly open membranous barriers and improve drug delivery. *Biochim. Biophys. Acta Biomembr.* **2009**, *1788*, 892–910. [CrossRef] [PubMed]
73. Thanou, M.; Nihot, M.T.; Jansen, M.; Verhoef, J.C.; Junginger, H.E. Mono-N-carboxymethyl chitosan (MCC), a polyampholytic chitosan derivative, enhances the intestinal absorption of low molecular weight heparin across intestinal epithelia in vitro and in vivo. *J. Pharm. Sci.* **2001**, *90*, 38–46. [CrossRef]
74. Upadhyaya, L.; Singh, J.; Agarwal, V.; Tewari, R.P. The implications of recent advances in carboxymethyl chitosan based targeted drug delivery and tissue engineering applications. *J. Control. Release* **2014**, *186*, 54–87. [CrossRef] [PubMed]
75. Jayakumar, R.; Prabaharan, M.; Nair, S.V.; Tokura, S.; Tamura, H.; Selvamurugan, N. Novel carboxymethyl derivatives of chitin and chitosan materials and their biomedical applications. *Prog. Mater. Sci.* **2010**, *55*, 675–709. [CrossRef]
76. Chen, X.-G.; Park, H.-J. Chemical characteristics of O-carboxymethyl chitosans related to the preparation conditions. *Carbohydr. Polym.* **2003**, *53*, 355–359. [CrossRef]
77. Vikhoreva, G.A.; Gal'braikh, L.S. Rheological properties of solutions of chitosan and carboxymethylchitin. *Fibre Chem.* **1997**, *29*, 287–291. [CrossRef]
78. An, N.T.; Dung, P.L.; Thien, D.T.; Dong, N.T.; Nhi, T.T.Y. An improved method for synthesizing N,N'-dicarboxymethylchitosan. *Carbohydr. Polym.* **2008**, *73*, 261–264. [CrossRef]
79. An, N.T.; Thien, D.T.; Dong, N.T.; Dung, P.L. Water-soluble N-carboxymethylchitosan derivatives: Preparation, characteristics and its application. *Carbohydr. Polym.* **2009**, *75*, 489–497. [CrossRef]
80. Upadhyaya, L.; Singh, J.; Agarwal, V.; Tewari, R.P. Biomedical applications of carboxymethyl chitosans. *Carbohydr. Polym.* **2013**, *91*, 452–466. [CrossRef] [PubMed]
81. Ge, H.-C.; Luo, D.-K. Preparation of carboxymethyl chitosan in aqueous solution under microwave irradiation. *Carbohydr. Res.* **2005**, *340*, 1351–1356. [CrossRef] [PubMed]

82. Di Colo, G.; Zambito, Y.; Burgalassi, S.; Nardini, I.; Saettone, M.F. Effect of chitosan and N-carboxymethylchitosan on intraocular penetration of topically applied ofloxacin. *Int. J. Pharm.* **2004**, *273*, 37–44. [CrossRef] [PubMed]
83. Prabaharan, M.; Gong, S. Novel thiolated carboxymethyl chitosan-g-β-cyclodextrin as mucoadhesive hydrophobic drug delivery carriers. *Carbohydr. Polym.* **2008**, *73*, 117–125. [CrossRef]
84. Bernkop-Schnürch, A.; Brandt, U.M.; Clausen, A.E. Synthesis and in vitro evaluation of chitosan-cysteine conjugates. *Sci. Pharm.* **1999**, *67*, 196–208.
85. Kast, C.E.; Frick, W.; Losert, U.; Bernkop-Schnürch, A. Chitosan-thioglycolic acid conjugate: A new scaffold material for tissue engineering? *Int. J. Pharm.* **2003**, *256*, 183–189. [CrossRef]
86. Bernkop-Schnürch, A.; Hornof, M.; Zoidl, T. Thiolated polymers—Thiomers: Synthesis and in vitro evaluation of chitosan–2-iminothiolane conjugates. *Int. J. Pharm.* **2003**, *260*, 229–237. [CrossRef]
87. Schmitz, T.; Grabovac, V.; Palmberger, T.F.; Hoffer, M.H.; Bernkop-Schnürch, A. Synthesis and characterization of a chitosan-*N*-acetyl cysteine conjugate. *Int. J. Pharm.* **2008**, *347*, 79–85. [CrossRef] [PubMed]
88. Kafedjiiski, K.; Krauland, A.H.; Hoffer, M.H.; Bernkop-Schnürch, A. Synthesis and in vitro evaluation of a novel thiolated chitosan. *Biomaterials* **2005**, *26*, 819–826. [CrossRef] [PubMed]
89. Kafedjiiski, K.; Föger, F.; Werle, M.; Bernkop-Schnürch, A. Synthesis and in vitro evaluation of a novel chitosan-glutathione conjugate. *Pharm. Res.* **2005**, *22*, 1480–1488. [CrossRef] [PubMed]
90. Bernkop-Schnürch, A.; Schwarz, V.; Steininger, S. Polymers with thiol groups: A new generation of mucoadhesive polymers. *Pharm. Res.* **1999**, *16*, 876–881. [CrossRef] [PubMed]
91. Li, J.; Shu, Y.; Hao, T.; Wang, Y.; Qian, Y.; Duan, C.; Sun, H.; Lin, Q.; Wang, C. A chitosan-glutathione based injectable hydrogel for suppression of oxidative stress damage in cardiomyocytes. *Biomaterials* **2013**, *34*, 9071–9081. [CrossRef] [PubMed]
92. Yin, L.; Ding, J.; He, C.; Cui, L.; Tang, C.; Yin, C. Drug permeability and mucoadhesion properties of thiolated trimethyl chitosan nanoparticles in oral insulin delivery. *Biomaterials* **2009**, *30*, 5691–5700. [CrossRef] [PubMed]
93. Sakloetsakun, D.; Hombach, J.M.R.; Bernkop-Schnürch, A. In situ gelling properties of chitosan-thioglycolic acid conjugate in the presence of oxidizing agents. *Biomaterials* **2009**, *30*, 6151–6157. [CrossRef] [PubMed]
94. Martien, R.; Loretz, B.; Thaler, M.; Majzoob, S.; Bernkop-Schnürch, A. Chitosan-thioglycolic acid conjugate: An alternative carrier for oral nonviral gene delivery? *J. Biomed. Mater. Res. Part A* **2007**, *82A*, 1–9. [CrossRef] [PubMed]
95. Barthelmes, J.; Perera, G.; Hombach, J.; Dünnhaupt, S.; Bernkop-Schnürch, A. Development of a mucoadhesive nanoparticulate drug delivery system for a targeted drug release in the bladder. *Int. J. Pharm.* **2011**, *416*, 339–345. [CrossRef] [PubMed]
96. Soler, R.; Bruschini, H.; Martins, J.R.; Dreyfuss, J.L.; Camara, N.O.; Alves, M.T.; Leite, K.R.; Truzzi, J.C.; Nader, H.B.; Srougi, M.; et al. Urinary glycosaminoglycans as biomarker for urothelial injury: Is it possible to discriminate damage from recovery? *Urology* **2008**, *72*, 937–942. [CrossRef] [PubMed]
97. Grabovac, V.; Guggi, D.; Bernkop-Schnürch, A. Comparison of the mucoadhesive properties of various polymers. *Adv. Drug Deliv. Rev.* **2005**, *57*, 1713–1723. [CrossRef] [PubMed]
98. Langoth, N.; Kahlbacher, H.; Schöffmann, G.; Schmerold, I.; Schuh, M.; Franz, S.; Kurka, P.; Bernkop-Schnürch, A. Thiolated chitosans: Design and in vivo evaluation of a mucoadhesive buccal peptide drug delivery system. *Pharm. Res.* **2006**, *23*, 573–579. [CrossRef] [PubMed]
99. Dünnhaupt, S.; Barthelmes, J.; Hombach, J.; Sakloetsakun, D.; Arkhipova, V.; Bernkop-Schnürch, A. Distribution of thiolated mucoadhesive nanoparticles on intestinal mucosa. *Int. J. Pharm.* **2011**, *408*, 191–199. [CrossRef] [PubMed]
100. Guggi, D.; Kast, C.E.; Bernkop-Schnürch, A. In vivo evaluation of an oral salmon calcitonin-delivery system based on a thiolated chitosan carrier matrix. *Pharm. Res.* **2003**, *20*, 1989–1994. [CrossRef] [PubMed]
101. Krauland, A.H.; Leitner, V.M.; Grabovac, V.; Bernkop-Schnürch, A. In vivo evaluation of a nasal insulin delivery system based on thiolated chitosan. *J. Pharm. Sci.* **2006**, *95*, 2463–2472. [CrossRef] [PubMed]
102. Koo, S.H.; Lee, J.-S.; Kim, G.-H.; Lee, H.G. Preparation, characteristics, and stability of glutathione-loaded nanoparticles. *J. Agric. Food Chem.* **2011**, *59*, 11264–11269. [CrossRef] [PubMed]
103. Moghaddam, F.A.; Atyabi, F.; Dinarvand, R. Preparation and in vitro evaluation of mucoadhesion and permeation enhancement of thiolated chitosan-pHEMA core-shell nanoparticles. *Nanomedicine* **2009**, *5*, 208–215. [CrossRef] [PubMed]

104. Jin, X.; Xu, Y.; Shen, J.; Ping, Q.; Su, Z.; You, W. Chitosan-glutathione conjugate-coated poly(butyl cyanoacrylate) nanoparticles: Promising carriers for oral thymopentin delivery. *Carbohydr. Polym.* **2011**, *86*, 51–57. [CrossRef]
105. Mei, D.; Mao, S.; Sun, W.; Wang, Y.; Kissel, T. Effect of chitosan structure properties and molecular weight on the intranasal absorption of tetramethylpyrazine phosphate in rats. *Eur. J. Pharm. Biopharm.* **2008**, *70*, 874–881. [CrossRef] [PubMed]
106. Mao, S.; Shuai, X.; Unger, F.; Wittmar, M.; Xie, X.; Kissel, T. Synthesis, characterization and cytotoxicity of poly(ethylene glycol)-graft-trimethyl chitosan block copolymers. *Biomaterials* **2005**, *26*, 6343–6356. [CrossRef] [PubMed]
107. Bernkop-Schnürch, A.; Steininger, S. Synthesis and characterisation of mucoadhesive thiolated polymers. *Int. J. Pharm.* **2000**, *194*, 239–247. [CrossRef]
108. Krauland, A.H.; Guggi, D.; Bernkop-Schnürch, A. Oral insulin delivery: The potential of thiolated chitosan-insulin tablets on non-diabetic rats. *J. Control. Release* **2004**, *95*, 547–555. [CrossRef] [PubMed]
109. Föger, F.; Schmitz, T.; Bernkop-Schnürch, A. In vivo evaluation of an oral delivery system for P-gp substrates based on thiolated chitosan. *Biomaterials* **2006**, *27*, 4250–4255. [CrossRef] [PubMed]
110. Dünnhaupt, S.; Barthelmes, J.; Rahmat, D.; Leithner, K.; Thurner, C.C.; Friedl, H.; Bernkop-Schnürch, A. S-protected thiolated chitosan for oral delivery of hydrophilic macromolecules: Evaluation of permeation enhancing and efflux pump inhibitory properties. *Mol. Pharm.* **2012**, *9*, 1331–1341. [CrossRef] [PubMed]
111. Dünnhaupt, S.; Barthelmes, J.; Thurner, C.C.; Waldner, C.; Sakloetsakun, D.; Bernkop-Schnürch, A. S-protected thiolated chitosan: Synthesis and in vitro characterization. *Carbohydr. Polym.* **2012**, *90*, 765–772. [CrossRef] [PubMed]
112. Dünnhaupt, S.; Barthelmes, J.; Iqbal, J.; Perera, G.; Thurner, C.C.; Friedl, H.; Bernkop-Schnürch, A. In vivo evaluation of an oral drug delivery system for peptides based on S-protected thiolated chitosan. *J. Control. Release* **2012**, *160*, 477–485. [CrossRef] [PubMed]
113. Hakimi, S.; Mortazavian, E.; Mohammadi, Z.; Samadi, F.Y.; Samadikhah, H.; Taheritarigh, S.; Tehrani, N.R.; Rafiee-Tehrani, M. Thiolated methylated dimethylaminobenzyl chitosan: A novel chitosan derivative as a potential delivery vehicle. *Int. J. Biol. Macromol.* **2017**, *95*, 574–581. [CrossRef] [PubMed]
114. Davidovich-Pinhas, M.; Bianco-Peled, H. Novel mucoadhesive system based on sulfhydryl-acrylate interactions. *J. Mater. Sci. Mater. Med.* **2010**, *21*, 2027–2034. [CrossRef] [PubMed]
115. Davidovich-Pinhas, M.; Bianco-Peled, H. Alginate-PEGAc: A new mucoadhesive polymer. *Acta Biomater.* **2011**, *7*, 625–633. [CrossRef] [PubMed]
116. Eshel-Green, T.; Bianco-Peled, H. Mucoadhesive acrylated block copolymers micelles for the delivery of hydrophobic drugs. *Colloids Surf. B* **2016**, *139*, 42–51. [CrossRef] [PubMed]
117. Štorha, A.; Mun, E.A.; Khutoryanskiy, V.V. Synthesis of thiolated and acrylated nanoparticles using thiol-ene click chemistry: Towards novel mucoadhesive materials for drug delivery. *RSC Adv.* **2013**, *3*, 12275–12279. [CrossRef]
118. Ma, G.; Zhang, X.; Han, J.; Song, G.; Nie, J. Photo-polymeriable chitosan derivative prepared by Michael reaction of chitosan and polyethylene glycol diacrylate (PEGDA). *Int. J. Biol. Macromol.* **2009**, *45*, 499–503. [CrossRef] [PubMed]
119. Shitrit, Y.; Bianco-Peled, H. Acrylated chitosan for mucoadhesive drug delivery systems. *Int. J. Pharm.* **2017**, *517*, 247–255. [CrossRef] [PubMed]
120. Albarkah, Y.A.; Green, R.J.; Khutoryanskiy, V.V. Probing the mucoadhesive interactions between porcine gastric mucin and some water-soluble polymers. *Macromol. Biosci.* **2015**, *15*, 1546–1553. [CrossRef] [PubMed]
121. Smart, J.D. The basics and underlying mechanisms of mucoadhesion. *Adv. Drug Deliv. Rev.* **2005**, *57*, 1556–1568. [CrossRef] [PubMed]
122. Qin, C.; Li, H.; Xiao, Q.; Liu, Y.; Zhu, J.; Du, Y. Water-solubility of chitosan and its antimicrobial activity. *Carbohydr. Polym.* **2006**, *63*, 367–374. [CrossRef]
123. Palazzo, C.; Trapani, G.; Ponchel, G.; Trapani, A.; Vauthier, C. Mucoadhesive properties of low molecular weight chitosan- or glycol chitosan- and corresponding thiomer-coated poly(isobutylcyanoacrylate) core-shell nanoparticles. *Eur. J. Pharm. Biopharm.* **2017**, *117*, 315–323. [CrossRef] [PubMed]
124. Trapani, A.; Sitterberg, J.; Bakowsky, U.; Kissel, T. The potential of glycol chitosan nanoparticles as carrier for low water soluble drugs. *Int. J. Pharm.* **2009**, *375*, 97–106. [CrossRef] [PubMed]
125. Uchegbu, I.F.; Carlos, M.; McKay, C.; Hou, X.; Schätzlein, A.G. Chitosan amphiphiles provide new drug delivery opportunities. *Polym. Int.* **2014**, *63*, 1145–1153. [CrossRef]

126. Uchegbu, I.F.; Andreas, G.S.; Laurence, T.; Alexander, I.G.; Julieann, S.; Soryia, S.; Erasto, M. Polymeric chitosan-based vesicles for drug delivery. *J. Pharm. Pharmacol.* **1998**, *50*, 453–458. [CrossRef] [PubMed]
127. Siew, A.; Le, H.; Thiovolet, M.; Gellert, P.; Schatzlein, A.; Uchegbu, I. Enhanced oral absorption of hydrophobic and hydrophilic drugs using quaternary ammonium palmitoyl glycol chitosan nanoparticles. *Mol. Pharm.* **2012**, *9*, 14–28. [CrossRef] [PubMed]
128. Qu, X.; Khutoryanskiy, V.V.; Stewart, A.; Rahman, S.; Papahadjopoulos-Sternberg, B.; Dufes, C.; McCarthy, D.; Wilson, C.G.; Lyons, R.; Carter, K.C.; et al. Carbohydrate-based micelle clusters which enhance hydrophobic drug bioavailability by up to 1 order of magnitude. *Biomacromolecules* **2006**, *7*, 3452–3459. [CrossRef] [PubMed]
129. Bonferoni, M.C.; Sandri, G.; Ferrari, F.; Rossi, S.; Larghi, V.; Zambito, Y.; Caramella, C. Comparison of different in vitro and ex vivo methods to evaluate mucoadhesion of glycol-palmitoyl chitosan micelles. *J. Drug Deliv. Sci. Technol.* **2010**, *20*, 419–424. [CrossRef]
130. Martin, L.; Wilson, C.G.; Koosha, F.; Tetley, L.; Gray, A.I.; Senel, S.; Uchegbu, I.F. The release of model macromolecules may be controlled by the hydrophobicity of palmitoyl glycol chitosan hydrogels. *J. Control. Release* **2002**, *80*, 87–100. [CrossRef]
131. Cho, I.S.; Park, C.G.; Huh, B.K.; Cho, M.O.; Khatun, Z.; Li, Z.; Kang, S.-W.; Choy, Y.B.; Huh, K.M. Thermosensitive hexanoyl glycol chitosan-based ocular delivery system for glaucoma therapy. *Acta Biomater.* **2016**, *39*, 124–132. [CrossRef] [PubMed]
132. Cho, I.S.; Cho, M.O.; Li, Z.; Nurunnabi, M.; Park, S.Y.; Kang, S.-W.; Huh, K.M. Synthesis and characterization of a new photo-crosslinkable glycol chitosan thermogel for biomedical applications. *Carbohydr. Polym.* **2016**, *144*, 59–67. [CrossRef] [PubMed]
133. Akiyama, Y.; Lueβen, H.L.; de Boer, A.G.; Verhoef, J.C.; Junginger, H.E. Novel peroral dosage forms with protease inhibitory activities. II. Design of fast dissolving poly(acrylate) and controlled drug-releasing capsule formulations with trypsin inhibiting properties. *Int. J. Pharm.* **1996**, *138*, 13–23. [CrossRef]
134. Bernkop-Schnürch, A.; Kast, C.E. Chemically modified chitosans as enzyme inhibitors. *Adv. Drug Deliv. Rev.* **2001**, *52*, 127–137. [CrossRef]
135. Watanabe, S.-I.; Takeuchi, T.; Chey, W.Y. Mediation of trypsin inhibitor-induced pancreatic hypersecretion by secretin and cholecystokinin in rats. *Gastroenterology* **1992**, *102*, 621–628. [CrossRef]
136. Song, Y.; Huang, Z.; Song, Y.; Tian, Q.; Liu, X.; She, Z.; Jiao, J.; Lu, E.; Deng, Y. The application of EDTA in drug delivery systems: Doxorubicin liposomes loaded via NH_4EDTA gradient. *Int. J. Nanomed.* **2014**, *9*, 3611–3621. [CrossRef]
137. Grießinger, J.A.; Hauptstein, S.; Laffleur, F.; Netsomboon, K.; Bernkop-Schnürch, A. Evaluation of the impact of multivalent metal ions on the permeation behavior of Dolutegravir sodium. *Drug Dev. Ind. Pharm.* **2016**, *42*, 1118–1126. [CrossRef] [PubMed]
138. Netsomboon, K.; Suchaoin, W.; Laffleur, F.; Prüfert, F.; Bernkop-Schnürch, A. Multifunctional adhesive polymers: Preactivated thiolated chitosan-EDTA conjugates. *Eur. J. Pharm. Biopharm.* **2017**, *111*, 26–32. [CrossRef] [PubMed]
139. Bernkop-Schnürch, A.; Scerbe-Saiko, A. Synthesis and in vitro evaluation of chitosan-EDTA-protease-inhibitor conjugates which might be useful in oral delivery of peptides and proteins. *Pharm. Res.* **1998**, *15*, 263–269. [CrossRef] [PubMed]
140. Bernkop-Schnürch, A.; Krajicek, M.E. Mucoadhesive polymers as platforms for peroral peptide delivery and absorption: Synthesis and evaluation of different chitosan–EDTA conjugates. *J. Control. Release* **1998**, *50*, 215–223. [CrossRef]
141. Kim, K.; Kim, K.; Ryu, J.H.; Lee, H. Chitosan-catechol: A polymer with long-lasting mucoadhesive properties. *Biomaterials* **2015**, *52*, 161–170. [CrossRef] [PubMed]
142. Ryu, J.H.; Lee, Y.; Kong, W.H.; Kim, T.G.; Park, T.G.; Lee, H. Catechol-functionalized chitosan/pluronic hydrogels for tissue adhesives and hemostatic materials. *Biomacromolecules* **2011**, *12*, 2653–2659. [CrossRef] [PubMed]
143. Kim, K.; Ryu, J.H.; Lee, D.Y.; Lee, H. Bio-inspired catechol conjugation converts water-insoluble chitosan into a highly water-soluble, adhesive chitosan derivative for hydrogels and LbL assembly. *Biomater. Sci.* **2013**, *1*, 783–790. [CrossRef]
144. Ryu, J.H.; Hong, S.; Lee, H. Bio-inspired adhesive catechol-conjugated chitosan for biomedical applications: A mini review. *Acta Biomater.* **2015**, *27*, 101–115. [CrossRef] [PubMed]
145. Lee, H.; Scherer, N.F.; Messersmith, P.B. Single-molecule mechanics of mussel adhesion. *Proc. Natl. Acad. Sci. USA* **2006**, *103*, 12999–13003. [CrossRef] [PubMed]

146. Patel, M.M.; Smart, J.D.; Nevell, T.G.; Ewen, R.J.; Eaton, P.J.; Tsibouklis, J. Mucin/poly(acrylic acid) interactions: A spectroscopic investigation of mucoadhesion. *Biomacromolecules* **2003**, *4*, 1184–1190. [CrossRef] [PubMed]
147. Riley, R.G.; Smart, J.D.; Tsibouklis, J.; Dettmar, P.W.; Hampson, F.; Davis, J.A.; Kelly, G.; Wilber, W.R. An investigation of mucus/polymer rheological synergism using synthesised and characterised poly(acrylic acid)s. *Int. J. Pharm.* **2001**, *217*, 87–100. [CrossRef]
148. Mortazavi, S.A.; Carpenter, B.G.; Smart, J.D. A comparative study on the role played by mucus glycoproteins in the rheological behaviour of the mucoadhesive/mucosal interface. *Int. J. Pharm.* **1993**, *94*, 195–201. [CrossRef]
149. Muzzarelli, R.A.A.; Ilari, P.; Tomasetti, M. Preparation and characteristic properties of 5-methyl pyrrolidinone chitosan. *Carbohydr. Polym.* **1993**, *20*, 99–105. [CrossRef]
150. Muzzarelli, R. Methyl Pyrrolidinone Chitosan, Production Process and Uses Thereof. WO1992009635A1, 11 June 1992.
151. Rinaudo, M.; Desbrières, J.; Le Dung, P.; Thuy Binh, P.; Dong, N.T. NMR investigation of chitosan derivatives formed by the reaction of chitosan with levulinic acid. *Carbohydr. Polym.* **2001**, *46*, 339–348. [CrossRef]
152. Kurita, Y.; Isogai, A. Reductive N-alkylation of chitosan with acetone and levulinic acid in aqueous media. *Int. J. Biol. Macromol.* **2010**, *47*, 184–189. [CrossRef] [PubMed]
153. Sandri, G.; Rossi, S.; Ferrari, F.; Bonferoni, M.C.; Muzzarelli, C.; Caramella, C. Assessment of chitosan derivatives as buccal and vaginal penetration enhancers. *Eur. J. Pharm. Sci.* **2004**, *21*, 351–359. [CrossRef] [PubMed]
154. Kim, C.-K.; Hong, M.-S.; Kim, Y.-B.; Han, S.-K. Effect of penetration enhancers (pyrrolidone derivatives) on multilamellar liposomes of stratum corneum lipid: A study by UV spectroscopy and differential scanning calorimetry. *Int. J. Pharm.* **1993**, *95*, 43–50. [CrossRef]
155. Sasaki, H.; Kojima, M.; Mori, Y.; Nakamura, J.; Shibasaki, J. Enhancing effect of pyrrolidone derivatives on transdermal penetration of 5-fluorouracil, triamcinolone acetonide, indomethacin, and flurbiprofen. *J. Pharm. Sci.* **1991**, *80*, 533–538. [CrossRef] [PubMed]
156. Auzély-Velty, R.; Rinaudo, M. Chitosan derivatives bearing pendant cyclodextrin cavities: Synthesis and inclusion performance. *Macromolecules* **2001**, *34*, 3574–3580. [CrossRef]
157. Venter, J.P.; Kotzé, A.F.; Auzély-Velty, R.; Rinaudo, M. Synthesis and evaluation of the mucoadhesivity of a CD-chitosan derivative. *Int. J. Pharm.* **2006**, *313*, 36–42. [CrossRef] [PubMed]
158. Chaleawlert-umpon, S.; Nuchuchua, O.; Saesoo, S.; Gonil, P.; Ruktanonchai, U.R.; Sajomsang, W.; Pimpha, N. Effect of citrate spacer on mucoadhesive properties of a novel water-soluble cationic β-cyclodextrin-conjugated chitosan. *Carbohydr. Polym.* **2011**, *84*, 186–194. [CrossRef]
159. Yostawonkul, J.; Surassmo, S.; Iempridee, T.; Pimtong, W.; Suktham, K.; Sajomsang, W.; Gonil, P.; Ruktanonchai, U.R. Surface modification of nanostructure lipid carrier (NLC) by oleoyl-quaternized-chitosan as a mucoadhesive nanocarrier. *Colloids Surf. B Biointerfaces* **2017**, *149*, 301–311. [CrossRef] [PubMed]
160. Thanou, M.; Florea, B.I.; Langemeÿer, M.W.E.; Verhoef, J.C.; Junginger, H.E. N-trimethylated chitosan chloride (TMC) improves the intestinal permeation of the peptide drug buserelin in vitro (Caco-2 Cells) and in vivo (rats). *Pharm. Res.* **2000**, *17*, 27–31. [CrossRef] [PubMed]
161. Pardeshi, C.V.; Belgamwar, V.S. Controlled synthesis of N,N,N-trimethyl chitosan for modulated bioadhesion and nasal membrane permeability. *Int. J. Biol. Macromol.* **2016**, *82*, 933–944. [CrossRef] [PubMed]
162. Kast, C.E.; Valenta, C.; Leopold, M.; Bernkop-Schnürch, A. Design and in vitro evaluation of a novel bioadhesive vaginal drug delivery system for clotrimazole. *J. Control. Release* **2002**, *81*, 347–354. [CrossRef]
163. Bernkop-Schnürch, A.; Guggi, D.; Pinter, Y. Thiolated chitosans: Development and in vitro evaluation of a mucoadhesive, permeation enhancing oral drug delivery system. *J. Control. Release* **2004**, *94*, 177–186. [CrossRef] [PubMed]
164. Xu, J.; Strandman, S.; Zhu, J.X.X.; Barralet, J.; Cerruti, M. Genipin-crosslinked catechol-chitosan mucoadhesive hydrogels for buccal drug delivery. *Biomaterials* **2015**, *37*, 395–404. [CrossRef] [PubMed]
165. Xu, J.; Tam, M.; Samaei, S.; Lerouge, S.; Barralet, J.; Stevenson, M.M.; Cerruti, M. Mucoadhesive chitosan hydrogels as rectal drug delivery vessels to treat ulcerative colitis. *Acta Biomater.* **2017**, *48*, 247–257. [CrossRef] [PubMed]

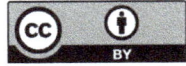

© 2018 by the authors. Licensee MDPI, Basel, Switzerland. This article is an open access article distributed under the terms and conditions of the Creative Commons Attribution (CC BY) license (http://creativecommons.org/licenses/by/4.0/).

MDPI
St. Alban-Anlage 66
4052 Basel
Switzerland
Tel. +41 61 683 77 34
Fax +41 61 302 89 18
www.mdpi.com

Polymers Editorial Office
E-mail: polymers@mdpi.com
www.mdpi.com/journal/polymers

www.ingramcontent.com/pod-product-compliance
Lightning Source LLC
LaVergne TN
LVHW070728100526
838202LV00013B/1194